Dementia and Language

Bringing together cutting-edge research from a group of international scholars, this innovative volume examines how people with dementia interact with others in a variety of social contexts, ranging from everyday conversation to clinical settings. Drawing on methods from conversation analysis, it sheds light on how people with dementia accomplish relevant goals in interaction, as well as how changes in an individual's discursive abilities may affect how conversationalists negotiate a world in common and continue to build their social relationships. By exploring interaction, this book breaks new ground in challenging the commonplace assumptions about what constitutes typical or atypical interactions in communication involving people with dementia, and further demonstrates the unique and creative strategies all speakers employ to facilitate better and more collaborative communication. It is essential reading for academic researchers and advanced students across sociolinguistics, interactional linguistics, and conversational analysis, as well as health care practitioners.

PETER MUNTIGL is Adjunct Professor at the Faculty of Education, Simon Fraser University, Canada. His recent publications include *Interaction in Psychotherapy* (2023, Cambridge University Press).

CHARLOTTA PLEJERT is Senior Associate Professor at the Department of Biomedical and Clinical Sciences, Linköping University, Sweden. Notable publications include *Multilingual Interaction and Dementia* (Plejert, Lindholm & Schrauf, 2017, Multilingual Matters).

DANIELLE JONES is Associate Professor at the Centre for Applied Dementia Studies, University of Bradford, UK. She is a medical sociologist with 20 years' experience of using Conversation Analysis to explore communication between people living with dementia, their families, and medical professionals.

Studies in Interactional Sociolinguistics

FOUNDING EDITOR
John J. Gumperz (1922–2013)
EDITORS
Paul Drew, Rebecca Clift, Lorenza Mondada, Marja-Leena Sorjonen

1. *Discourse Strategies* John J. Gumperz
2. *Language and Social Identity* edited by John J. Gumperz
3. *The Social Construction of Literacy* Jenny Cook-Gumperz
4. *Politeness: Some Universals in Language Usage* Penelope Brown and Stephen C. Levinson
5. *Discourse Markers* Deborah Schiffrin
6. *Talking Voices: Repetition, Dialogue, and Imagery in Conversational Discourse* Deborah Tannen
7. *Conducting Interaction: Patterns of Behaviour in Focused Encounters* Adam Kendon
8. *Talk at Work: Interaction in Institutional Settings* edited by Paul Drew and John Heritage
9. *Grammar in Interaction: Adverbial Clauses in American English Conversations* Cecilia E. Ford
10. *Crosstalk and Culture in Sino-American Communication*, Linda W. L. Young (with foreword by John J. Gumperz),
11. *AIDS Counselling: Institutional Interaction and Clinical Practice* Anssi Perakyla
12. *Prosody in Conversation: Interactional Studies* edited by Elizabeth Couper-Kuhlen and Margret Selting
13. *Interaction and Grammar* edited by Elinor Ochs, Emanuel A. Schegloff and Sandra A. Thompson
14. *Credibility in Court: Communicative Practices in the Camorra Trials* Marco Jacquemet
15. *Interaction and the Development of Mind* A. J. Wootton
16. *The News Interview: Journalists and Public Figures on the Air* Steven Clayman and John Heritage
17. *Gender and Politeness* Sara Mills
18. *Laughter in Interaction* Philip Glenn
19. *Matters of Opinion: Talking about Public Issues* Greg Myers
20. *Communication in Medical Care: Interaction between Primary Care Physicians and Patients* edited by John Heritage and Douglas Maynard
21. *In Other Words: Variation in Reference and Narrative* Deborah Schiffrin
22. *Language in Late Modernity: Interaction in an Urban School* Ben Rampton
23. *Discourse and Identity* edited by Anna De Fina, Deborah Schiffrin and Michael Bamberg

24 *Reporting Talk: Reported Speech in Interaction* edited by Elizabeth Holt and Rebecca Clift
25 *The Social Construction of Literacy*, 2nd Edition edited by Jenny Cook-Gumperz
26 *Talking Voices*, 2nd Edition by Deborah Tannen
27 *Conversation Analysis* edited by Jack Sidnell
28 *Impoliteness: Using Language to Cause Offence* Jonathan Culpeper
29 *The Morality of Knowledge in Conversation* edited by Tanya Stivers, Lorenza Mondada and Jakob Steensig
30 *Conversational Repair and Human Understanding* edited by Makoto Hayashi, Geoffrey Raymond and Jack Sidnell
31 *Grammar in Everyday Talk: Building Responsive Actions* by Sandra A. Thompson, Barbara A. Fox, and Elizabeth Couper-Kuhlen
32 *Multimodal Conduct in the Law: Language, Gesture and Materiality in Legal Interaction* by Gregory Matoesian and Kristin Enola Gilbert
33 *The Suspect's Statement: Talk and Text in the Criminal Process* Martha Komter
34 *How Mediation Works: Resolving Conflict Through Talk* Angela Cora Garcia
35 *Action Ascription in Interaction* edited by Arnulf Depperman and Michael Haugh
36 *Encounters at the Counter: The Organization of Shop Interactions* edited by Barbara Fox, Lorenza Mondada, and Marja-Leena Sorjonen
37 *Dementia and Language: The Lived Experience in Interaction* edited by Peter Muntigl, Charlotta Plejert, and Danielle Jones

Dementia and Language
The Lived Experience in Interaction

Edited by
Peter Muntigl
University of Ghent and Simon Fraser University

Charlotta Plejert
Linköping University

Danielle Jones
University of Bradford

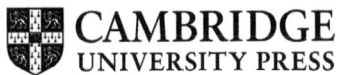

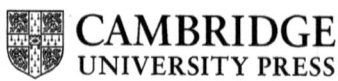
CAMBRIDGE
UNIVERSITY PRESS

Shaftesbury Road, Cambridge CB2 8EA, United Kingdom

One Liberty Plaza, 20th Floor, New York, NY 10006, USA

477 Williamstown Road, Port Melbourne, VIC 3207, Australia

314–321, 3rd Floor, Plot 3, Splendor Forum, Jasola District Centre, New Delhi – 110025, India

103 Penang Road, #05–06/07, Visioncrest Commercial, Singapore 238467

Cambridge University Press is part of Cambridge University Press & Assessment, a department of the University of Cambridge.

We share the University's mission to contribute to society through the pursuit of education, learning and research at the highest international levels of excellence.

www.cambridge.org
Information on this title: www.cambridge.org/9781108424530
DOI: 10.1017/9781108339377

© Peter Muntigl, Charlotta Plejert and Danielle Jones 2024

This publication is in copyright. Subject to statutory exception and to the provisions of relevant collective licensing agreements, no reproduction of any part may take place without the written permission of Cambridge University Press & Assessment.

When citing this work, please include a reference to the
DOI 10.1017/9781108339377

First published 2024

A catalogue record for this publication is available from the British Library

Library of Congress Cataloging-in-Publication Data
Names: Muntigl, Peter, editor. | Plejert, Charlotta, editor. | Jones, Danielle (Medical sociologist), editor.
Title: Dementia and language : the lived experience in interaction / edited by Peter Muntigl, Charlotta Plejert, Danielle Jones.
Other titles: Studies in interactional sociolinguistics ; 37.
Description: Cambridge, United Kingdom ; New York, NY : Cambridge University Press, 2024. | Series: Studies in interactional sociolinguistics ; 37 | Includes bibliographical references and index.
Identifiers: LCCN 2024008193 (print) | LCCN 2024008194 (ebook) | ISBN 9781108424530 (hardback) | ISBN 9781108442053 (paperback) | ISBN 9781108442053 (epub)
Subjects: MESH: Dementia | Social Interaction | Communication
Classification: LCC RC521 (print) | LCC RC521 (ebook) | NLM WM 220 | DDC 616.8/31–dc23/eng/20240318
LC record available at https://lccn.loc.gov/2024008193
LC ebook record available at https://lccn.loc.gov/2024008194

ISBN 978-1-108-42453-0 Hardback

Cambridge University Press & Assessment has no responsibility for the persistence or accuracy of URLs for external or third-party internet websites referred to in this publication and does not guarantee that any content on such websites is, or will remain, accurate or appropriate.

Contents

List of Figures	page x
List of Tables	xi
List of Contributors	xii
Transcript Notation Key	xiv

Part 1 Introduction

1. Interaction Research and Dementia   3
   PETER MUNTIGL, DANIELLE JONES, AND
   CHARLOTTA PLEJERT

Part 2 Dementia and Diagnostics

2. Good Reasons for Non-standardization in the Administration of Cognitive Assessments   25
   DANIELLE JONES, CLARE JACKSON AND RAY WILKINSON

3. (Mis)alignment at Dementia Diagnosis: A Window into Differing Expectations, Perceptions and Agendas in the Memory Clinic   50
   JEMIMA DOOLEY AND ROSE MCCABE

4. The Role of Applied Conversation Analysis to Enhance Equity in Care for People with Dementia from Minority Ethnic Groups   73
   CHARLOTTA PLEJERT

Part 3 Dementia and Conversational Strategies

5. Using "Now What" to Discursively Compensate for Frontotemporal Dementia-related Challenges: A Longitudinal Case Study   103
   LISA MIKESELL

6. Being Sociable: A Case Study of a Man with Vascular Dementia Singing in Conversation   128
ROY M. G. L. W. FOSTER

7. On the Use of Tag Questions by Co-participants of People with Dementia: Asymmetries of Knowledge, Power and Interactional Competence   151
JACQUELINE KINDELL, JOHN KEADY AND RAY WILKINSON

8. Initiating and Pursuing a Topical Agenda with Limited Communicative Resources   175
ANNE MARIE DALBY LANDMARK AND JAN SVENNEVIG

Part 4   Dementia and Epistemics

9. Identifying Family Members in Photographs: Practical Epistemic and Deontic Challenges for a Person with Frontotemporal Dementia   197
PETER MUNTIGL AND STEPHANIE HÖDL

10. 'You Know This Better': Interactional Challenges for Couples Living with Dementia when the Epistemic Status Regarding Shared Past Events Is Uncertain   226
ANNA EKSTRÖM, ELIN NILSSON AND ALI REZA MAJLESI

11. Maintaining Personhood and Authority in Everyday Talk of a Family Living with Dementia   249
LYNDSAY M. LINDLEY

Part 5   Communicative Challenges in Everyday Social Life

12. Language and Cognition in Conversations with a Person with Alzheimer's Disease   269
DANIELLE JONES

13. Using Digital Communication Support in Interaction Involving People with Dementia: Interactional Strategies to Facilitate Participation and Engagement   292
CHRISTINA SAMUELSSON AND ANNA EKSTRÖM

14. "It's More than Eating, It's a Social Situation": Video Analysis and Professional Vision in Dementia Care   316
CAMILLA LINDHOLM AND TUULA TYKKYLÄINEN

15. Social Quizzes for People Living with Dementia: How Enactment
    Impacts Interaction 336
    JOE WEBB

Index 356

Figures

13.1 Screenshot from CIRCA showing the different categories. *page* 297
13.2 Screenshot from CIRCUS showing different personal
     categories. 298

Tables

3.1	People with dementia: characteristics	*page* 52
5.1	Frequency of "now what" across eight 62-minute intervals	109
9.1	Epistemic positions compared for seeking information vs. exam questions	205
11.1	Participants' demographic information	251
13.1	Number and length of recordings with CIRCA and CIRCUS for the dyads	300

Contributors

JEMIMA DOOLEY (Sir Henry Wellcome Building for Mood Disorders Research, University of Exeter, UK)

ANNA EKSTRÖM (Department of Biomedical and Clinical Sciences (BKV), Linköping University, Sweden)

ROY M. G. L. W. FOSTER (Medical Policy Unit, Colorado Department of Labor and Employment, USA; University of Colorado School of Medicine, USA)

STEPHANIE HÖDL (Department of Neurology, Ghent University Hospital, Belgium)

CLARE JACKSON (Department of Sociology, University of York, UK)

DANIELLE JONES (Centre for Applied Dementia Studies, University of Bradford, UK)

JOHN KEADY (Division of Nursing, Midwifery and Social Work, University of Manchester, UK)

JACQUELINE KINDELL (Division of Psychology, Communication & Human Neuroscience, University of Manchester, UK)

ANNE MARIE DALBY LANDMARK (Department of Educational Science, University of Oslo, Norway)

CAMILLA LINDHOLM (Faculty of Information Technology and Communication Sciences, Tampere University, Finland)

LYNDSAY M. LINDLEY (School for Business and Society, University of York, UK)

ROSE MCCABE (Centre for Mental Health Research, City, University London, UK)

ALI REZA MAJLESI (Department of Education, Stockholm University, Sweden)

List of Contributors

LISA MIKESELL (School of Communication and Information, Rutgers University, USA)

PETER MUNTIGL (Faculty of Education, Simon Fraser University, Canada; Department of Translation, Interpretation and Communication, Ghent University, Belgium)

ELIN NILSSON (Department of Culture and Society, Linköping University, Sweden)

CHARLOTTA PLEJERT (Department of Biomedical and Clinical Sciences (BKV), Linköping University, Sweden)

CHRISTINA SAMUELSSON (Department of Clinical Science, Intervention and Technology, Karolinska Institute, Sweden)

JAN SVENNEVIG (Department of Nordic and Media Studies, University of Agder, Norway)

TUULA TYKKYLÄINEN (Faculty of Education, Helsinki University, Finland

JOE WEBB (School for Policy Studies, University of Bristol, UK)

RAY WILKINSON (Division of Human Communication Sciences, School of Allied Health Professions, Nursing and Midwifery, University of Sheffield, UK)

Transcript notation key

Transcription Notation

Symbol	Meaning	Symbol	Meaning
[	starting point of overlapping talk	↓word	markedly downward shift in pitch
]	endpoint of overlapping talk	↑word	markedly upward shift in pitch
(1.5)	silence measured in seconds	.hhh	audible inhalation, # of h's indicate length
(.)	silence less than 0.2-s		
.	falling intonation at end of utterance	hhh	audible exhalation, # of h's indicate length
,	continuing intonation at end of utterance	heh/huh/ hah/hih	laugh particles
?	rising intonation at end of utterance	wo(h)rd	laugh particle/outbreath inserted within a word
¿	medium (falling-) rising intonation (a dip and a rise)	(word)	uncertain
( )	inaudible section	.hh hx	sigh
wor-	truncated, cut-off speech	~word~	tremulous/wobbly voice through text
wo:rd	prolongation of sound	.snih	sniff
word=word	latching (no audible break between words)	huhh.hhihHuyuh	sobbing
<word>	stretch of talk slower, drawn out	>hhuh<	sobbing – produced at a faster rate
>word<	stretch of talk rushed, compressed	↑hhuh<	sobbing – if sharply inhaled or exhaled
°word°	stretch of talk spoken quietly	((cough))	audible non-speech sounds
<u>word</u>	emphasis	*word*	non-verbal behavior represented in italics on a separate tier below verbal conduct

(cont.)

Transcription Notation			
Symbol	Meaning	Symbol	Meaning
WORD	markedly loud	'# #', '* *'	symbols indicating onset and termination of non-verbal conduct with respect to verbal conduct
@	the speaker is smiling	£	smiley voice/suppressed laughter

Part 1

Introduction

1 Interaction Research and Dementia

Peter Muntigl, Danielle Jones, and Charlotta Plejert

1.1 Introduction

Dementia is a syndrome (a group of related symptoms) associated with an ongoing decline of brain functioning (NHS, 2020). Dementia is currently the seventh leading cause of death and one of the major causes of disability and dependency among older people globally. According to the Office for National Statistics (ONS) in the UK, "'dementia and Alzheimer's disease' were the leading cause of death in 2022. Collectively they accounted for 65,967 deaths (11.4% of the total), up from 61,250 (10.4%) in 2021" (Alzheimer's Research UK, 2023). It is estimated that approximately 55 million people live with dementia worldwide, with almost 10 million people developing dementia each year (WHO, 2023). The most frequent cause of dementia, present in over half of the cases, is Alzheimer's disease (AD). Other types include frontotemporal dementia, vascular dementia, and dementia with Lewy Bodies (Alzheimer's Society, 2023).

It is suggested that approximately three quarters of people with dementia have not received a formal diagnosis, and therefore do not have access to treatment, care, and organized support, which places a greater burden on family care. There is an increasing need for timely diagnosis and early intervention in order to reduce this "treatment gap" and raise public awareness of dementia-related disorders. The social ramifications of dementia are highly significant, with the symptoms of dementia being perceived differently in different parts of the world, and indeed within different cultural, social, and religious groups (Alzheimer Europe, 2018). Better public awareness and understanding could reduce the stigma associated with dementia for the people living with the condition, their family, and other caregivers (ADI, 2019).

The changes to memory, cognitive abilities, social conduct, and personality detected in people with dementia are generally assessed using clinical criteria (i.e., tests of cognitive and executive function) that are performed in institutional settings. However, there is an emerging field of research examining how these cognitive and social changes are interactively realized and negotiated in the many relevant social contexts in which people with dementia regularly take part. These include exploring the interactions of people being assessed for dementia (Elsey et al., 2015; Jones et al., 2016, 2020; Majlesi & Plejert, 2018) and being diagnosed with dementia (Dooley et al., 2018), as well as people with dementia and their families engaging in everyday interactions (Jones, 2015; Kindell et al., 2013; Mikesell, 2009; Nilsson, 2022) and within social care contexts (Lindholm, 2015; Österholm & Samuelsson, 2015; Webb et al., 2020). These studies have begun to explore how social relations are affected, and potentially put at risk, as they are negotiated *in situ* in the everyday social contexts in which people with dementia co-construct their lives with others.

This volume aims to bring together new advances in the field, creating a collection of papers that examine how people with dementia interact with others in a variety of social contexts ranging from clinical to everyday settings. It will focus on four highly relevant themes in dementia research: *Dementia and Diagnostics*, *Dementia and Conversational Strategies*, *Dementia and Epistemics*, and *Communicative Challenges in Everyday Social Life*. It aims to shed more light on how persons with dementia accomplish relevant goals in interaction, and also how changes in an individual's discursive abilities may impact on how conversationalists negotiate a world in common and continue to build their social relationships. All contributions for this edited volume draw on the methods of Conversation Analysis (CA), an approach to social interaction that provides a detailed view of the moment-by-moment accomplishment of social life (Heritage, 1984; Levinson, 2006; Sacks, 1995; Schegloff, 2006; Sidnell, 2012; Sidnell & Stivers, 2013). All transcriptions presented in the chapters draw from the transcription notation originally developed by Gail Jefferson and certain chapters also include notations for non-verbal conduct taken from Mondada (2018) (set out at the beginning of this book). By exploring interactional practices through the lens of CA, this volume seeks to explore interactions involving people with dementia in a variety of contexts, pointing to both the interactional difficulties that often arise and also the creativity and collaboration within these interactional encounters.

1.2   Conversational Strategies: Abilities vs. Deficits

Traditional analyses of language and dementia derive from cognitive and experimental sciences and have been based on speech samples elicited in clinical settings by psycholinguists, neurolinguists, and speech pathologists using questionnaires (Neumann et al., 1999), test batteries (Appell et al., 1982; Bayles, 2003; Blair et al., 2007), or proxy reports from relatives and carers (Logsdon et al., 2002; Sweeting & Gillhooly, 1997). These experimental studies largely focused on word-finding difficulties (anomia) symptomatic of the communicative decline predominantly associated with AD. Other dementias were largely absent from this early research. Language or communicative difficulties were attributed to the "patient'," situated inside the individual psyche and conceived as a product of internal mental mechanisms. Thus, much of the earlier research in the field adopted a *deficit*-focused approach underpinned by the biomedical model of dementia (Hydén et al., 2014).

Early attempts to move away from the experimental paradigm and establish a "personal research approach" came from Kitwood's psychosocial theories of dementia (1988, 1990, 1997). He argued that his approach goes "far beyond the measurement of indices or the codification of behaviors" found in the objective, depersonalized approach of experimental science (1988:176). Kitwood (1997) points out that "in society there has been a tendency to perceive people with dementia, because of their memory and communication problems, as less than human, and their experiences, views and rights to choose have not been recognized. Such views are embedded within the established and authoritative biomedical model of dementia, where psychosocial aspects of care have been marginalized" (in Aggarwal et al., 2003:187). It has been suggested that despite cognitive impairment, "personhood" survives, and may be dependent both on our attitudes towards people with dementia and our treatment of them as people (Crisp, 1999). This shift in perspective gave rise to more person-centered approaches to dementia research, reflecting the increasing need to maintain a connection to the contexts in which people are valued, and in which one's experiences are shared. Researchers began to realize the need to "preserve the wealth of living reality" (Sabat, 1991a: 16). During the late twentieth century researchers challenged the somewhat linear assumption of traditional experimental perspectives that communicative disorder merely results from cognitive impairment. It is instead necessary to observe and closely describe patterns that emerge from naturally occurring interactions that allow us to formulate an understanding of the underlying mechanism contributing to dysfunction.

Conversational interaction involving persons with dementia has been analyzed from a variety of theoretical and methodological perspectives, including discourse analysis (Sabat & Harré, 1992; Temple et al., 1999), systematic functional linguistics (Müller & Wilson, 2008), and narrative analysis (Hydén & Örulv, 2009; Örulv & Hydén, 2006). This shift also saw a rise in studies using CA to explore communication involving people living with dementia (Guendouzi & Müller, 2006; Hamilton, 1994; Mikesell, 2009, 2010; Perkins et al., 1998). Ripich et al. (1991) noted that much of the early literature failed to report on the discourse of the *other* participants who accompany people living with dementia. They suggest that "knowledge of partner's discourse features is crucial since communication is reciprocal with each participant shaping the interaction" (332). Rather than studying single utterances and isolated language products, CA researchers focus on "uncovering the *socially organized features of talk in context*, with a major focus on action sequences" (Heritage & Atkinson 1984:5). CA research involving people with dementia began to investigate the central features of talk such as repair (Watson et al., 1999), questions (Hamilton, 1994; Jones, 2006; Mikesell, 2009), and misunderstandings of sequential aims in conversation (Mikesell, 2009). Research in the field acknowledged the need for longitudinal analysis exploring communication and cognition over time (Bayles, 1984; Hamilton, 1994; Jones, 2012; Mikesell, 2010; Nilsson, 2018), and valued the exploration of single case studies (Hamilton, 1994, 2008; Jones, 2012, 2015; Müller & Guendouzi, 2005; Müller & Wilson, 2008), adopting an individualistic approach in order to provide a heightened understanding of interactional influence on language as it relates to dementia.

Jones (2015:556) acknowledged that "along with this focus on interaction, there was increasingly a shift in perspective, away from communicative disorder as solely situated in the limitations of a person's cognitive impairments, towards a wider focus on communication as a joint, collaborative achievement. It is important to view any impairment in communicative functioning or interaction as contextually situated and collaboratively produced." Studies found that, in the presence of cognitive deficit, people with dementia are competent, skillful, and co-operative conversationalists (Hamilton, 1994; Müller & Wilson, 2008; Sabat, 1991b). Hamilton's (1994) longitudinal sociolinguistic study, spanning over four years, detailed her conversations with a single person with AD (Elsie). Hamilton noted that even in Elsie's final stage of interactional ability, in which she had a limited communicative repertoire, she was still able to achieve a range of interactional functions including requesting clarification, turn-taking, and orienting to personal topics. Furthermore, through their conversation analytic investigation of the functional aspects of laughter during conversations with an individual with dementia, Wilson et al. (2007:1002) detailed the conversational strategies employed by people with dementia during interaction. Despite the progressive nature of the disease, they discovered that individuals retain the social proficiency that permits them to contribute to conversation as a social action in meaningful and contextually appropriate ways, being competent conversational partners. Research moved from focusing on language deficits, that is word and sentence level analysis, to studying communication and communicative competency more widely. There was a greater concern in the emerging conversation analytic research to address the notion of interactional and pragmatic *ability* as an emergent phenomenon in the field of dementia research.

In the early part of the twenty-first century, further theoretical and policy developments saw another shift in understanding dementia as a disability. Dementia is recognized as a disability both under UK domestic law (Equality Act 2010) and international convention (UN Convention on the

Rights of Persons with Disabilities 2007). In 2010 (reviewed in 2017) the Dementia Action Alliance created the National Dementia Declaration, a set of seven expectations or statements of what life should be like for people with dementia. These were co-created by people with dementia and were used to inform the UK Prime Minister's Challenge on Dementia (DoH, 2012). Importantly, related to research, people identified "We have the right to know about and decide if we want to be involved in research that looks at cause, cure and care for dementia and be supported to take part" (Alzheimer's Society, 2023). Increasingly, a right-based approach to understanding dementia as a disability has been adopted, in which the voices of people with dementia are included in policy development, as well as health and social care service design and research. The social model of disability, which views people as being disabled primarily by barriers in society, not by their impairment or difference, started to influence dementia research, and indeed CA affords a promising tool for understanding social interaction and the mechanisms people use to conduct social life.

There has been a long tradition in the field of CA to "brand" the communication of those with conditions such as autism, aphasia, and more recently dementia as "atypical" (see Wilkinson, 2019). Although many of these studies have identified competency in the communicative practices of those with these conditions, atypicality based on diagnostic categories reinforces a medical model, perpetuating the "us" and "them" dichotomy – people are "atypical" by virtue of their condition. There is evidence to suggest that the interaction of some people with dementia and their interlocutors, within certain contexts, is "atypical." For example, Jones et al. (2016) and Elsey et al. (2015) formed interactional profiles which differentiate between those with dementia and those without. When people in the memory clinic without dementia could routinely answer questions about their memory problems, independently and in great detail, people with dementia often could not. In circumstances where people who had a dementia diagnosis could not answer questions about their age, for example, and had to seek help from their companion to answer, this clearly is atypical – demonstrating both a cognitive incapacity and interactional deficit. However, branding a whole population of individuals under the banner of "atypicality" no longer fits with the social model of disability. After all, there are situations in which "neurotypical" individuals breach the norms of social interaction to achieve certain interactional goals.

Within this volume, researchers have started to challenge the binary notions of normal versus abnormal, typical versus atypical, competency versus incompetency, deficit versus ability. Mikesell (Chapter 5 this volume) demonstrates how a person with dementia can use compensatory strategies within interaction that simultaneously illuminate both trouble and a demonstration of resourcefulness in navigating such troubles. Mikesell argues that such practices point to both deficit *and* skill and suggest that a dichotomous framework – identifying a practice or behavior as *either* a deficit *or* skill – is unlikely to accurately capture the social engagement of those diagnosed with neurological disorders. Jones (Chapter 12 this volume) also suggests that "While conversation analytic research has played an important role in changing perceptions about the *abilities* of people with dementia (and the collaborative nature of interaction), perhaps these binary concepts (competence *versus* incompetence) are not useful in defining our analysis of complex cognitive issues and interactional events, and possibly do not reflect the complexities of these social encounters." Dooley and Webb (2024) have encouraged CA researchers to ensure research in the field is inclusive, diverse, and equal, and challenge the common assumptions of condition-specific atypicality.

1.3 Epistemics and Deontics

The terms *epistemics* and *deontics*, as used in this volume, are concepts that are grounded in CA work (for a brief overview see Stevanovic & Svennevig, 2015). In broad terms, epistemics refers to knowledge and how various dimensions of knowing are important for understanding how people interact with each other. Deontics, on the other hand, refers generally to persons' authority or capacity to control courses of actions, such as getting others to do things or directing interactional agendas.

Epistemics in conversation goes back at least to Sacks' writings in the 1960s (1995) on *entitlements* of experience. He noted, for example, that people who have experienced something first-hand generally have greater rights to talk about (and also be affected by) these events than people with only second-hand knowledge of what took place. Later on, Labov and Fanshel (1977) discussed what they termed A-events vs. B-events, in which speakers uttering an A-event action (e.g., statement) have greater knowledge than their interlocutors, and lesser knowledge if uttering a B-event action (e.g., information or confirmation-seeking question). Pomerantz (1980) then introduced the notion of Type 1 vs. Type 2 knowables. Whereas the former knowable involves what a speaker is obligated to know (e.g., aspects of one's own biography, what one did the previous day or earlier in the day), the latter involves knowledge that is occasioned (e.g., knowledge of others, events experienced second-hand).

More recently, epistemics has been conceptualized within an elaborate framework involving three interconnected levels or dimensions: epistemic domains, epistemic status, and epistemic stance (Heritage, 2012a, 2012b). Epistemic domain (also termed *territories of knowledge*, Heritage, 2012b) refers to types of knowledge to which a person has special/expert access or rights. This may include biographical knowledge (i.e., Type 1 knowables) or field-specific knowledge such as a medical doctor's expert knowledge of "medicine," acquired through training and experience. Thus, epistemic domains tend to be populated by certain people, and in social interactions, differences in knowledge status amongst people may and do become apparent. For example, in a medical consultation doctors will have greater medical knowledge than patients. The degree of knowledge between persons is by no means absolute, however, but instead involves a gradient (Heritage, 2012a). Although some patients may have virtually no knowledge of an ailment, other patients may be in possession of detailed information (they have read about the ailment, have a relative who is a doctor, may themselves be a doctor, etc.) or they may be seen as having expert knowledge of their own experiences – compare Mishler's (1984) distinction between "medicine" and "lifeworld." Differences in epistemic status concerning a subject may, therefore, be very pronounced or even negligible. Finally, epistemic domains and epistemic status are not seen as fixed constructs, but are rather achieved and negotiated through interaction. What this means is that being an expert in an area is not taken as given. Rather, expert knowledge must be displayed and also ratified by the other conversational participants. For this reason, what is said and how it is said will work to position someone as knowing (or not knowing). Using language in certain ways thus works to build what is commonly called an epistemic stance, as someone who has greater or lesser knowledge on a given matter. A stance is very much an in-the-moment display of one's degree of access and rights to knowledge, in which [K^+] denotes greater and [K^-] lesser rights and access to knowledge. Numerous epistemic stance resources – for example, declarative syntax to inform (A-event) vs. declarative syntax to seek confirmation (B-event) – are perpetually deployed in conversation to negotiate epistemic status (Heritage, 2012a). Stance may also be put into the service of accomplishing transformations. Recipients of talk need not accept how others have positioned them with respect to knowledge; that is, interpretations may be challenged, and new facts may be brought to light.

Deontics is generally interpreted in terms of deontic status and stance, which parallels the organizational structure found in epistemic work (Stevanovic & Peräkylä, 2014; Stevanovic & Svennevig, 2015). Deontic status concerns a person's capacity to influence actions and agendas, whereas deontic stance involves a speaker's in-the-moment accomplishment of "control" (getting others to do things) or lack thereof. As with epistemics, deontic status is not fixed but negotiable, and stance resources will play an important role in either having a speaker accept the status quo or challenge it.

These concepts are of fundamental importance in dementia research for a number of reasons. The noted "cognitive decline" in persons with dementia may influence what people are able to recall or what knowledge they are able to display in conversation. In epistemic terms, the territory of knowledge of a person with dementia will likely diminish over time, and so that person's epistemic authority may no longer be taken for granted (see, for example, Landmark, 2021; Schrauf, 2020). As far as conversations go, this may influence what may be considered a B-event utterance. For example, can it be expected that persons with dementia will be able to take up a [K$^+$] position when asked what they did yesterday or this morning? Or similarly, do persons with dementia become somehow restricted in their ability to initiate A-event utterances, in which they make authoritative, epistemic displays of important events in their lives? As already stated, the focus of this volume is not solely on identifying knowledge deficits. Rather, attention is given to both limitations *and* capabilities, and – even more importantly – how knowledge issues arising within the interactions are addressed and managed: the chapters in Part 3 of this volume specifically address these points. Further, epistemic limitations do not translate into persons necessarily displaying a position of "not knowing." What many of the chapters in this volume show is that persons with dementia may also develop strategies to somehow compensate for their diminished territories of knowledge. This attests to the creativity and resourcefulness of persons with dementia in their efforts to adjust to and make up for their changing circumstances.

Dementia has also been noted to affect the deontic aspect of social interaction. As has been noted especially for frontotemporal dementia (behavioral variant), people tend not to initiate conversational sequences, thus severely limiting their ability to set or control topical agendas, placing their interlocutors in the position of having to do so in order to keep the conversation going (Muntigl & Hödl Chapter 9 this volume; Smith, 2010). Another consequence of not initiating sequences is that people then tend to be placed in "recipient" roles, that is in a deontically weaker position. Thus, rather than getting others to do things, they must constantly react to (comply with) others' requests, directives, proposals, and so on.

An examination of the epistemic and deontic challenges associated with social interactions in which persons with dementia are conversational participants sheds considerable light on the changing relationships between them and others. Losing authority and autonomy to know and act in social situations can diminish perceptions that one is a competent social actor. This can further lead to a negative self-image, threatening the *face* of the person with dementia (Goffman, 1967). Various chapters in the volume also deal with face and facework in relation to dementia. These potentially negative consequences make it especially important to examine where diminished authority/autonomy surfaces within conversational sequences, with an eye towards understanding how these threats to face may be managed in an emotionally supportive and empathic way.

1.4 Applications: Applied Conversation Analysis

There is an emerging field of conversation analytic research which aims to effect change and which uses CA findings to inform interventions to enhance the quality of life and care of people with dementia. Whereas it is of great importance to use CA to capture experiences and thoroughly document how dementia has an impact on the everyday life of those concerned, it is equally important to use such findings as evidence that can contribute to the development of best practices in care, and inform education, guidelines, and policies. When CA is used for such purposes, it is labelled *applied CA* (see Antaki, 2011 for an overview). Applied CA is commonly associated with discourse that in one way or the other takes place in institutional settings, for example interactions in health care (e.g., dementia assessment and diagnosis, psychotherapy, suicide helpline calls), business talk, or in the classroom.

For applied CA to be effective, it should ideally be conducted in close collaboration with those directly concerned: people with dementia, partners and relatives, care-providing staff, and clinicians, to mention a few. A commonly recognized challenge is that CA methods (and the benefits of using such methods) may be difficult to understand and might seem inaccessible for some stakeholders. This can be due to a range of issues (see O'Reilley & Lester, 2019). One potential issue is that anecdotal evidence may lead to practitioner perceptions that CA is too technical and time-consuming, or that the method does not provide results that are based on quantitative measurements, which may not be well-generalizable. Another issue may be that the professionals, whose interactions are to be investigated by means of CA, are concerned that they are to be evaluated, and errors and faults will be detected and criticized. It is important to point out that this is by no means the aim of applied CA, in which the focus ordinarily is to scrutinize, as objectively as possible, how interaction in a specific setting and activity is organized and how it unfolds, with the purpose of identifying structures that can be utilized for developing best practices. To build trust is key in this context, and several visits to a setting might be needed before informants are comfortable with video recordings being made of their practices and activities (Tsekleves & Keady, 2021). Providing feedback to those who engage in the project is also a very important part of the applied approach (see Lindholm & Tykkyläinen, Chapter 14 this volume; Plejert, Chapter 4 this volume).

Even though some methodological and practical challenges are highlighted above, researchers conducting applied CA are mainly experiencing recognition and appreciation, and find themselves working fruitfully together with other professions on a mutually identified problem area or a common goal of bringing about positive change and development. Several examples are found in the present volume that connect to the approach denoted "interventionist"

CA (e.g., Lindholm & Tykkyläinen, Chapter 14 this volume; Plejert, Chapter 4 this volume; see also Antaki, 2011; Stokoe, 2011). In this approach, CA results shed light on the organization of interaction in a specific setting – for example, dementia diagnosis, interaction in residential care, the use of communication aids, and so on – and analysis is conducted with the underlying idea or goal that some kind of intervention is to be developed to promote aspects such as patient safety and the well-being of everyone involved. Such interventions include educational healthcare interventions (see, for example Pilnick et al., 2018) and Artificial Intelligence (AI) digital doctors. Underpinned by CA findings, these can be used to assess a person for dementia, with the aim of accelerating dementia diagnostic pathways (Mirheidari et al., 2019). Other applied CA research that is emerging is the exploration of how people with dementia use assistive technologies and smart home devices to conduct daily activities at home (see Samuelsson & Ekström, Chapter 13 this volume). CA has the potential to help inform the development of such devices to ensure they are user-friendly for people with disabilities like dementia (Albert, 2021; Ingebrand, 2023).

Applied CA is about collaboration between researchers and various participants, who may gain from the specific advantages of the method's rigorous aim not to make claims beyond what can be based on evidence from the material or data at hand. Even if applied CA is viewed as a discipline in its own right, it is becoming increasingly common that it is used in multidisciplinary projects. This used to be problematic, from a more orthodox CA-stance (see Antaki, 2011; Plejert, Chapter 4 this volume), as scholars were concerned that combining CA with other methods (for example, an observer's view on context or participants' retrospective accounts of an event) would dissolve the method's original, emic ambition. However, use of applied CA allows collection of evidence to support interventions that become ecologically valid in a way that is not possible through experimental trials. Through this qualitative method, the reflexive relationship between micro and macro is illuminated (Boden & Zimmerman, 1991; Heritage & Clayman, 2011). Within the area of dementia research, applied CA thus offers the unique opportunity to provide information about details of the organization of interaction that are not so easily detectable, or even possible to obtain, by other methods.

1.5   Outline of This Book

Each Part of this volume addresses one aspect of human interaction and dementia. Part 2: Dementia and Diagnostics examines how CA can shed light on diagnostic activities involving people with dementia. Negotiating the diagnostic pathway and receiving a dementia diagnosis is arguably one of the most significant points in a person's journey through dementia. There is growing importance being placed on achieving timely diagnosis, and improving the rate and quality of diagnosis for those with dementia. Furthermore, interaction analysts are beginning to demonstrate how communication can play a vital role in the success and quality of diagnostic encounters. Chapter 2 (Jones et al.) examines some of the practical challenges associated with administering standardized tests (i.e., Addenbrooke's Cognitive Examination/ACE-III) to people with dementia. Drawing from the CA concept of *recipient design*, which basically means that an utterance's design features will be tailored to its addressee, they argue that physicians generally have "good interactional reasons" for deviating from the requirement of offering standardized questions as they are formulated in ACE-III. Their chapter highlights the contingent nature of testing situations and that physicians sometimes may need to make adjustments to question formats in order to properly accommodate the needs and abilities of people with dementia. Chapter 3 (Dooley and McCabe) also explores an aspect of clinical assessment by examining conversations that involve diagnostic feedback. In particular, they focus on episodes of *misalignment*, in which doctors and patients explore divergent conversational agendas: for example, when doctors attempt to provide specific feedback concerning the dementia diagnosis and patients instead pursue a different, contrasting agenda. Their work not only delves into some of the, often face-saving, strategies from doctors, but also suggests ways of improving the "diagnosis experience" for the people taking part in the feedback conversation. Finally, Chapter 4 (Plejert) takes an *applied, conversation analytic* view of the testing situation (Antaki, 2011). By examining an episode from a video-recorded, interpreter-mediated dementia assessment, she is able to pinpoint moments of interactional trouble that arise from the interpretation process and how such trouble is oriented to or "missed" due to the complexities of three-way communication in which one of the participants does not (fully) understand what is being said. The chapter then also discusses how this applied study may offer various types of "interventions" that can benefit professionals, stakeholders, and, importantly, persons with dementia.

Part 3: Dementia and Conversational Strategies explores unique interactional practices or patterns involving people with dementia that are commonly found in a variety of conversational contexts. People with dementia, their family members, and caregivers are found to develop interactional strategies that are highly functional and may sometimes serve to compensate for other resources that have been lost. Chapter 5 (Mikesell) examines the interactions over time of Robert, a person with the behavioral variant of frontotemporal dementia (bvFTD). This longitudinal study focuses on the evolving discursive functions of a single interactional practice – the use of the phrase "now what" – that is strategically and innovatively used to recruit assistance from interlocutors. However, his later uses of "now what" are notably less effective and interlocutors often do not respond. One of the chapter's unique contributions is that it blurs the distinction between deficits (the challenges individuals face) and skillfulness (the creative navigation of challenging environments) by showing how "now what" may work as a compensatory strategy that orients to both the troubles Robert faces while simultaneously demonstrating his resourcefulness in navigating the trouble. Chapter 6 (Foster) is a study of a man (Dan) with vascular dementia who sometimes sings in everyday interactions with his family, and focuses on what Dan accomplishes by singing in those interactions. His singing is responsive to prior talk, gets a range of interactional tasks done (such as complimenting, complaining, requesting, and doing humor), and makes relevant a co-participant response. Thus, the analysis of this discursive practice provides insight into communication by people with dementia and how they use these practices to accomplish everyday social goals. Chapter 7 (Kindell et al.) examines the repeated use of tag questions by spouses/carers when talking to a person with semantic dementia. They analyze the form and uses of tag questions in these interactions and explore how they can constitute a fruitful conversational device for those talking to a person with dementia. They explore the implications of these findings in terms of how use of tag questions can be seen as an example of how those habitually interacting with people with dementia may adapt their style of talking, and how it may facilitate the participation of the person with dementia in conversation. This practice has the added benefit of minimizing the disruption to the conversation brought about by the cognitive and linguistic impairments associated with dementia. Finally, Chapter 8 (Landmark and Svennevig) highlights a person with dementia's creativity in influencing courses of action despite his limited conversational resources. They found that the person in question, Koki, was able to take topical initiative in two ways: first, by expressing his unique understanding of a given situation, and second, by making decisions about how to pursue practical problems. This study places the spotlight on Koki's resourcefulness in the face of real-word interactional challenges.

Part 4: Dementia and Epistemics includes a series of chapters on the topic of knowledge or knowledge states (epistemics) in interaction, regarding how people with dementia and their families demonstrate or negotiate what they know. People with dementia are often unable to demonstrate epistemic authority due to problems with memory, comprehension, and understanding, and so it is extremely important to investigate how dementia impacts epistemic abilities during social interaction. Chapter 9 (Muntigl and Hödl) focuses on the practical epistemic organization of a common household activity in which people with FTD regularly take part: viewing family photos. In this context, the activity of viewing photos involved family members and caregivers directing the person with FTD to identify people in photographs. Epistemic stances taken up by the participants were found to index the person with FTD's "reduced" epistemic domain with respect to her ability in recognizing family members in photos. For example, interrogative action formats were used when answering, which suggests "guessing," and family members would often provide hints, encouragement, and positive assessments (after correct guesses). However, people with FTD often assume a position of epistemic authority when asserting who is *not* on the picture. Finally, it seems easier for persons with FTD to recognize co-present persons. This suggests that recognition may be facilitated by additional features such as voice and the cotemporal setting. Chapter 10 (Ekström et al.) focuses on how the management of telling about troubles relates to living with dementia. In the chosen excerpts for this study, the spouse without dementia is the speaker of a story in which the person with dementia is the main character. This is a challenging situation wherein the speaker balances getting the story about their partner's disease across while not imposing on their partner's rights to knowledge and experience. The analysis shows that the spouse without dementia, when disclosing sensitive matters regarding the spouse with dementia, orients to differences in epistemic status between the speakers, and also commonly makes use of multimodal resources such as touch and gaze, as well as laughter, potentially in relation to the management of face and distress in situations of memory loss. Finally, Chapter 11 (Lindley) reveals some highly sophisticated practices of demonstrating epistemic authority by a person with AD. The analysis of interactive episodes demonstrates how a person with AD uses conversational practices to help position herself as an expert in her own autobiographical events and also to be able to offer advice on a variety of subjects.

Part 5: Communicative Challenges in Everyday Social Life sets out how certain troubles may arise during interactions involving people with dementia and how these troubles are managed throughout the ensuing interaction. Chapter 12 (Jones) explores the intersection between cognition and interaction by longitudinally analyzing the cognitive abilities of a person with dementia (May) (and the change in those abilities over time), examining how memory loss is reflected in verbal conduct during everyday family communication. Chapter 13 (Samuelsson and Ekström) contributes to the understanding of the possibilities and pitfalls of using personalized communication applications installed on tablet computers to support communication by people with dementia and their conversational partners. By examining video-recorded conversations between people with dementia and their carers, using digital communication for the purpose of asking questions or managing the content of the application (e.g., deciding which photo to view), they identified a range of practices that may have either greater or lesser benefits for supporting conversation. The aim of this chapter is to further the understanding of carer strategies to promote participation and involvement for persons living with dementia. Chapter 14 (Lindholm and Tykkyläinen) examines an intervention designed for professional caregivers to enhance the quality of mealtime interactions between people with dementia and their communication partners. Through detailed analyses of the verbal and embodied practices during mealtimes, it is demonstrated how the staff members' view of mealtimes change during the intervention. The chapter ends with a discussion of what can be achieved by an interaction-oriented approach to accomplishing routine caregiving tasks, focusing on both the well-being of the residents and dementia care employees' satisfaction. Finally, Chapter 15 (Webb) investigates how different quiz formats facilitate or impede participation and social interaction in group quizzes. People with dementia frequently attend groups that provide opportunities for engaging in activities, often facilitated through organized games such as quizzes. Webb found that social quizzes impose an interactional framework composed of a three-part sequence (question – answer – evaluation), marking this activity as institutional. This chapter outlines not only how quizzes may be enacted in various ways, but also demonstrates how these different forms of enactment may have interactional (and social) consequences for all participants. Special attention is given to how face threats may be realized and oriented to in these contexts.

References

Aggarwal, N., Vass, A. A., Minardi, H. A., Ward, R., Garfield, C. and Cybyk, B. (2003) 'People with dementia and their relatives: personal experiences of Alzheimer's and of the provision of care.' *Journal of Psychiatric and Mental Health Nursing*, 10: 187–197.

Albert, S. (2021) Virtual Assistants and Personal Assistants in Homecare Interactions: A Conversation Analytic Case Study (Blog, 20 October). Available: https://saulalbert.net/blog/virtual-assistants-and-personal-assistants-in-homecare-interactions-conversational-user-interfaces-as-assistive-technologies/.

Alzheimer's Disease International (ADI) (2019) World Alzheimer's report. Available: www.alzint.org/u/WorldAlzheimerReport2019.pdf.

Alzheimer Europe (2018) The Development of Intercultural Care and Support for People with Dementia from Minority Ethnic Groups. Available: www.alzheimer-europe.org/sites/default/files/alzheimer_europe_ethics_report_2018.pdf.

Alzheimer's Research UK (2023) Dementia Leading Cause of Death in 2022. 12 April. Available: www.alzheimersresearchuk.org/dementia-leading-cause-of-death-in-2022/#:~:text=The%20Office%20for%20National%20Statistics,61%2C250%20(10.4%25)%20in%202021.

Alzheimer's Society (2023) Types of Dementia. Available www.alzheimers.org.uk/about-dementia/types-dementia. access

Antaki, C. (2011) *Applied Conversation Analysis. Intervention and Change in Institutional Talk*. Basingstoke: Palgrave Macmillan.

Appell, J., Kertesz. A. and Fisman, M. (1982) 'A study of language functioning in Alzheimer patients.' *Brain and Language*, 17(1): 73–91.

Bayles, K. A. (1984) 'Language and dementia.' In A. Holland (ed.) *Language Disorders in Adults: Recent Advances.* San Diego: College-Hill Press, pp. 209–244.

(2003) 'Effects of working memory deficits on the communicative functioning of Alzheimer's dementia patients.' *Journal of Communication Disorders*, 36: 209–219.

Blair, M., Marczinski, C. A., Davis-Faroque, N. and Kertesz, A. (2007) 'A longitudinal study of language decline in Alzheimer's disease and frontotemporal dementia.' *Journal of the International Neuropsychological Society*, 13(2): 237–245.

Boden, D., and Zimmerman, D. H. (eds.) (1991) *Talk and Social Structure: Studies in Ethnomethodology and Conversation Analysis.* University of California Press.

Crisp J. (1999) 'Towards a partnership in maintaining personhood.' In T. Adams and C. L. Clarke (eds.) *Dementia Care. Developing Partnerships in Practice.* London: Ballière Tindall, pp. 95–119.

Department of Health (DoH) (2012) Prime Minister's challenge on dementia: Delivering major improvements in dementia care and research by 2015. Available: https://assets.publishing.service.gov.uk/government/uploads/system/uploads/attachment_data/file/215101/dh_133176.pdf.

Dooley, J., and Webb, J. (2024) 'Atypical interactions in healthcare: A state-of-the-art review of conversation-analytic research, with reflections on equity, diversity and inclusion.' *Research on Language and Social Interaction* 57(1), 109–126.

Dooley, J., Bass, N. and McCabe, R. (2018) 'How do doctors deliver a diagnosis of dementia in memory clinics?' *British Journal of Psychiatry*, 212(4): 239–245.

Elsey, C., Drew, P., Jones, D., Blackburn, D., Wakefield, S., Harkness, K. and Reuber, M. (2015) 'Towards diagnostic conversational profiles of patients presenting with dementia or functional memory disorders to memory clinics.' *Patient Education and Counselling*, 98(9): 1071–1077.

Equality Act 2010 (England, Wales, Scotland). Available: www.legislation.gov.uk/ukpga/2010/15/contents.

Goffman, E. (1967) *Interaction Ritual: Essays on Face-to-Face Interaction.* New York: Pantheon Books.

Guendouzi, J. A. and Müller, N. (2006) *Approaches to Discourse in Dementia.* Mahwah, NJ: Lawrence Erlbaum Associates.

Hamilton, H. E. (1994) *Conversations with an Alzheimer's Patient: An Interactional Sociolinguistic Study.* Cambridge: Cambridge University Press.

(2008) 'Language and dementia: Sociolinguistic aspects.' *Annual Review of Applied Linguistics*, 28: 91–110.

Heritage, J. (1984) *Garfinkel and Ethnomethodology.* Cambridge: Polity Press.

(2012a) 'Epistemics in Action: Action Formation and Territories of Knowledge.' *Research on Language and Social Interaction*, 45(1): 1–29, https://doi.org/10.1080/08351813.2012.646684.

(2012b) 'The epistemic engine: Sequence organization and territories of knowledge.' *Research on Language and Social Interaction*, 45(1): 30–52, https://doi.org/10.1080/08351813.2012.646685.

Heritage, J. and Atkinson, J. M. (1984) 'Introduction.' In J. M. Atkinson and J. Heritage (eds.) *Structures of Social Action: Studies in Conversation Analysis.* Cambridge: Cambridge University Press, pp. 1–16.

Heritage, J. and Clayman, S. (2011) *Talk in Action: Interactions, Identities, and Institutions*. Hoboken: John Wiley and Sons.

Hydén, L. C. and Örulv, L. (2009) 'Narrative and identity in Alzheimer's disease: A case study.' *Journal of Aging Studies*, 23(4): 205–214.

Hydén, L. C., Lindemann, H. and Brockmeier, J. (2014) *Beyond Loss. Dementia, Identity, Personhood*. New York: Oxford University Press.

Ingebrand, E. (2023) *Dementia and Learning: The Use of Tablet Computers in Joint Activities*. Doctoral dissertation, Department of Culture and Society, Linköping University, Sweden. Available: https://liu.diva-portal.org/smash/record.jsf?pid=diva2%3A1754837&dswid=-7156.

Jones, D. (2006) 'Please can I come home: Conversations with an Alzheimer's patient.' BA (Hons) dissertation, Department of Sociology, University of York, UK.

(2012) 'Conversations with a person with Alzheimer's disease: A conversation analytic study.' Unpublished Ph.D. dissertation. University of York, UK.

(2015) 'A family living with Alzheimer's disease: The communicative challenges.' *Dementia: The International Journal of Social Research and Practice*, 14(5): 555–573.

Jones, D., Drew, P., Elsey, C., Blackburn, D., Wakefield, S., Harkness, K. and Reuber, M. (2016) 'Conversational assessment in memory clinic encounters: Interactional profiling for differentiating dementia from functional memory disorders.' *Aging and Mental Health*, 20(5): 500–509.

Jones, D., Wilkinson, R., Jackson, C. and Drew, P. (2020) 'Variation and interactional non-standardization in neuropsychological tests: The case of the Addenbrooke's cognitive examination.' *Qualitative Health Research*, 30(3): 458–470.

Kindell, J., Sage, K., Keady, J. and Wilkinson, R. (2013) 'Adapting to conversation with semantic dementia: Using enactment as a compensatory strategy in everyday social interaction.' *International Journal of Language and Communication Disorder*, 48(5): 497–507.

Kitwood, T. (1988) 'The technical, the personal, and the framing of dementia.' *Social Behaviour*, 3: 161–179.

(1990) 'The dialectics of dementia: With particular reference to Alzheimer's disease.' *Ageing and Society*, 10: 177–196.

(1997) *Dementia Reconsidered – the Person Comes First*. Buckingham: Open University Press.

Labov, W. and Fanshel, D. (1977) *Therapeutic Discourse: Psychotherapy as Conversation*. New York: Academic Press.

Landmark, A. (2021) 'Couples living with dementia managing conflicting knowledge claims.' *Discourse Studies*, 23(2): 191–212.

Levinson, S. (2006) 'On the human "interaction engine".' In N.J. Enfield and S.C. Levinson (eds.) *Roots of Human Sociality: Culture, Cognition and Interaction*. Oxford: Berg Publishers, pp. 39–69.

Lindholm, C. (2015) 'Parallel realities: the interactional management of confabulation in dementia care encounters.' *Research on Language and Social Interaction*, 48(2): 176–199.

Logsdon, R. G., Gibbons, L. E., McCurry, S. M. and Teri, L. (2002) 'Assessing quality of life in older adults with cognitive impairment.' *Psychosomatic Medicine*, 64: 510–519.

Majlesi, A. R., and Plejert, C. (2018) 'Embodiment in tests of cognitive functioning: A study of an interpreter-mediated dementia evaluation.' *Dementia*, 17(2): 138–163, https://doi.org/10.1177/1471301216635341.

Mikesell, L. (2009) 'Conversational practices of a frontotemporal dementia patient and his interlocutors.' *Research on Language and Social Interaction*, 42(2): 135–162.

(2010) 'Repetitional responses in frontotemporal dementia discourse: Asserting agency or demonstrating confusion?' *Discourse Studies*, 12(4): 465–500.

Mishler, E. G. (1984) *The Discourse of Medicine: Dialectics of Medical Interviews*. Norwood, NJ: Ablex Publishing Corporation.

Mirheidari, B., Blackburn, D., Walker, T., Reuber, M. and Christensen, H. (2019) 'Dementia detection using automatic analysis of conversations.' *Computer Speech & Language*, 53: 65–79.

Mondada, L. (2018) 'Multiple temporalities of language and body in interaction: Challenges for transcribing multimodality.' *Research on Language and Social Interaction*, 51(2): 85–106. https://doi.org/10.1080/08351813.2018.1413878.

Müller, N. and Guendouzi, J. A. (2005) 'Order and disorder in conversation: Encounters with dementia of the Alzheimer's type.' *Clinical Linguistics & Phonetics*, 19(5):393–404.

Müller, N. and Wilson, B. T. (2008) 'Collaborative role construction in a conversation with dementia: An application of systemic functional linguistics.' *Clinical Linguistics & Phonetics*, 22(10–11): 767–774.

Neumann, P. J., Kuntz, K. M., Leon, J., Araki, S. S., Hermann, R. C., Hsu, M. and Weinstein, M. C. (1999) 'Health utilities in Alzheimer's disease: a cross-sectional study of patients and caregivers.' *Medical Care*, 37(1): 27–32.

NHS (2020) Dementia Guide [online]. Available: www.nhs.uk/conditions/dementia/.

Nilsson, E. (2018) Facing dementia as a *we*: Investigating couples' challenges and communicative strategies for managing dementia. Linköping University, Doctoral Dissertation. Available: http://liu.diva-portal.org/smash/get/diva2:1201944/FULLTEXT01.pdf.

(2022) 'Framing dementia experiences in a positive light: Conversational practices in one couple living with dementia.' *Dementia*, 21(3): 830–850.

Örulv, L. and Hydén, L. C. (2006) 'Confabulation: Sense-making, self-making and world-making in dementia.' *Discourse Studies*, 8(5): 647–678.

Österholm, J. and Samuelsson, C. (2015) 'Orally positioning persons with dementia in assessment meetings.' *Ageing & Society*, 35(2): 367–388, https://doi.org/10.1017/S0144686X13000755.

Perkins, L., Whitworth, A. and Lesser, R. (1998) 'Conversing in dementia: A conversation analytic approach.' *Journal of Neurolinguistics*, 11(1–2): 33–53.

Pilnick, A., Trusson, D., Beeke, S., O'Brien, R., Goldberg, S. and Harwood, R. H. (2018) 'Using conversation analysis to inform role play and simulated interaction in communications skills training for healthcare professionals.' *BMC Medical Education*, 18, https://bmcmededuc.biomedcentral.com/articles/10.1186/s12909-018-1381-1.

Pomerantz, A. (1980) 'Telling my side: "Limited access" as a "fishing" device.' *Sociological Inquiry*, 50(3–4): 186–198, https://doi.org/10.1111/j.1475-682X.1980.tb00020.x.

O'Reilly, M. and Lester, J. (2019) 'Applied conversation analysis for counselling and psychotherapy researchers.' *Counselling & Psychotherapy Research*, 19: 97–101.

Ripich, D., Vertes, D., Whitehouse, P., Fulton, S. and Ekelman, B. (1991) 'Turn-taking and speech act patterns in the discourse of senile dementia of the Alzheimer's type patients.' *Brain and Language*, 40: 330–343.

Sabat, S. (1991a) *The Experience of Alzheimer's Disease: Life Through a Tangled Veil.* Oxford: Blackwell.

(1991b) 'Turn-taking, turn-giving and Alzheimer's disease: A case study in conversation.' *Georgetown Journal of Language and Linguistics*, 2: 161–175.

Sabat, S. R. and Harré, R. (1992) 'The construction and deconstruction of self in Alzheimer's disease.' *Ageing and Society*, 12: 443–461.

Sacks, H. (1995) *Lectures on Conversation, Volumes 1 & 2.* Edited by G. Jefferson. Oxford: Wiley-Blackwell.

Schegloff, E. A. (2006) 'Interaction: The infrastructure for social institutions, the natural ecological niche for language, and the arena in which culture is enacted.' In N. J. Enfield and S.C. Levinson (eds.) *Roots of Human Sociality: Culture, Cognition and Interaction.* Oxford: Berg Publishers, pp. 70–96.

Schrauf, R. W. (2020) 'Epistemic responsibility – labored, loosened, and lost: Staging Alzheimer's disease.' *Journal of Pragmatics*, 168: 56–68.

Sidnell, J. (2012) 'Basic conversation analytic methods.' In J. Sidnell and T. Stivers (eds.) *The Handbook of Conversation Analysis.* Chichester: Wiley-Blackwell, pp. 77–99.

Sidnell, J. and Stivers, T. (eds.) (2013) *The Handbook of Conversation Analysis.* Oxford: Wiley-Blackwell.

Smith, M. S. (2010) 'Exploring the moral basis of frontotemporal dementia through social action.' In A. W. Mates, L. Mikesell and M. S. Smith (eds.) *Language, Interaction and Frontotemporal Dementia: Reverse Engineering the Social Mind.* London: Equinox, pp. 49–83.

Stevanovic, M. and Peräkylä, A. (2014) 'Three orders in the organization of human action: On the interface between knowledge, power, and emotion in interaction and social relations.' *Language in Society*, 43(2): 185–207, https://doi.org/10.1017/S0047404514000037.

Stevanovic, M. and Svennevig, J. (2015) 'Introduction: Epistemics and deontics in conversational directives.' *Journal of Pragmatics*, 78: 1–6, https://doi.org/10.1016/j.pragma.2015.01.008.

Stokoe, E. (2011) 'Simulated interaction and communication skills training: The "conversation-analytic role-play method".' In C. Antaki (ed.) *Applied Conversation Analysis.* Basingstoke: Palgrave Macmillan, pp. 119–139.

Sweeting, H. and Gilhooly, M. (1997) 'Dementia and the phenomenon of social death.' *Sociology of Health & Illness*, 19(1): 93–117.

Temple, V., Sabat, S. and Kroger, R. (1999) 'Intact use of politeness in the discourse of Alzheimer's sufferers.' *Language & Communication*, 19: 163–180.

Tsekleves, E. and Keady, J. (2021) *Design for People Living with Dementia: Interactions and Innovations.* Abingdon: Routledge.

United Nations Convention on the Rights of Persons with Disabilities. Available: www.un.org/development/desa/disabilities/convention-on-the-rights-of-persons-with-disabilities.html.

Watson, C. M., Chenery, H. J. and Carter, M. S. (1999) 'An analysis of trouble and repair in the natural conversations of people with dementia of the Alzheimer's type.' *Aphasiology*, 13(3): 195–218.

Webb, J., Lindholm, C. and Williams, V. (2020) 'Interactional strategies for progressing through quizzes in dementia settings.' *Discourse Studies*, 22(4): 503–522, https://doi.org/10.1177/1461445620914673.

Wilkinson, R. (2019) 'Atypical interaction: Conversation analysis and communicative impairments.' *Research on Language and Social Interaction*, 52(3): 281–299, https://doi.org/10.1080/08351813.2019.1631045.

Wilson, B. T., Müller, N. and Damico, J. S. (2007) 'The use of conversational laughter by an individual with dementia.' *Clinical Linguistics & Phonetics*, 21(11–12): 1001–1006.

World Health Organization (WHO) (2023) Dementia: Fact Sheet. Available: www.who.int/news-room/fact-sheets/detail/dementia.

Part 2

Dementia and Diagnostics

2 Good Reasons for Non-standardization in the Administration of Cognitive Assessments

Danielle Jones, Clare Jackson and Ray Wilkinson

2.1 Introduction

Cognitive assessment tools are a key component of the diagnostic process, and aim to facilitate identification of cognitive impairment, its severity and the cognitive domains affected (Panegyres et al., 2016). The outcome of these tests is an important basis for early access to therapeutic care and management. Measuring cognitive function is, therefore, one of the most important assessments clinicians make (Alzheimer's Society, 2015). A wide range of cognitive screening and assessment tools designed to test different aspects of cognitive functionality (e.g., recall, reasoning, abstract thinking, visuospatial and verbal skills) are available, for example the Addenbrooke's cognitive examination (ACE-III), the Montreal Cognitive assessment (MOCA), the Six-item Cognitive Impairment Test (6CIT) and the Mini-Mental State Exam (MMSE).[1] The ACE-III, examined in this chapter, has reportedly good diagnostic specificity (Hsieh et al., 2013) that is sensitive to the early stages of dementia (Bruno & Schurmann Vignaga, 2019), and has been recommended in the UK by the Department of Health and the Alzheimer's Society for use in specialist memory services (Alzheimer's Society, 2015). However, a recent Cochrane Review (Beishon et al., 2019) raises questions about the quality of research that underpins estimates of the utility of the ACE-III. Significantly, Beishon et al. point to a lack of information about how the test was carried out in relevant studies.

Clinicians are aided in the administration of the ACE-III by a guide which helps to ensure standard procedures are followed. The implementation of tests matters because interpretation of outcomes relies on normative scores derived from the assumed standardization of the testing process. If the correct administrative procedures are not followed, the test is 'not useful in indicating whether

---

[1] It is also notable that the ACE-III, in common with the other tests listed, is designed for speakers of English. For people with a diverse linguistic and cultural background, the Cross-cultural Neuropsychological Test Battery (CNTB) and Rowland Universal Dementia Assessment (RUDAS) have proven more useful for major populations than the above-mentioned tests (e.g. Nielsen et al., 2019).

[a patient's] score falls in the normal or pathological range' (Venneri, 2005: 97) and, therefore, could affect a clinician's ability to make an accurate diagnosis. Despite the basic requirement for standardization of procedures, specialist clinicians anecdotally report having received no formal training on the administration of the ACE-III. Furthermore, the guidance document is not always clear; there are no instructions on how to introduce the test, and some questions have verbatim instruction whilst other questions are *quasi*-scripted and do not require the practitioner to use specific wording. These inconsistencies enable interactional variation in the administration of the test (Jones et al., 2020).

In common with most cognitive assessment tools, the ACE-III is implemented by means of talk-in-interaction (Drew et al., 2006). All talk is locally occasioned and contingent; hence it unavoidably introduces non-standardized elements to the testing process. There is a body of Conversation Analysis (CA) research exploring standardization-in-interaction in a range of different settings: for example surveys (Houtkoop-Steenstra, 2000; Maynard et al., 2002), education (Marlaire & Maynard, 1990; Maynard & Turowetz, 2017) and healthcare (Jones et al., 2020). This research is predominantly interested in the 'interactional substrate' – the social organization of talk during standardized examinations and survey interviews. Much as in the delivery of standardized cognitive assessments, standardization in surveys focuses on reducing interviewer variability and thus on improving reliability, so that different interviewers act according to interviewing rules. However, such research has revealed that: 'Standardization in survey research or any other realm is not guaranteed by its rules and procedures. Standardization has to be achieved according to the variegated circumstances that impinge on any attempt to follow those rules and procedures' (Maynard & Schaeffer, 2006: 27).

Maynard and Marlaire (1992) suggest that the interactional practices testers employ when administering psychoeducational standardized examinations can influence recipients' responses, and their experience of 'being tested'. Ultimately, they showed that test scores are collaborative products of the testing process rather than reflecting the (ostensibly) neutral qualities of the instrument. Some interviewers/testers, for instance, opt for a more conversational approach by changing the scripted, 'neutrally' formulated standardized questions (Houtkoop-Steenstra, 1997) because the rigidities of standardization can lead to contrived interactions. Similarly, in an ethnographic study of memory clinics, Swallow and Hillman (2018: 229) illustrate practitioners' 'tinkering' practices in 'carefully choreograph[ing] the consultation process' (Swallow and Hillman, 2018: 234) in a number of practical ways. These include actively omitting test items and going off-script to provide reassurance and encouragement. Swallow and Hillman suggest these practices are mechanisms for taking care of the vulnerabilities of the diagnostic encounter: that is, active ad hoc redesigning of test implementation, stepping away from standardization, occurs to prioritize recipiency and emotional labour.

The rigidities of standardized surveys/interviews are often overcome by interviewers revising the original questions to include more natural or *recipient-designed* formulations (Houtkoop-Steenstra, 1995; Houtkoop-Steenstra & Antaki, 1997; Maynard & Schaeffer, 2006). Recipient design is a conversation analytic concept developed by Sacks (1992) to refer to the ways that speakers adapt talk for co-participants. This is a normative feature of interaction such that interlocutors hold each other accountable for failing to orient to what they know about each other and the particular circumstances of the interaction. Underpinned by Goffman's (1967) work on *face*, Houtkoop-Steenstra and Antaki (1997: 286) show how interviewers use recipient design to encourage 'face-protective responses in environments that are marked by interactional troubles', that is they change the question to help the respondent to answer successfully. In medical assessments, where strict administrative procedure is required, there appears to be a tension between standardization (underpinned by institutional constraints) and recipient design (see Heritage, 2002).

The above findings suggest a need for fine-grained analysis of the situated implementation of cognitive assessments. In an earlier paper (Jones et al., 2020), we reported findings based on video recordings of clinicians and patients doing the ACE-III, showing a variety of ways that test implementation in practice is neither fixed nor standardized. For example, we demonstrated variation in the way clinicians introduce the test to patients as part of the ongoing activities in a consultation. To some extent, this variation might be expected as there is no administrative guidance for practitioners in how to prepare patients for the test. However, the different methods the practitioners used appeared to be consequential for how patients received and understood the testing activity. Our earlier work also demonstrated deviations from the standardized instructions that the ACE-III does provide. For example, practitioners might vary the design of questions and/or introduce elements of reassurance that are not present in the guidance.

This chapter continues and extends our earlier work. Following a description of our methods (Section 2.2), we return to the matter of variation in test introduction (Section 2.3.1) and extend our previous analysis by suggesting a possible association with practitioners' working diagnoses. We then return to the evident non-standardization of the delivery of test questions, including elements of recipient design (Section 2.3.2). Finally, we introduce entirely new analyses of practitioner utterances that are positioned after a patient has answered (or attempted to answer) a question – that is, in the third turn (Section 2.3.3). In this work we are not aiming to highlight particular issues with the ACE-III as a problematic assessment, nor the testers as incompetent;

rather, we are pointing to more general issues about the social nature of tests of cognitive functioning, and the competing demands clinicians face in (1) trying to carry out the test in line with the instructions, that is in a standardized way and (2) doing so in a manner which takes into account how the patients are responding or might respond. By exploring some of the ways in which the administration of the ACE-III differs from standard procedures in clinical guidance – including ways in which elements of the consultation are recipient-designed – we show there are often 'appropriate' interactional reasons for non-standard administration of cognitive examination.

2.2 Methods

The data are video recordings of 105 initial assessment consultations in a specialist neurology-led memory service in the UK. Patients have predominantly been referred by their General Practitioners and these initial consultations typically comprise history-taking, followed by the ACE-III and sometimes a mood questionnaire, and then a brief physical examination. Further diagnostic testing, including a neuropsychology battery and Magnetic Resonance Imaging (MRI) are completed in a later appointment. The ACE-III is scored out of 100, with the higher score denoting better cognitive function and the cut-off for dementia being 82–88/100 (Crawford et al., 2012). Previous research has focused on the history-taking conversations before patients take the formal cognitive test (Elsey et al., 2015; Jones et al., 2016; Reuber et al., 2018). The current research focuses on the administration of the ACE-III. There were 92 recorded occurrences of the ACE-III being administered between October 2012 and October 2014, from which a sample of 40 cases were randomly selected for detailed analysis. The administration of the test takes on average 15 minutes (the full initial consultation lasts on average approximately 35 minutes). In the sample consultations, patients (represented as Pat in the transcripts) are interacting with five different clinicians – three neurologists and two neurology registrars (Neu in transcripts). The interactions were transcribed in detail, according to the conventions used in CA.

There is now an established body of CA research in medical settings (Heritage & Maynard, 2006; Stivers, 2007; Robinson & Heritage, 2014; Leydon & Barnes, 2020) which has identified patterns of language and interaction that inform practice (Heritage et al., 2007; Wilkinson, 2013), medical assessment (Heritage & Stivers, 1999; Reuber et al., 2009) and treatment recommendations (Stivers, 2002; Stivers & Barnes, 2018; Toerien, 2021). CA is also used to examine closely the various communicative formats used to 'deliver' medically relevant actions, such as diagnosis (Heath, 1992; Peräkylä, 1998; Maynard, 2017) – including dementia diagnoses (Dooley et al., 2018) – as well as to explore linguistic and interactional patterns that can help clinicians to establish differential diagnosis (Elsey et al., 2015; Jones et al., 2016; Reuber et al., 2018). In this study, we draw on CA methods to examine recordings of clinicians and patients completing the ACE-III.

2.3 Analysis

Our earlier work (Jones et al., 2020) revealed interactional *variations* in the administration of the ACE-III (e.g., in the ways that clinicians introduce the test), and *deviations* from the (quasi-)scripted guidance designed to ensure standardization. We showed that clinicians appear to design the questions in ways that reflect or account for patients' perceived abilities. Here, as outlined above, we will start by further exploring interactional variation and deviation during the introduction to the test.

2.3.1 *Interactional Variation: Introduction of the Memory Assessment*

There is *variation* in the manner in which clinicians transition from the history-taking phase of the consultation to administering the ACE-III (Jones et al., 2020). History-taking involves between 10 to 20 minutes of clinician-led questions in order to understand the person's background and their current concerns. There is no guidance on how to introduce the test and each clinician completes this differently. Furthermore, as Jones et al. (2020) showed, variations in the introduction of the test appear to have implications for patients' understanding, with some patients displaying uncertainty, as is evident from their embodied or verbal reactions. For example, some clinicians do not mention the test explicitly during the consultation itself, saying, for instance, 'We'll just run through a few quick questions, then I'll examine you' immediately before the test commences. Utterances of this kind, coming at the end of what is already a substantial period of questioning (during the history-taking), do not clearly convey that the upcoming questions are part of a discrete test, and this can therefore create confusion for patients. Other patients appear to be fully aware of the expectations for the next phase of the consultation when the clinician adopts a different approach: explicitly naming the test, providing information about the questions within it and how the test was validated (see Jones et al., 2020, for a full analysis).

Extract 1 shows another version of test introduction from a different clinician (not explored in Jones et al., 2020). In this version, the clinician introduces the upcoming test by both marking and naming a change of activity, characterizing it as a 'memory test' but without furnishing details.

Extract 1
```
01   Neu1:   Erm:: So >I'm gonna> do:: (.) a
02           memory test on you now.=Is that okay:,
03   Pat:    Yeah.
04   Neu1:   Er: So what day: is it today:,
```

In Extract 1, the clinician tells the patient that they are going to be subject to a memory test (lines 1–2). The turn design conveys the clinician's high deontic and epistemic authority (see Stevanovic & Peräkylä, 2012; Muntigl, this volume) to decide about what happens next ('I'm going to...'; notwithstanding the tag at the end of line 2) and expertise to conduct this test 'on' the patient (line 2). The test itself is characterized as a memory test, but no further details are given. The patient confirms they are okay to continue – 'Yeah' (line 3) – thus claiming (but not displaying) understanding of what is coming next.

Extract 2 shows the moment of transition from history-taking to testing involving the same clinician and another patient. Here, the hierarchical stance is more collaborative with the clinician's proposal that 'we'll do a memory test now' (line 1) suggesting more of a joint activity for the clinician and the patient.

Extract 2
```
01   Neu1:   OK. So we'll do a memory test now.=Okay:?
02   Pat:    Yeah.
03   Neu1:   So what day is it toda:y?
```

It is interesting to note that this clinician (Neu1) is the only one (of the five clinicians recorded) to routinely seek consent or permission from the patient to begin the testing phase of the consultation – 'Is that okay?' (Extract 1, line 2) and 'Okay?' (Extract 2, line 1), thus introducing further variation. Notably, though, in both these cases the clinician does not lift his gaze to the patient when seeking this consent, thus giving it a tokenistic quality. Instead, the clinician is engaged in gathering the test paperwork from a cupboard behind him and attaching the patient's information to the test paper.

Further to exploring variation between the individual clinicians' styles of introducing the formal cognitive assessment, we found that clinicians would alter their own practice for different patients. The clinicians in the memory clinic informed us during informal discussions that they generally form an initial impression of the patients' abilities during the history-taking phase. They reported that within the first five minutes of talking to the patient they have generally formed a 'working diagnosis'. Clinicians often use an initial 'gut feeling' as part of their clinical decision-making (Lindeberg et al., 2019) and the accuracy of this clinical impression on determining a correct diagnosis has been positively assessed (Pond et al., 2013). With this in mind, we suggest that clinicians may be adapting their administration of the cognitive assessment tool according to their working diagnosis. That is, in these interactions clinicians can be seen to be (re)designing aspects of the test to suit the patient's abilities or undertaking extra interactional work to prepare some patients for the potentially difficult nature of the test. This concept of recipient design (Sacks, 1992) relates to the relationship between the tester and recipient of the test. This was particularly evident during the introduction of the test.

The two patients in Extracts 1 and 2 were given a working diagnosis of non-progressive memory problems (which may be summarized under the term functional cognitive disorder (FCD)) after the initial consultation and subsequently received a formal diagnosis of FCD (Pennington, et al., 2015). In contrast, the patients in Extracts 3 and 4) both received a dementia diagnosis from the same clinician (Neu1). Prior to the conversation in Extract 3, the patient had been asked a series of questions requiring her to recall several details regarding her family's medical history, which she was struggling to remember, and she informed the clinician that he was 'asking difficult questions'.

Extract 3

```
01   Neu1:  So I'm gonna do a memory test on you
02          now.=Okay,
03   Pat:   °Yeah°..shih((sniff))
04          (0.4)
05   Neu1:  So these are (.) designed to be a
06          bit tricky a[n::.st] retch your memory,
07   Pat:              [Yeah.   ]
08   Neu1:  So it'd be (similar to-) (.) but even
09          harder questions unfortunately for you:,
10          (.)
11   Neu1:  Erm: so, (.) what day is it today?
```

Extract 3 begins in a very similar manner to the previous two extracts, with the clinician informing the patient that a memory test will ensue (line 1), and (nominally) seeking consent, 'Okay' (line 2). Although the patient confirms readiness/willingness to perform the test – 'Yeah' (line 3) – this is said very quietly and is followed by an audible sniff. Sniffing can be interactionally relevant (Hepburn, 2004; Hoey, 2020), though, to our knowledge, systematic analysis has not been conducted in this sequential environment. Together with the quietly spoken agreement, we speculate that this sniff is perhaps a display of unsureness or apprehension. Rather than commencing the test, as in the previous two examples, the clinician first orients to the patient's possible 'unsureness'. 'So' (line 4), in turn-initial position, could be seen to be 'other-attentive' (Bolden, 2006). In stating that the test is 'designed to be a bit tricky and stretch your memory' (lines 5–6), the clinician could be both orienting to his perception of the patient's cognitive difficulties as well as to the patient's lack of conviction in her confirmation to proceed with the test. The clinician is working here to absolve the patient should she find the test difficult by characterizing it as designedly difficult. The sense that the clinician is orienting to an already formed working diagnosis of more severe cognitive difficulties is supported further when he states that the questions would be 'even harder questions unfortunately for you' (lines 8 and 9). The questions may be designedly tricky, but here the clinician is expressing that the patient (with her particular cognitive deficits) would find them even harder to answer. The clinician here is engaging in additional interactional work to prepare the patient for the task ahead and, in expressing regret about the difficulty of the questions with 'unfortunately' (line 9), he is working to build solidarity and set (perhaps low) expectations. This introduction is therefore designed for this particular patient in this particular interaction.

Extract 4, again with the same clinician (Neu1), shows very similar features.

Extract 4
```
01   Neu1:   Okay. So I'm going to do a memory test with
02           you now.= If that's oka:y,
03           (0.2) ((Dr looks at Patient))
04   Pat:    .hhh HH[Hhhh]
05   Neu1:          [I kno]w these
06           aren'[t (.) particularl]y nice:,
07   Pat:         [(I've  haven't) ]
08   Pat:    °um hmm°
09   Neu1:   >But they're okay,<.hh So what da:y is it
10           today,
```

Similar to the collaborative introduction to the test in Extract 2 ('we'll do a memory test now' (line 1)), here the clinician declaratively introduces the test by stating 'So I'm going to do a memory test with you now' (lines 1–2). He follows it up again with a tag question seeking consent to proceed, 'If that's okay' (line 2). Apart from the slight change in formation from doing a test 'on you' (Extracts 1 and 3) to 'with you' (Extract 4), and the tag question being formulated with either 'is that okay' (Extract 1), 'Okay' (Extracts 2 and 3) and 'If that's okay' (Extract 4), these are all very similar introductions to the test. Unlike in the other extracts, however, here the patient does not confirm that it is okay to proceed. The tag question's format invites a polar response from the patient, but her response is not type-conforming (Raymond, 2003), suggesting potential disaffiliation. Possible resistance on the part of the patient is first adumbrated by a gap (line 3) followed by an audible sigh (line 4). Hoey (2013) suggests that sighing has an indexical relationship with emotion – specifically negative emotion. Here the patient could be audibly using the sigh to convey some level of distress. In both these extracts, the patients use of non-lexical tokens the sniff (Extract 3) and the sigh (Extract 4) to (possibly) display some problem with the proposed course of action.

Again, the clinician orients to the patient's negative stance by displaying his awareness of the disagreeable nature of the memory test – 'I know these aren't particularly nice' (lines 5 and 6) – before reassuring the patient that 'they're ok' (line 9). Here the extra interactional work appears to arise more out of the contingencies of the patient's response, rather than that clinician's perception of their ability. However, it is worth noting the contrast between the ways the test is introduced for patients with likely FCD (Extracts 1 and 2) and those with likely dementia (Extracts 3 and 4). Furthermore, when the clinician has a working diagnosis of dementia (Extracts 3 and 4), he gazes up at the patient when seeking consent to complete the memory test. He does not give this level of attention to the patients with FCD.

In summary, we have explored variation in the way that clinicians introduce the formal cognitive examination. We have further shown through analysing cases from a single clinician (Neu1) with different patients how the introduction to the test is often recipient-designed, with the clinician adapting interactional practices when patients have more severe cognitive difficulties. This alteration may either be contingent on the patient's negative response to the course of action proposed by the clinician or orients to the clinician's perception of the patient's ability. In the consultations where the clinician has formed a working diagnosis of dementia during the history-taking phase, they often amended their introduction to include more attention (in their gaze patterns) and convey some of the difficulty the test may pose for the patient. These alterations suggest that there may be good reasons for variation in the introduction to the test.

2.3.2 Interactional Non-standardization and Recipient Question Design

There are other elements of the test that show evidence of recipient design. Different clinicians deviate from the parameters of the test to design questions in ways that function to 'help' the patient establish the correct answer. This is evident for both questions that have verbatim instruction, as well as for quasi-scripted questions. Jones et al. (2020: 465–466) showed how clinicians help the patient with the more basic questions, like identifying the season of the year. Extract 5 demonstrates how the question ordinarily runs off.

Extract 5
```
01   Neu2:   And what season of the year is it,=
02   Pat:    =Autumn.
03           (0.4)
04   Neu2:   .hhh Where are we,=What's the name of this
05           place,
```

This extract shows an unproblematic question–answer sequence which follows the standard administrative procedure for the test, continuing with the next question (line 4). This extract is taken from someone who reported subjective cognitive complaints. In contrast, in Extract 6 the clinician engages in extra interactional work, orienting to the patient's difficulty in responding to the question and helping the patient to establish the correct answer.

Extract 6

```
01   Neu3:   Erm, what erm, what season of the year are
02           we in? Is it spring, summer, autumn, winter?
03           What season is it?
04   Pat:    Erm. (0.4)
05   Neu3:   £I know it's hard to tell at the
06           moment. Huh huh huh huh
07   Pat:    Yeah.=
08   Neu3:   =What would you say?
09   Pat:    Erm, (0.4) Autumn.
10   Neu3:   Oh okay. That's great.
```

The patient in Extract 6 displayed extreme levels of cognitive decline during history-taking (he did not know his age or why he was at the clinic). He subsequently scored only 31 out of 100 on the ACE-III, which is highly indicative of dementia. In the test immediately before this question about the season the patient said the wrong day, did not know the date, replied with 'Monday' when asked the month, and replied with the name of the country when asked what year it was. Here the clinician is again asking, 'what season of the year are we in' (lines 1 and 2), and then proceeds to produce candidate options for the patient (line 2). Given the patient had just responded with the name of the country when asked the year, the clinician is here mobilizing recipient design by restricting the category of responses the patient can produce. This kind of anticipatory work – anticipating trouble and explicating possible answers for the patient deviates from the guidance. Trouble in responding is confirmed when the patient utters a marker of hesitation and pauses (line 4). Instead of moving on or reasserting the same question (which is a more typical course of action when a patient's response is delayed), the clinician states, 'I know it's hard to tell at the moment' (lines 5–6). This implies that the current weather condition, which is visible from the window, is atypical for the season they are in, thus assisting the patient to determine the correct answer (e.g., if it was snowing, and the weather was atypical, one might deduce that it was perhaps spring or summer). It could also work to excuse the patient for his displayed lack of knowledge – helping to *save face* – placing the blame for his inability to respond on the atypical weather rather than his failing cognition (Goffman, 1955). The clinician further prompts for a reply with 'what would you say' (line 8) – this implies that a guess based on this information may be acceptable. Despite this extra interactional work, the patient incorrectly responds with 'autumn' (line 9) (when in fact it is spring). The clinician offers a receipt for the incorrect response with 'Oh okay' (line 10), a turn in which the oh-prefacing is the only indicator that the response was in some way unexpected (Heritage, 1998).

Jones et al. (2020) also showed how clinicians deviate from the administrative guide during the 'attention–subtraction' task, which states, 'Ask the participant to subtract 7 from 100, record the answer, and then ask the participant to keep subtracting 7 from each new number until you ask them to stop' (Right Decisions Service, 2017). This ordinarily runs off as shown in Extract 7:

Extract 7
```
01   Neu4:   Can you subtract seven from one hundred,
02   Pat:    Ninety-three.
03   Neu4:   And then keep taking seven from the
04           number that you get.
05           (0.4)
06   Pat:    Eigh::ty-four::,(0.6)s:: seventy-s:even,
07           (0.2) seventy,(0.6) s:ixty-three:,
08   Neu4:   Good.
```

In Extract 7 the clinician does not offer any further guidance to the patient and does not attempt to support the patient's handling of the calculations. However, Jones et al. (2020) showed that some clinicians alter this sequence by repeating the patient's response after each subtraction within the design of the next sum, meaning the number of origin is repeated back to the patient: for example, 'and seven away from ninety-three' (Jones et al., 2020: 465). We suggested that this showed evidence of co-construction, where the clinician appears to be helping the patients by adding information into the question and thus placing less of a burden on the patient's attention skills to independently remember the numbers. These different designs demonstrate a divergence from the standardized test requirements given in the guidance and also places differential 'cognitive load' (Chandler & Sweller, 1991; Majlesi & Plejert, 2018) on patients.

We have also found occasions when the same question is amended, or as in the next case (Extract 8) abandoned by the clinician when it is clear that the patient is unable to complete it accurately. The patient in Extract 8 scored 65 out of 100 on the ACE-III and was diagnosed with dementia. Again, the patient had displayed interactional signs of dementia during history-taking (Jones et al., 2016; Reuber et al., 2018) and was given a working diagnosis of dementia by the clinician after the initial consultation. The scoring guide states that clinicians should 'not stop the participant if they make a mistake. Allow them to carry on and check subsequent answers for scoring' (Right Decisions Service, 2017), as the patients can score up to five points on this question, one for each correct subtraction. For example, in Extract 7, the patient got the first subtraction correct (line 2) but all the subsequent subtractions wrong (lines 6–7), so would have scored 1 for this question (although notably the error arises from the first incorrect answer because the remaining answers are correct in terms of subtracting seven each time). Even though the patient got the second subtraction wrong, the clinician allowed them to continue with the course of the question. In Extract 8 the clinician administers this question quite differently:

Extract 8
```
01    Neu4:    Can you subtract seven from a hundred,
02             (1.2)
03    Pat:     .hh Er:::(0.2) ninety-two:.
04             (0.6)
05    Neu4:    Okay what we'll do is- er: can you spell me
06             the word 'world',
```

The patient projects trouble in answering, with a long gap (line 2) and the turn initial delay, 'er' (line 3) before producing the wrong answer 'Ninety-two' (line 3) (albeit only incorrect by one number). The clinician then starts to narrate the next course of action he is going to take, which departs from pursuing further answers from the patient ('Okay what we'll do is', line 5). Instead of completing this phrase with something like 'move to the next question', the clinician proceeds to actually produce the next question: 'can you spell me the word "world"' (lines 5–6). The clinician is here orienting to the patient's troubles, and perhaps his own working diagnosis of the patient's abilities, and is choosing not to follow the administrative and scoring guidance by abandoning the question. This is another way in which the clinicians design and administer the assessment for particular patients.

We have shown how clinicians vary the administration of the ACE-III, both in the manner in which it is introduced within the initial consultation and regarding the design of certain questions by deviating from the scripted or quasi-scripted guidance that is meant to ensure that standard administrative procedures are followed. There is evidence of recipient design, which is often locally occasioned in the interaction itself, for example when patients display some trouble with the course of action or in responding to a particular question. These troubles may also be predicted by clinicians based on their perception of 'how the patient is doing' in the consultation more generally and the working diagnosis they have formed. Clinicians do extra interactional work to orient to these troubles and work to help the patients with the questions. We now move to show how this 'special attention' appears in different sequential locations within the administration of the ACE-III, notably in the clinician's third-turn responses (Sacks, 1992; Schegloff, 1992; Schegloff, 2007).

2.3.3   Recipient Design in the Third Turn: FCD

Another place where clinicians demonstrate some additional interactional attention to the patient is in the third turn. Elaborations after a potentially completed sequence of talk has been widely discussed in CA literature (Schegloff, 2007), identifying different purposes for third-turn utterances in different interactional environments, such as in everyday interaction (Beach, 1993), courtrooms (Atkinson and Drew, 1979), job interviews (Button, 1987), news interviews (Clayman, 1988; Clayman & Heritage, 2002; Clayman et al., 2020), classrooms (McHoul, 1978; Koole, 2010) and survey interviews (Houtkoop-Steenstra, 2000; Maynard & Schaeffer, 2006). Expansion in the third turn might be designed to be either minimal or non-minimal (Schegloff, 2007). Non-minimal post expansions project further talk, such as repair. Minimal expansions represent one further turn at talk following the second pair part and do not project further talk; hence they are also known as 'sequence-closing thirds' (Schegloff, 2007: 118). Minimal post-expansions accomplish a range of actions, including receipts of information using tokens such as 'okay' (Beach, 1993), minimal confirmatory/assessing responses such as 'good' (Maynard & Marlaire, 1992) and what survey methodologists characterise as feedback (Houtkoop-Steenstra, 1997; Maynard & Schaeffer, 2006). Interviewers can use this third-turn position not only to acknowledge a response, but also to convey evaluations of it for the purpose of providing reassurance and motivation (Swallow and Hillman, 2018). However, interviewing protocols often advise administrators to produce 'neutral' acknowledgements only, thus refraining from indicating whether a response is correct or incorrect (Mehan et al., 1986). Maynard and Marlaire (1992) demonstrated how acknowledgments (such as smiling and nodding following a correct response) do not necessarily affect an individual answer but may have a cumulative influence on performance.

Importantly, the ACE-III administrative guide has no advice on how clinicians should respond to answers. In our dataset, there appear to be different approaches adopted by different clinicians and for different patients and their abilities. That is, we see a distinction in the interactional uses of third turns depending on whether the patient has FCD or dementia. Extracts 9–11 exemplify routine practice when a patient has a working diagnosis of FCD and Extracts 12–15 (Section 2.3.4) feature patients with dementia. We found that when there is a working diagnosis of FCD, clinicians generally do not produce third-turn responses or, if they are produced, they are typically minimal – either 'okay' or 'good' – and appear at the end of a task sequence rather than between individual question–answer sequences. The focal sequence within Extracts 9–14 is taken from an 'attention–orientation' task in the ACEIII, which is scored out of 5 (Extract 15 deals with a different question). On the test paper clinicians are told: 'Ask: which – No./Floor, Street/Hospital, Town, County, Country'. The test then moves to an 'attention–registration' task where the participants are asked to repeat and remember three words.

In our first example (Extract 9), the clinician uses no post-expansion in the third turn.

Extract 9
```
01   Neu4:   An- Where are we,=What's the name of this place,
02   Pat:    ((City name)).
03           (0.8)
04   Neu4:   Um- th- the name of this specific building,
05   Pat:    Er ((Hospital name)).
06   Neu4:   And >do you know what< floor we're on,
07   Pat:    (Floor letter)
08   Neu4:   And what county is ((City name)) in,
09   Pat:    ((County name)).
10   Neu4:   And what country is, n- do we live in,
11   Pat:    England.
12   Neu4:   .hh I'm going to give you the name of three
13           things I want you to remember,
```

After each response the clinician moves to the next question in the sequence, even when the task is changing (line 12). Looking across the dataset, this lack of minimal post-expansion is typical when the patient has FCD. However, there is often some ambiguity in the initial question in this section: 'what's the name of this place?' (line 1). As Schegloff (1972) shows, a range of possibly correct answers are relevant in response to such a question (e.g., the specific room, the building, city and so on). In this case the patient responds with the name of the city (line 2) (other patients provide alternative place terms including more generic responses such as 'a hospital'). The test is here seeking the name of the specific hospital as the 'correct' response and therefore, in the third turn (line 4), the clinician repairs the question to be more specific: 'the name of the specific building'. Although this is not prefaced by an explicit marker of repair, for example 'I mean' (see Schegloff, 1992), following a gap (line 3) and turn-initial delay the clinician partially repeats her prior turn ('the name of the') before replacing the ambiguous term 'place' with the more particular locational formulation 'this building'. This attends to the lack of specificity inherent in the initial question as set out in the test papers. That is, in order to gain a point on the test, the patient needs to produce the name of the building in response to this question. Following the reformulated question, the patient does produce the required response (line 5) and the clinician moves on with no further elaboration or acknowledgment.

Extract 10 is very similar, in that the initial question requires some revision. However, here the clinician acknowledges the end of the task sequence before moving to a new activity ('Good' – line 13).

Extract 10
```
01   Neu1:   What building are we in,
02   Pat:    Hospital.
```

```
03   Neu1:   What's the na:me of the hospital,
04   Pat:    ((Hospital name))
05   Neu1:   And what floor are we on,
06   Pat:    ((Floor letter)).
07   Neu1:   And what town,
08   Pat:    ((City name))
09   Neu1:   And the county,
10   Pat:    ((County name)).
11   Neu1:   And the country,
12   Pat:    England.
13   Neu1:   Good.
14           (0.2)
15   Neu1:   >Now I'm g-< I'm going to ask you to repeat
16           three words...
```

The clinician's initial question here is a little more constrained than in Extract 9, asking 'what building are we in?' (Extract 10, line 1). Despite needing to identify a 'building' (Extract 10) instead of a 'place' (Extract 9), the patient does not respond with the name of the hospital, but labels the type of building, that is a 'hospital' (line 2). Again, the clinician attends to the test requirements for a more specific locational formulation by asking the patient 'What's the name of the hospital' (line 3). Although this may not be interactionally salient to the patient, analysing the data in relation to the external requirements of a standardized test reveals the clinician's orientation to be more specific. Reformulating the question enables the patient to produce the 'correct' locational formulation to gain a point on the test. As noted, this question appears to be a source of trouble in many of the interactions we have examined, suggesting a need for further advice to clinicians regarding the specificities of this question. In this case, the patient goes on to produce the required response (line 4) and the clinician moves forward, notably using *and*-prefaced questions (Heritage & Sorjonen, 1994), which was not a feature of the revised question at line 3. This further suggests that the question at line 3 was not the next in a sequence of questions, but rather a clarification of the earlier question. There is no overt acknowledgment of the patient's responses until the end of the task sequence – 'Good' (line 13). This minimal post-expansion is designed to close the prior sequence before initiating the next (Beach, 1993; Schegloff, 2007). It could also be audibly assessing the prior responses as being accurate, hence providing the patient with reassurance (Swallow & Hillman, 2018).

We see something similar in Extract 11, where 'Okay' (line 12) is used to receipt the answer and to close the sequence before moving to the next task.

Extract 11
```
01   Neu2:   A::nd can you tell me the name of the
02           building we're in,
03   Pat:    .tch .hh ((Hospital name))
04   Neu2:   And the floor that we're on,
```

```
05    Pat:     Er:((letter)) floor.
06    Neu2:    And the:: city,
07    Pat:     (City name)=
08    Neu2:    =The county,
09    Pat:     ((City name)) is ((county)) isn't[it,]
10    Neu2:                                  [And] country,
11    Pat:     UK. Huh hh
12    Neu2:    Okay.=And just repeat these three words...
```

Merritt (1980: 144) suggests that 'Okay' acts as a 'bridge, a linking device between two stages or phases of the [service] encounter'. Furthermore, as Maynard and Schaeffer (2006) suggest, 'okay' signifies the boundaries of related questions in that interviewers withhold third-turn acknowledgments when a subsequent question links to the topic of its predecessor, and produce acknowledgments when the next question shifts topic. In Extract 11, 'Okay' (line 12) bridges topics and shifts between two discrete tasks on the ACE-III. Clinicians also do not appear to confirm the responses of patients with FCD, even if patients seek confirmation. For example, the patient in Extract 11 is uncertain of the county but nevertheless gives the correct response, followed by a confirmation check 'isn't it' (line 9). The clinician does not confirm that the patient has given the correct response and instead continues with the next question.

In sum, when there is a working diagnosis of FCD, clinicians generally do not produce third-turn responses, or if they are produced, they are typically minimal, either 'okay' or 'good', and appear at the end of a task sequence rather than between individual question–answer sequences. The third turn can also be used to address a lack of specificity within the design of the initial question as required by the test. Clinicians use this turn to restrict the range of place terms to a specific locational formulation to enable a patient to score a point on the test. Third-turn utterances often look different when clinicians interact with people with a working diagnosis of dementia, as discussed in Section 2.3.4.

2.3.4   Recipient Design in the Third Turn: Dementia

When clinicians have established a working diagnosis of dementia based on a patient's 'performance' during history-taking, they often conduct the ACE-III differently. Some clinicians do not require these patients to be as specific in their responses (as compared with Extracts 9 and 10). Also, they do not use the third turn to seek a more specific, and thus correct response. For example, in Extract 12 the patient responds to the question about the 'name of the building you're in' (lines 1 and 2) with 'Hospital' (line 4). As we have seen above (Extract 10), this locational formulation is not accurate and requires further revision to receive a point on the test. Here, the patient has a working diagnosis of dementia and the clinician does not alter the question in the third turn; instead, they appear to accept this more general locational formulation and move to the next question (although it is not clear if the patient received a point for this question on the test paper).

Extract 12

```
01   Neu4:   Okay.= Can you tell me the name of the
02           building you're in,
03           (0.2)
04   Pat:    Hospital.
05   Neu4:   A:nd the floor that you're on,
```

Extract 13 also demonstrates the clinician's lack of orientation to eliciting a full and correct response to this question. For the purpose of the transcript in Extract 13 we have used the pseudonym 'Sandington' for the hospital name.

Extract 13

```
01   Neu1:   What building are we in at the moment,
02   Pat:    Pardon,
03   Neu1:   What's the name of this building,
04   Pat:    Oh it's er a- Sa- Sa- Sa- (0.4) hhh it's
05           got S (0.6) um::, (0.4) tch I've been
06           here (.) many times. Sadn- Sandi- Sandi-
07           (0.4) HHH Sa- Sadding- or something like that.
08   Neu1:   That's right.= Yeah. The Sandington.=
09   Pat:    SANDington. Yeah.
10   Neu1:   >°Good°. And wha-< do you know what floor we're on,
11   Pat:    Yes:.
12   Neu1:   What floor is it,
13           (0.2)
14   Pat:    ((Floor letter))
15   Neu1:   Very good. What's the name of the town we're in,
16   Pat:    ↑Well it's ((City name))↑.
17   Neu1:   And the county,
18   Pat:    Er:: ((County name)).
19   Neu1:   And the: country,
20           (0.2)
21   Pat:    And the country, (0.2) erm::: ye- the whole
22           of it, erm: ↑I don't know↑,
23           (0.4)
24   Com:    .hhhhh hhhh
25           (0.6)
26   Pat:    No, it goes, you see,
27   Neu1:   Okay. Can you repeat after me these three words:
```

Despite the patient only partially and somewhat incorrectly establishing the first sounds of the hospital name, 'Sandi-' and 'Sadding' (lines 6–7), the clinician confirms this as being correct – 'that's right. Yeah' (line 8) – and provides the correct name for the patient – 'The Sandington' (line 8).

Clinicians thus seem to offer more leeway in what counts as accurate response when a person has dementia; in the recording of this session the clinician can be seen to be ticking the box on the sheet following this response.

Clinicians also appear to 'help' and reassure patients by using the third turn to explicitly confirm responses as being correct, for example 'that's right' (Extract 13, line 8), or to offer a reassuring assessment of their performance when they get a question right, for example 'very good' (Extract 13, line 15). The extract ends with the clinician closing the task sequence with 'okay' (Extract 13, line 27). Maynard and Marlaire (1992) demonstrate that administrators typically use 'good' when an answer is correct and 'okay' when it is incorrect. In Extract 13, 'good' (line 10) and 'very good' (line 15) are used when the individual question is (accepted as) correct, and 'okay' (line 27) is used following an incorrect response. Although further systematic analysis is required, it appears to be the case, certainly with people with dementia, that 'good' is often used when a response is correct and 'okay' when it is incorrect (also see Extract 14).

Extract 14 demonstrates this pattern of clinicians using 'okay' more frequently throughout each task sequence following incorrect answers. On these occasions clinicians are more likely to excuse the patient's inability and reassure them, for example 'Okay. Not to worry' (Extract 14, line 11).

Extract 14

```
01    Neu3:    Um:: a few quick questions about where
02             we are:, right now,=Do you know what this
03             building is,=What's this place that we're in,
04             (0.2)
05    Pat:     Um: (0.2) your, your job. Huh[huh huh ]
06    Neu3:                                [Yeah, W-] What's
07             this building,=whe- what is it, er, (0.2) do
08             you know what it's called, (.) ↑this building
09             that we're in at the moment,↑
10    Pat:     No:, not at the moment.
11    Neu3:    Okay,=Not to worry. .hh Um ((coughs)) >excuse me,<
12             Do you know what floor we're on,=What floor of
13             the building we're on,
14    Pat:     Third I think.
15    Neu3:    Okay, no worries. Oka:y:., Do you know what town
16             we're in?
17    Pat:     Pard[on.]
18    Neu3:        [Whi] ch- which to:wn: or which city are
19             we in at the moment,
20             (0.2)
21    Pat:     Um:: (0.2) tch (1.2) No.
22    Neu3:    O:kay:, don't wor[ry.]
23    Pat:                      [Sho]uld be- I should be-
24    Neu3:    ↑No it's alrig[ht↑,]
25    Pat:                   [Bu- ]
```

```
26   Neu3:   You've been moving around a bit. That's okay, Um:
27           do you know what county we're in,
28   Pat:    ((County name)).
29   Neu3:   Yes:, ABSolutely. [= Good.]
30   Pat:                     [huh huh] huh
31   Neu3:   That's good. And do you know what country we're in?
32   Pat:    England.
33   Neu3:   Yeah,=I know it sounds daft doesn't it.=Bu[t er ] we
34   Pat:                                              [Yeah.]
35   Neu3:   have to check these things.=Okay, now I'm just
36           going to mention three objects...
```

Interestingly in this extract the clinician does reformulate the first question about the name of the building. The patient's response 'your job' (line 5) is not 'close enough' to being correct to enable the clinician to accept it as an adequate response and therefore he reissues it – 'what's this building' (lines 6–7) – then reformulates it – 'do you know what it's called this building' (lines 7–8). The patient then answers 'no' (line 10) and continues to suggest that not knowing is temporary – 'not at the moment' (line 10). The clinician expands this sequence with 'Okay' (line 11) and then offers the patient some reassurance that he should not worry about not knowing – 'Not to worry' (line 11). The third-turn utterances across this extract – including 'okay' + reassurance, for example 'not to worry' (line 11), 'no worries' (line 15), 'don't worry' (line 22) – occur after all three of the incorrect responses in the task sequence. Following the patient's two correct responses in this task sequence, when correctly identifying the county (line 28) and country (line 32), the clinician uses the third turn to confirm the response and positively and emphatically assess it: 'Yes. ABSolutely. Good' (line 29) and 'Yeah' (line 33). This illustrates how clinicians are far more likely to use the third turn in these question–answer sequences when the patient has dementia.

Furthermore, clinicians sometimes use post-expansion sequences to do extra interactional work to account for a patient's inability to answer correctly. The patient in Extract 14 is unable to identify the town or city, and further audibly implies that he should be able to do so: 'I should be-' (line 23) (although he stops before completing this phrase, which could be heading for 'I should be able to...'). The clinician again offers a reassuring response – 'No it's alright' (line 24) – and then continues, working to *save face*, with a reasonable account of why the patient legitimately cannot respond: 'You've been moving around a bit. That's okay' (line 26). In Extract 15, this extra interactional work is also evident when the patient is unable to name the president of America who was assassinated in the 1960s.

Extract 15

```
01   Neu3:   Can you tell me, who was the:: um the
02           president of t- of America that was assassinated
03           back in the nineteen-sixties,
```

```
04              (0.6)
05    Neu3:     He was the President of th- of the United States
06              that was assassinated in the sixties,=Can you
07              remember who that was,
08    Pat:      No.=I didn't even know. (    ) huhuhu
09    Neu3:     °No°, it was a long time ago,
```

In the third turn the clinician accounts for the patient's inability to answer, mitigating the 'fault' or inability from the patient and instead suggesting it is legitimate to *not* know the answer given the time period since the indexed event's occurrence, that is 'it was a long time ago' (line 9). It is interesting to note here that the clinician asks the patient if he can *remember* the event (line 7). The patient resists the implication that his not answering is because of his cognitive inability to remember, but instead imbues this with an epistemic dimension, asserting that he did not possess the knowledge in the first place – 'I didn't even know' (line 8). Nevertheless, clinicians can work to account for an incorrect response and reassure the patient in more-than-minimal expansion of the sequence. This type of expansion and inability account is not generally seen in relation to people with FCD.

2.4 Discussion and Conclusion

We have continued our earlier work (Jones et al., 2020), further demonstrating variation and non-standard administration of the ACE-III in clinical practice. We have shown, for example, that clinicians actively redesign test implementation, stepping away from standardization, to prioritize recipiency and emotional labour (Swallow & Hillman, 2018), that is they incorporate elements of recipient design within the questions they ask (e.g., Extract 6). While this variation in administration may undermine standard assessment procedures, it could be seen to be an important component for enhancing patient experience. Furthermore, we have drawn an important distinction within clinician conduct when testing patients with a 'working diagnosis' of FCD as compared to those with a dementia diagnosis. Clinicians appear to orient to the patients' needs and abilities when introducing the test and seeking consent, working harder to set expectations, provide reassurance and prepare patients with suspected dementia for the task ahead. Clinicians often deviate from the parameters of the test to design questions in ways that function to 'help' patients with suspected dementia.

We have also demonstrated variation in clinical practice when administering the ACE-III in how clinicians respond to patients' answers and how they expand question–answer sequences. When patients have FCD, clinicians either do not use the third turn at all or do so only minimally to close the task sequence. Third turns are also used to orient to the need for the patient to produce a more specific response to achieve a mark in the test. However, when a patient has dementia, clinicians often use the third turn more frequently within each task sequence either to confirm and assess a correct response (using 'good' or even 'very good'), to reassure a patient following an incorrect response (for example, 'don't worry') or to provide a legitimate account for why the patient may not be able to provide the correct answer, thus absolving them of 'fault' in their inability to correctly answer a question. Clinicians are also less likely to pursue specific responses from people with dementia, for example a specific locational formulation, accepting a wider range of formulations as being correct. Some clinicians do not always appear to hold patients with dementia to the same standards to acquire a point on the test as those with FCD. These tests shine a light on people's cognitive difficulties, exposing them in the consultation, which can create a significant emotional burden on the people undertaking them (Cheston et al., 2000; Cahill et al., 2008). Akin to the work of Houtkoop-Steenstra and Antaki (1997), we show how clinicians use recipient design to help patient's *save face* in environments that are marked by both interactional and (perceived) cognitive troubles. Clinicians work harder in their interaction with patients they suspect have dementia to provide support and reassurance during administration of the tests.

This raises the question of why patients with FCD receive a more 'standard' approach to testing. The ACE-III in this context follows history-taking, during which the patient's social and interactional competence (or 'incompetence') has begun to be exposed (Elsey et al., 2015; Jones et al., 2016). Clinicians report forming a working diagnosis during these interactions, and perhaps respond to this clinical expertise by choosing to follow standard procedure for patients they perceive to be cognitively competent. In turn, for those patients who have struggled to respond to basic questions during history-taking, clinicians adapt their delivery of the ACE-III. Aside from the larger structure of the consultation, these adaptations are also, in part, generated within the sequential unfolding of the interaction itself: for example, clinicians reacting with reassurance when a patient displays some distress during the introduction to the test. This raises inherent tension between the demands for clinicians to follow the standard administrative procedures on one hand and the demands of recipient design on the other. It can be suggested, therefore, that there are often good interactional reasons for non-standard administration of cognitive assessments.

References

Alzheimer's Society (2015) Helping you to assess cognition: A practical toolkit for clinicians. Available at: www.wamhinpc.org.uk/sites/default/files/dementia-practical-toolkit-for-clinicians.pdf.

Atkinson, M. and Drew, P. (1979) *Order in Court: The Organization of Verbal Interaction in Judicial Settings*. London: The Macmillan Press.

Beach, W. A. (1993) 'Transitional regularities for 'casual' "Okay" usages'. *Journal of Pragmatics*, 19: 325–352.

Beishon, L. C., Batterham, A. P., Quinn, T. J., Nelson, C. P., Panerai, R. B., Robinson, T. and Haunton, V. J. (2019) 'Addenbrooke's Cognitive Examination III (ACE-III) and mini-ACE for the detection of dementia and mild cognitive impairment'. *Cochrane Database of Systematic Reviews* (12) CD013282. https://doi.org/10.1002/14651858.CD013282.pub2.

Bolden, G. (2006) 'Little words that matter: Discourse markers "so" and "oh" and the doing of other-attentiveness in social interaction'. *Journal of Communication*, 56(4): 661–688.

Bruno, D. and Schurmann Vignaga, S. (2019) 'Addenbrooke's cognitive examination III in the diagnosis of dementia: A critical review'. *Neuropsychiatric Disease and Treatment*, 15(15): 441–447.

Button, G. (1987) 'Answers as interactional products: Two sequential practices used in interviews'. *Social Psychology Quarterly*, 50(2): 160–171.

Cahill, S. M., Gibb, M., Bruce, I., Headon, M. and Drury, M. (2008) '"I was worried coming in because I don't really know why it was arranged': The subjective experience of new patients and their primary caregivers attending a memory clinic'. *Dementia*, 7(2): 175–189.

Chandler, P. and Sweller, J. (1991) 'Cognitive load theory and the format of instruction'. *Cognition and Instruction*, 8(4): 293–332.

Cheston, R., Bender, M. and Byatt, S. (2000) 'Involving people who have dementia in the evaluation of services: A review'. *Journal of Mental Health*, 9(5): 471–479.

Clayman, S. E. (1988) 'Displaying neutrality in television news interviews'. *Social Problems*, 35(4): 474–492.

Clayman, S. E. and Heritage, J. (2002) *The News Interview: Journalists and Public Figures on the Air*. Cambridge, UK: Cambridge University Press.

Clayman, S. E., Heritage, J. and Hill, A. M. J. (2020) 'Gender matters in questioning presidents'. *Journal of Language and Politics*, 19(1): 125–143.

Crawford, S., Whitnall, L., Robertson, J. and Evans, J. J. (2012) 'A systematic review of the accuracy and clinical utility of the Addenbrooke's Cognitive Examination and the Addenbrooke's Cognitive Examination-Revised in the diagnosis of dementia'. *International Journal of Geriatric Psychiatry*, 27: 659–669.

Dooley, J., Bass, N. and McCabe, R. (2018) 'How do doctors deliver a diagnosis of dementia in memory clinics?' *British Journal of Psychiatry*, 212(4): 239–245.

Drew, P., Raymond, G. and Weinberg, D. (eds.) (2006) *Talking Research: Language and Interaction in Sociological Methodology*. London: Sage.

Elsey, C., Drew, P., Jones, D., Blackburn, D., Wakefield, S., Harkness, K. and Reuber, M. (2015) 'Towards diagnostic conversational profiles of patients presenting with dementia or functional memory disorders to memory clinics'. *Patient Education and Counselling*, 98(9): 1071–1077.

Goffman, E. (1955) 'On face-work'. *Psychiatry*, 18(3): 213–231.

—— (1967) *Interaction Ritual: Essays on Face-to-Face Behavior*. New York: Doubleday Anchor.

Heath, C. (1992) 'The delivery and reception of diagnosis in the general-practice consultation'. In P. Drew and J. Heritage (eds.) *Talk at Work: Interaction in Institutional Settings*. Cambridge, UK: Cambridge University Press, pp. 235–267.

Hepburn, A. (2004) 'Crying: Notes on description, transcription, and interaction'. *Research on Language and Social Interaction*, 37(3): 251–290.
Heritage, J. (1998) 'Oh-prefaced responses to inquiry'. *Language in Society*, 27: 291–334.
   (2002) 'Ad hoc inquiries: Two preferences in the design of routine questions in an open context'. In D. W. Maynard, H. Houtkoop-Steenstra, N. C. Schaeffer and H. van der Zouwen (eds.) *Standardization and Tacit Knowledge Interaction and Practice in the Survey Interview*. New York: Wiley, pp. 313–333.
Heritage, J. and Maynard, D. W. (2006) *Communication in Medical Care*. Cambridge, UK: Cambridge University Press.
Heritage, J. and Sorjonen, M. L. (1994) 'Constituting and maintaining activities across sequences: And-prefacing as a feature of question design'. *Language in Society*, 23(1): 1–29.
Heritage, J. and Stivers, T. (1999) 'Online commentary in acute medical visits: A method of shaping patient expectations'. *Social Science & Medicine*, 49: 1501–1517.
Heritage, J., Robinson, J., Elliott, M., Veckett, M. and Wilkes, M. (2007) 'Reducing patients' unmet concerns in primary care: The difference one word can make'. *Journal of General Internal Medicine*, 22: 1429–1433.
Hoey, E. M. (2013) 'Do sighs matter? Interactional perspectives on sighing'. *Berkeley Linguistics Society* 61–74, https://doi.org/10.3765/bls.v39i1.3870.
   (2020) 'Waiting to inhale: On sniffing in conversation'. *Research on Language and Social Interaction*, 53(1): 118–139.
Houtkoop-Steenstra, H. (1995) 'Meeting both ends: Between standardization and recipient design in telephone survey interviews'. In P. Ten Have and G. Psathas (eds.) *Situated Order: Studies in the Social Organization of Talk and Embodied Activities*. Washington, DC: University Press of America pp. 91–107.
   (1997) 'Being friendly in survey interviews'. *Journal of Pragmatics*, 28: 591–623.
   (2000) *Interaction and the Standardized Survey Interview. The Living Questionnaire*. Cambridge, UK: Cambridge University Press.
Houtkoop-Steenstra, H. and Antaki, C. (1997) 'Creating happy people by asking yes-no questions'. *Research on Language and Social Interaction*, 30(4): 285–313.
Hsieh, S., Schubert, S., Hoon, C., Mioshi, E. and Hodges, J. R. (2013) 'Validation of the Addenbrooke's Cognitive Examination III in frontotemporal dementia and Alzheimer's disease'. *Dementia and Geriatric Cognitive Disorders*, 36(3–4): 242–250.
Jones, D., Drew, P., Elsey, C., Blackburn, D., Wakefield, S., Harkness, K. and Reuber, M. (2016) 'Conversational assessment in memory clinic encounters: interactional profiling for differentiating dementia from functional memory disorders'. *Aging & Mental Health*, 20(5): 500–509.
Jones, D., Wilkinson, R., Jackson, C. and Drew, P. (2020) 'Variation and interactional non-standardization in neuropsychological tests: The case of the Addenbrooke's Cognitive Examination'. *Qualitative Health Research*, 30(3): 458–470.
Koole, T. (2010) 'Displays of epistemic access: Student responses to teacher explanations'. *Research on Language and Social Interaction*, 43(2): 183–209.
Leydon, G. M. and Barnes, R. K. (2020) 'Conversation Analysis'. In C. Pope and N. Mays (4 ed.) *Qualitative Research in Health Care*. Hoboken, NJ: Wiley Publications, pp. 135–150.

Lindeberg, S., Samuelsson, C. and Müller, N. (2019) 'Swedish clinical professionals' perspectives on evaluating cognitive and communicative function in dementia'. *Clinical Gerontologist*, 1–15, https://doi.org/10.1080/07317115.2019.1701168.

Majlesi, A. R. and Plejert, C. (2018) 'Embodiment in tests of cognitive functioning: A study of an interpreter-mediated dementia evaluation'. *Dementia*, 17(2): 138–163.

Marlaire, C. and Maynard, D. W. (1990) 'Standardized testing as an interactional phenomenon'. *Sociology of Education*, 63: 83–101.

Maynard, D. W. (2017) 'Delivering bad news in emergency care medicine'. *Acute Medicine & Surgery*, 4(1): 3–11.

Maynard, D. W. and Marlaire, C. L. (1992) 'Good reasons for bad testing performance: The interactional substrate of educational exams'. *Qualitative Sociology*, 15(2): 177–202.

Maynard, D. and Schaeffer, N. C. (2006) 'Standardization-in-interaction: The survey interview'. In P. Drew., G. Raymond. and D. Weinberg (eds.) *Talking Research: Language and Interaction in Sociological Methodology*. London: Sage, pp. 9–27.

Maynard, D. W. and Turowetz, J. (2017) 'Doing testing: How concrete competence can facilitate or inhibit performances of children with autism spectrum disorder'. *Qualitative Sociology*, 40: 467–491.

Maynard, D. W., Houtkoop-Steenstra, H., Schaeffer, N. C. and van der Zouwen, H. (2002) *Standardization and Tacit Knowledge Interaction and Practice in the Survey Interview*. New York: Wiley.

McHoul, A. (1978) 'The organization of turns at formal talk in the classroom'. *Language in Society*, 7: 183–213.

Mehan, H., Hertweck, A. and Meihls, J. L. (1986) *Handicapping the Handicapped: Decision-Making in Students' Educational Careers*. Stanford, CA: Stanford University Press.

Merritt, M. (1980) 'On the use of "OK" in service encounters'. In R. W. Shuy and A. Shnukal (eds.) *Language Use and the Uses of Language*. Washington, DC: Georgetown University Press, pp. 162–172.

Nielsen, T. R., Segers, K., Vanderaspoilden, V., Beinhoff, U., Minthon, L., Pissiota, A., Bekkhus-Wetterberg, P., Bjørkløf, G. H., Tsolaki, M., Gkioka, M. and Waldemar, G. (2019) 'Validation of a brief Multicultural Cognitive Examination (MCE) for evaluation of dementia'. *International Journal of Geriatric Psychiatry*, 34(7): 982–989.

Panegyres, P. K., Berry, R. and Burchell, J. (2016) 'Early dementia screening'. *Diagnostics*, 6(1): 6.

Pennington, C., Newson, M., Hayre, M. and Coulthard, E. (2015) 'Functional cognitive disorder: What is it and what to do about it?' *Practical Neurology*, 15(6): 436–444

Peräkylä, A. (1998) 'Authority and accountability: The delivery of diagnosis in primary health care'. *Social Psychology Quarterly*, 61: 301–320.

Pond, C. D., Mate, K. E., Phillips, J., Stocks, N. P., Magin, P. J., Weaver, N. and Brodaty, H. (2013) 'Predictors of agreement between general practitioner detection of dementia and the revised Cambridge Cognitive Assessment (CAMCOG-R)'. *International Psychogeriatrics*, 25(10): 1639–1647, https://doi.org/10.1017/S1041610213000884.

Raymond, G. (2003) 'Grammar and social organization: Yes/no interrogatives and the structure of responding'. *American Sociological Review*, 68(6): 939–967.

Reuber, M., Blackburn, D., Elsey, C., Wakefield, S., Ardern, K., Harkness, K., Venneri, A., Jones, D., Shaw, C. and Drew, P. (2018) 'An interactional profile to assist the differential diagnosis of neurodegenerative and functional memory disorders'. *Alzheimer Disease & Associated Disorders: An International Journal*, 32(3): 197–206.

Reuber, M., Monzoni, C., Sharrack, B. and Plug, L. (2009) 'Using interactional and linguistic analysis to distinguish between epileptic and psychogenic nonepileptic seizures: A prospective, blinded multirater study'. *Epilepsy & Behavior*, 16: 139–144.

Right Decisions Service (2017) ACE-III and M-ACE English Guide 2017. Available https://rightdecisions.scot.nhs.uk/media/vk2cizbp/ace-iii-scoring-guide-uk-2017.pdf.

Robinson, J. D. and Heritage, J. (2014) 'Intervening with conversation analysis: The case of medicine'. *Research on Language and Social Interaction*, 47(3): 201–218.

Sacks, H. (1992) *Lectures on Conversation* (Vol. II, G. Jefferson, ed.). Oxford: Blackwell.

Schegloff, E. A. (1972) 'Notes on a conversational practice: Formulating place'. In D. Sudnow (ed.) *Studies in Social Interaction*. New York: The Free Press, pp. 75–119.

(1992) 'Repair after next turn: The last structurally provided defense of intersubjectivity in conversation'. *American Journal of Sociology*, 97(5): 1295–1345.

(2007) *Sequence Organization in Interaction: A Primer in Conversation Analysis*, Volume 1. Cambridge, UK: Cambridge University Press.

Stevanovic, M. and Peräkylä, A. (2012) 'Deontic rights in interaction: The right to announce, propose, and decide'. *Research on Language & Social Interaction*, 45(3): 297–321.

Stivers, T. (2002) 'Participating in decisions about treatment: Overt parent pressure for antibiotic medication in pediatric encounters'. *Social Science & Medicine*, 54: 1111–1130.

(2007) *Prescribing under Pressure: Parent-Physician Conversations and Antibiotics*. London: Oxford University Press.

Stivers, T. and Barnes, R. (2018) 'Treatment recommendation actions, contingencies, and responses: An introduction'. *Health Communication*, 33(11): 1331–1334, https://doi.org/10.1080/10410236.2017.1350914.

Swallow, J. and Hillman, A. (2018) 'Fear and anxiety: Affects, emotions and care practices in the memory clinic'. *Social Studies of Science*, https://doi.org/10.1177/0306312718820965.

Toerien, M. (2021) 'When do patients exercise their right to refuse treatment? A conversation analytic study of decision-making trajectories in UK neurology outpatient consultations'. *Social Science and Medicine*, 290: 114278, https://doi.org/10.1016/j.socscimed.2021.114278.

Venneri, A. (2005) 'The promised land: The blooming business of neuropsychological assessment guidance books'. *Cortex*, 41: 96–98.

Wilkinson, R. (2013) 'The interactional organization of aphasia naming testing'. *Clinical Linguistics and Phonetics*, 27(10–11): 805–822.

3 (Mis)alignment at Dementia Diagnosis
A Window into Differing Expectations, Perceptions and Agendas in the Memory Clinic

Jemima Dooley and Rose McCabe

3.1 Background

Clinicians report a challenge in communicating a dementia diagnosis above that of other diagnoses that stems from an incongruence between the expectations of the person with dementia and the agenda in the memory clinic, which focuses on communicating the diagnosis, starting medication (if appropriate), and referring/signposting to relevant support services (Bailey et al., 2019). This is often attributed to the neurological effects of dementia leading to symptoms of memory loss and impaired insight (McGlynn & Schacter, 1989), but there are other important factors affecting a person's engagement in the diagnostic process. Dementia is a stigmatized condition, so people may be unwilling to discuss symptoms (Markova et al., 2014; Milne, 2010). Additionally, making negative public self-assessments is a delicate activity that is affected by the social need to save 'face', that is to maintain a positive self-identity (Clare et al., 2013; Mograbi et al., 2012). Furthermore, people often attend memory clinics because of concerns raised by family or friends, which may cause tension in those relationships and unwillingness to engage with professionals (Karnieli-Miller et al., 2012; Quinn et al., 2017).

This chapter will explore how contextual factors such as those presented above manifest in interactions in the memory clinic by microanalysing communication in diagnostic meetings, focusing on instances of misalignment between doctors and the person living with dementia. Conversation Analysis (CA) offers a method to explore and analyse alignment (and hence misalignment). CA explores social actions in conversation, analysing how turns in talk are designed to realize one or more actions. Social actions can happen in single turns of talk, or they can be built over several turns of talk in a more extended interactional project (Schegloff, 2007). The recipient can either align with this action or project, through orienting to its completion, or misalign by setting the action or project on an alternative path. For example, in the simple action of asking a question, the recipient can either align, by answering the question, or misalign, by avoiding answering or starting a different project. In the interactional project of recommending and prescribing treatment, patients can align by engaging in the treatment discussion and considering treatment prescription, or misalign by withholding acceptance or offering alternatives (Stivers, 2005).

CA studies have shown how focusing on misalignment in healthcare communication can help identify communication challenges and provide support on how to overcome these. For example, two studies identifying misalignment in clinical triage calls led to recommendations for where organisations should focus their training to decrease incorrect triage (Morgan & Muskett, 2020; Murdoch et al., 2015). Albury et al. demonstrated how, in a study of General Practitioners recommending weight loss services, a comparison of where alignment versus misalignment occurred provided the opportunity for a clear description of elements of the weight loss recommendations that were most successful (Albury et al., 2021). Voutilainen et al. explored a case of misalignment in psychotherapy, showing how both participants dealt with this and discussing its relevance to the concept of the therapeutic alliance (Voutilainen et al., 2010).

In this chapter we will build on this tradition to illustrate occurrences of misalignment across dementia diagnosis feedback consultations. Our aim is to explore and discuss what factors may be influencing misalignment, and the possible implications for improving the diagnosis experience for people receiving the diagnosis, their companions, and clinicians.

3.2   The Study

Data were collected for the ShareD study (Shared decision making in mild to moderate Dementia) (McCabe et al., 2019) in the form of 101 video recordings of diagnosis feedback meetings in two sites in the UK – Devon (Site A, rural and semi-rural) and London (Site B, urban). Details of data collection methods can be found in previous publications (Dooley et al., 2018; 2019; McCabe et al., 2019). In the UK, dementia assessment and diagnosis primarily take place in memory clinics, where people undergo cognitive assessment, brain scans, and history-taking prior to diagnosis feedback. At Site A, assessment and diagnosis took place on one day in a 4-hour hospital appointment, and at Site B this occurred over several appointments over the space of weeks or months. The primary goal of the diagnosis feedback meeting is to communicate the diagnosis, start medication if appropriate, and refer and signpost to relevant support services.

3.3   Participant Information

This chapter focuses on three cases. These were selected as typical representations of how misalignment can occur in these meetings after analysis of the entire dataset in the aforementioned publications.

Table 3.1 *People with dementia: characteristics*

	Meeting A	Meeting B	Meeting C
Pseudonym	Maggie	Judith	Bill
Age	84	82	83
Gender	Female	Female	Male
Diagnosis	Mixed Alzheimer's disease and vascular dementia	Mixed Alzheimer's disease and vascular dementia	Mixed Alzheimer's disease and vascular dementia
ACE-III score	72	67	58
Site where recruited	A	B	A
Accompanied by	Daughter	Daughter-in-law	Friend
Clinician type	Geriatrician	Psychiatrist	Psychiatrist

The three meetings are labelled A, B, and C. Participant details can be found in Table 3.1. All the people receiving a diagnosis of dementia were in their early to mid-eighties and received a diagnosis of mixed Alzheimer's and vascular dementia. Their ACE-III scores indicate mild to moderate impairment.

Maggie and Bill were from Site A, meaning they had their assessment and diagnosis in the same appointment. Judith was from Site B, meaning she had her assessments some weeks prior to the diagnostic meeting.

All these three people living with dementia came with companions: Maggie with her daughter, Judith with her daughter-in-law, and Bill with a friend. Maggie saw a geriatrician, and Judith and Bill saw different psychiatrists.

3.4 Analysis

We present a conversation analysis of these three diagnostic feedback meetings to demonstrate how and where misalignment between the doctor and person living with dementia materializes. In previous analyses (Dooley, 2017), we described the phases of dementia diagnostic feedback meetings: (1) elicitation of orientation to the purpose of the meeting, (2) feedback from brain scans and cognitive testing, (3) diagnosis delivery, and (4) discussions of treatment and support. We will present each meeting in turn with extracts illustrating how misalignment can occur at each stage.

Transcripts follow Jeffersonian transcript conventions (Hepburn & Bolden, 2013). Doctors are referred to as DR, people with dementia as their pseudonym, and companions as CN.

3 (Mis)Alignment at Dementia Diagnosis

3.4.1 Meeting A

An elicitation of patient orientation to the clinic purpose has not been described in diagnostic appointments in other conditions, suggesting that this is a result of clinicians expecting an initial misalignment about the meeting purpose (Dooley et al., 2018).

The doctor in this meeting directly asks Maggie what she was expecting from the clinic (line 1).

Extract 1: A1 : DR=doctor; MAG=Maggie
```
01   DR:    ↑what expectation did you have of coming here toda:y.
02          (1.5)
03   MAG:   somebody that would he:lp with my memory:,
04   DR:    oh:: ↑ri:ght .hh ye::s[ we:ll that' s] what- that' s what
05   MAG:                         [ kHHM         ]
06   DR     we do::,
```

After a pause, Maggie provides an answer aligning with the memory clinic agenda, illustrating awareness of her memory problems through expressing hope that she can receive 'help' (lines 2–3). The doctor's elongated and emphasized 'oh right' (line 4) indicates a change of state, registering Maggie's response as new knowledge and thus unexpected (Heritage, 1984). This may be because the doctor did not expect the patient to be aware of the clinic purpose (an expectation which is justified, as will be discussed below). This also could be the reason for their extended confirmation ('yes well that's what we do' lines 4–5), to fill a gap where they expected to be informing the patient. The consultation then progresses to the next stage, which involves feeding back test results.

As in diagnostic delivery in other conditions, test feedback in memory clinics is designed to achieve intersubjective understanding of the nature and extent of Maggie's memory difficulties. This allows the doctor to forecast the diagnostic news and thus calibrate Maggie's expectations in relation to the forthcoming diagnosis (Maynard, 2003). Extract 2 illustrates how the doctor approaches the test feedback gradually, starting with positive assessments of where Maggie performed well on the tests (lines 1–9).

Extract 2: A2
```
01   DR:    I've had a look at the:: the testing that you di:d (0.5)
02          with (psychologist),
03          (1)
04   DR:    and you did pretty well in some areas didn' t you
05          some things are fa- working: >pretty well aren' t they<
06          your: your numbers are very good a:nd .hh (.) um tch
07          (.) knowing: where you a:re and the things abou:t
08          what' s going on in the news and everything you' re
09          obviously up to da:te aren' t you¿
```

```
10   MAG:   °mhm.°
11   DR:    .hh um but there was >a couple of things that you fou-<
12          you struggled with the: (.) um learning new things was
13          (1.2)
14   DR:    were you: do you remember that?
15          (0.9) (MAG frowns and looks down)
16   DR:    the learning n- new addresses and things was [ a bit]
17   MAG:                                                [ye:s  ]
18   MAG:   quite possibly.
19   DR:    mm. .hh and then actually some of it you learned but
20          you had trouble getting it back out again [ so  ]
21   MAG:                                             [mhm]
22          (0.4)
23   DR:    there's a retrieval problem there >isn't there< like
24          finding na:mes and (0.5) remember where you put stuff I
25          gather that's been a bit of an issu:e.
26          (1.3)
27   DR:    tch um and I've had a look at your head scan as
28          well, (0.5) which er:m, (0.3) i- is oka:y it shows
29          (0.4) er: nothing horrible there >but it does show
30          that< (0.5) you' ve got a proble:m wi:th (0.6) tch a
31          little bit with circulation round the brain >round the
32          little blood vessels< (.) which you'd expect >because
33          you've had a lot of trouble< with (0.4)
34          ((MAG leans forward and starts nodding))
35          circulation >round other bits of you< haven't you with
36          the (0.3) pacemaker and the [(change with y-?)]
37   MAG:                                [ye:s with        ] the
38          hea:rt mm.
```

Throughout her positive feedback, the doctor encourages agreement from Maggie with multiple tag questions (lines 4, 5, and 9). Maggie responds to these with a single quiet acknowledgement token (line 10). This minimal response may be a result of the qualifications in this description ('*some* areas'), projecting that a negative assessment will follow. The doctor continues with a general statement that there were 'a couple of things' Maggie 'struggled' with (lines 11–13). The rising intonation invites a response, but Maggie does not react either verbally or non-verbally. On the doctor's pursuit of this (line 15), Maggie furrows her brow and looks down, and the doctor persists (line 17), this time outlining specific difficulties with the address-recall task. Maggie responds with a qualified agreement ('quite possibly' lines 18–19), and the doctor continues to describe Maggie's 'retrieval problem' (lines 24–26). Again, Maggie makes neither a verbal nor a non-verbal response (line 27).

This withheld response is important because it demonstrates a lack of affiliation with the interactional project that the doctor is trying to achieve – that of forecasting the upcoming diagnosis. A comparison with the discussion of the brain scan results shows how differently patients can react to test feedback (lines 28–36). There is a notable change in Maggie's involvement:

she nods vigorously, sits forward in her chair and agrees in overlap (line 38). Comparing Maggie's engagement with discussing the physical problem with her heart, that is both known to Maggie and less stigmatized as a condition, with the results of the cognitive testing shows how hard it is to face these results, even when she knows she needs help with her memory (Extract 1).

The diagnosis delivery follows, with the doctor directly telling Maggie she has Alzheimer's disease in lines 1–2 of Extract 3.

Extract 3: A3

```
01   DR:    well I think what you: >what you've got is you've got<
02          Alzheimer's disea:se.
03   MAG:   I ha:ve? ((leans forward, eyes widening))
04   DR:    m[m:m.]
05   MAG:    [tch H]
06          (0.3)
07   MAG:   oh: dear.
08          (1.7) ((DR nods))
09   MAG:   I'm not very pleased about tha:t.
10   DR:    no and I'm sure it's a difficult thing isn't it.
11   MAG:   mm.
12          (0.6)
13   DR:    you must have had a little th th thought about it
14          though at the back of your mi:nd [kn] owing
15   MAG:                                    [m ]
16   DR:    you were coming here today and how difficult it's been
17          for you recently=have you had a¿ (.) did you have an
18          inkli:ng?
19          (0.4)
20   DR:    did you have a little thought that that mi:ght be part
21          of [the problem?]
22   MAG:      [hhhh         ]
23          (2.3) (MAG looks away, mouth turned down)
24   MAG:   yes but then on the other hand I know I do things we:ll.
25   DR:    you do: ((exaggerated nodding))
26          (0.4)
27   DR:    ye:s
```

Maggie has an immediate negative reaction to the diagnosis. Her 'I have' is characteristic of 'ritualized disbelief' in 'surprise' sequences (Wilkinson & Kitzinger, 2006). This is accompanied by an exaggerated open-mouthed, wide-eyed expression (line 3), before Maggie tuts and breathes out loudly while closing her eyes and tilting her head back and to the side (line 5). Stoic, unmarked responses to diagnosis (e.g. 'mm') before quick progression to treatment discussions are the norm (Maynard, 2003), so this strong reaction is unusual in diagnosis settings. In the pause (line 8), Maggie is not moving and the doctor nods. Maggie disaffiliates by voicing her displeasure: 'I'm not very pleased' (line 9). After demonstrating understanding (line 10), the doctor challenges Maggie's surprise, suggesting that this diagnosis may have been anticipated (lines 13–21). Maggie sighs and looks away with a downturned mouth (lines 22–23). Her positive assessment of her abilities demonstrates misalignment with the diagnosis (line 24). This misalignment requires attention from the doctor before they can progress to treatment and management, which they do by responding with emphasized agreement, realigning and affiliating with the patient's viewpoint (lines 25–27).

Extract 4: A4

```
01    MAG:    so what is the situation do: I have to have treatment?
02            (0.5)
03    MAG:    or,
04            (0.6)
05    DR:     there are tablets you can take,
06    MAG:    m[hm]
07    DR:      [if] you would like to.
08    MAG:    yes.
09            (0.5)
10    DR:     we can certainly have a talk about tha:t.
11    MAG:    m:m.
12            (0.7)
13    DR:     there's some practical things that we ought to go over,
14            (.) especially while (daughter)'s here because
15            there's some practical issues where: we need to make
16            sure that you're safe.
17            (0.4)
18    DR:     and protected.
19            (0.3)
20            .hh um and then there's some:: um (.) ladies in the
21            community who would like to:, (0.7) say hello to you:
22            and you should know that they're there:
```

It is not typical for people receiving the diagnosis to initiate treatment discussions in these meetings. In doing so, Maggie is showing alignment with the interactional project of getting treatment that was also evident in Extract 1 where she asks for 'help with her memory'. In Extract 4, the doctor confirms that Maggie can have tablets but refrains from strongly endorsing them, only offering them to Maggie 'if you would like' (line 7). Maggie immediately accepts the doctor's recommendation (line 8). However, in neglecting to go into more detail on the medication, the doctor demonstrates that their focus is on Maggie receiving help with living at home (lines 13–22). Maggie's response to this is noticeably different: she withholds any verbal or non-verbal reply. She thus appears to align with and support further talk about treatment or medication but refrains from aligning with or supporting talk focused on other issues. The need for home support 'to make sure you're safe' is problematic for Maggie's self-assessment that she 'does things well' (Extract 3), and not aligning with this may be a mechanism to save face.

3 (Mis)Alignment at Dementia Diagnosis

In sum, Maggie comes to her diagnostic feedback wanting help with her memory. She does not engage with her negative results in the cognitive testing, which is common throughout the dataset. Her explicit demonstration of surprise when receiving a diagnosis is less common, with many people receiving dementia diagnoses adhering to the norm of reacting stoically to bad diagnostic news (Dooley et al., 2018). While Maggie is keen to receive medication, she does not engage with the suggestion of support in the home. This demonstrates how a person with dementia's alignment with the doctor's interactional project of diagnosis and treatment is connected to their self-presentation: Maggie demonstrates understanding that she has memory difficulties and medication can help, but disaffiliates with the diagnosis and idea that she has support needs.

The misalignment evident in Meeting B follows a different pattern, but also reflects the role of self-identity for the person receiving the diagnosis in these meetings.

3.4.2 Meeting B

As in Extract 1, the doctor in this meeting starts with a direct question to elicit orientation (line 1).

Extract 5: B1: DR=doctor; JUD=Judith

```
01   DR:    do you know why it is that you've come here today:.
02          (1.2)
03   JUD:   yeah:: (0.3) you wanna know: w- what medication I'm
04          taking.
05          (.)
06   DR:    yes:=
07   JUD:   =that's it yeah:.
08   DR:    yeah: >well that's certainly true we'll talk about<
09          tha:t.=.hh (.) um,
10          (0.5)
11   DR:    but the mai:n rea:son >for the appointment< (.) today:
12          was to follow up=to talk over a little bit abou:t (0.4)
13          u:m (0.5) the: (.) the problem that you talked with the
14          doctor about before:.=so that was arou:nd talking about
15          your memory:¿
16          (0.5)
17   JUD:   mm yeah: (.) mm.
```

After a delay, Judith responds to the doctor's question by stating that the doctor is going to check her medication (lines 3–4). It is worth noting that the referral letter does ask the patient to bring her medication, so Judith is partly correct. The doctor offers qualified agreement, with 'well' projecting a more complicated response (line 8) (Heritage, 2015). In describing the meeting as a 'follow up' and highlighting 'the problem that you talked with the doctor about before', it appears that Judith has already spoken with a clinician about her potential dementia (lines 11–15). The doctor clarifies the purpose of the current meeting, and the topic of the previous meeting, as 'memory', which prompts only a minimal acknowledgement from Judith (lines 16–17). This meeting is from Site B, where the cognitive testing appointment would have happened weeks previously, and it may be the case that Judith does not remember this. However, whatever the reason, this interaction starts with a mismatch between what the doctor and Judith expect to happen in the consultation.

Doctor B does not discuss the test results in as much detail as Doctor A did, instead simply forecasting a diagnosis, as shown in Extract 6 (lines 1–3). The 'that' in line 1 refers to the cognitive testing.

Extract 6: B2
```
01   DR:    °ah° the- the result of that >which was that< (0.8)
02          suggested I think that the memory loss has been a
03          little bit wor:se than we would expe:ct.
04          (.)
05   JUD:   yeah:: we:ll.
06          (1)
07   JUD:   I suppose you notice hh ↑heh heh °heh heh°
```

While this bad news is mitigated ('a little bit worse'), it is asserted directly with little facework. Judith's delayed, well-prefaced response, alongside her laughter, demonstrates discomfort (Haakana, 2001; Heritage, 2015). Her statement 'I suppose you notice', with the 'you' indicating what other people as opposed to what Judith herself notices, demonstrates misalignment and a possible differing perspective.

Judith, similar to Maggie in Extract 2, is more willing to engage in the results of the brain scan.

Extract 7: B3
```
01   DR:    the- the blood vesse:ls in the brain were: (.) >there was
02          a< °i:° a few areas where they weren't quite wor:king as
03          eh- (.) wo[rki]ng per[fectly]
04   JUD:             [oh ]        [ye:s  ]
05          (0.4)
06   DR:    now[that-]
07   JUD:      [I    ] know I've go:t (0.6) high blood press(h)ure
08          £a(h)[nd (h)everyth(h)ing] (h)else£
09   DR:         [oh ri::ght.         ]
10   DR:    ↑well qui:te yeah >I mean that's< (.) pr- that's one of
11          the: commonest (0.3) cau:ses of that sort of proble:m̰
```

The doctor states that the blood vessels are not 'working perfectly' (lines 1–3). Judith aligns with emphatic agreement in overlap (line 4). She displays existing knowledge of her vascular problems, downplaying them with a dismissive description 'and everything else' (lines 7–8). While aligning with the immediate action of discussing the results of the brain scan, this downplay of known symptoms indicates misalignment with the doctor's interactional project of a forecasted 'new diagnosis'. Her laughter is also likely to be a reflection of the delicacy of this misalignment (Haakana, 2001). The doctor's response is a direct reaction to this: with the 'well' projecting disagreement as they recharacterize the blood pressure issues as one of the 'causes' of her dementia symptoms (lines 10–11).

The test results are followed by delivery of the diagnosis as a 'mild form of a condition called dementia', which Judith responds to with a minimal acknowledgement (not shown). The doctor then elaborates, pursuing further response from Judith by explaining the different types of dementia. He finishes this at the start of Extract 8, defining Judith's dementia as Alzheimer's disease.

Extract 8: B4: CN=companion

```
01   DR:    an:d what I would say is (.) I think that probably i:s
02          the- the form of dementia that you ha:ve
03          (0.5)
04   DR:    this (.) [is Alzheim]er's Dis[ea:se.]
05   JUD:            [yeah::   ]         [and be]ing deaf doesn't
06          he:lp hh[hh heh heh hahaha       ] [ah hahaha] ha
07   DR:            [being deaf doesn't help]
08   CN:                                       [nh heh heh]
09   DR:    and having: a: and saying that you[had some] visual
10   JUD:                                     [yeah    ]
11   DR:    proble:ms as well that doesn't[help[    eith]er:.  ]
12   JUD:                                 [ah  [ hah hah] ha ha]
13   CN:                                       [yeah    ]
14   JUD:   hah haha[ haha] ha
15   DR:            [hmhm]
16   JUD:   .HH[yeah: ]
17   DR:       [but you] can be selectively deaf as
18          [we:ll  ]
19   CN:    [nh ↑heh] [↑hah hah   ]
20   DR:              [hoh hoh ↑hoh]
```

Judith misaligns with the diagnosis delivery by topicalising her hearing impairment (line 5). This could be read as Judith accounting for her test results as a basis for the diagnosis by claiming mitigating circumstances because of her deafness. Her laughter frames this as a joke, which the doctor acknowledges with a smile and an upgrade to include her 'visual problems' (lines 9–11), while the companion joins in the laughter. The doctor upgrades this further with a smile and a comment about Judith's 'selective' deafness (lines 17–18), appearing to make explicit Judith's lack of acknowledgement of the diagnosis. This co-constructed, light-hearted interchange works both to mitigate Judith's potential complaint and to align with her self-identity.

The discussion moves to treatment, where Judith challenges the doctor's recommendation to start medication.

Extract 9: B7 – CN=companion

```
01    DR:    I can give you a prescription today .h and then one of
02           our nurses will get in contact with you in about a
03           week's ti:me to see how things are going
04           (1.2)
05    JUD:   °↑oh:°
06           (.)
07    DR:    yeah:.
08           (.)
09    JUD:   ↑do you think I nee:d one (to CN)
10           (0.5)
11    CN:    we:ll what the doctor said (0.4) is that it will stop your
12           memory: (.) or hopefully: the idea is that it wi:ll (2.0)
13           [help        ] your memory:
14    DR:    [>should I<  ]
15           (.)
16           yeah: that's ri:ght it's [ a medicine ]
17                                    [it will help] it's .hh (1.1) I
18           w- if it was me: I would take it.
19           (1.0)
20    JUD:   oh: well it can't do any har:m >can it< ↑eh
21           [heh heh hah hah hah hah] ha ha
22    CN:    [indee:d it ca:n't.     ]
23    DR:    it nor- it w- it shouldn't do exactly:.
```

Judith's reaction to the suggestion of medication and follow up demonstrates misalignment with both the interactional project of medication prescription and also the diagnosis itself in her questioning of the need for treatment (line 9). This question is directed towards her companion. The companion's response invokes the doctor's expertise, and she looks towards the doctor as she answers (lines 11–13). The doctor begins to explain further, but the companion interrupts with a strong, persuasive endorsement (lines 17–18). Judith's reluctance is evident in her agreement on the basis 'it can't do any harm' (line 20), indirectly displaying her opinion that medication is not necessary. Her laughter again illustrates the delicacy of disagreeing with the doctor's recommendation. However, this time, the doctor and the companion do not join in; their agenda in encouraging Judith to take the medication is prioritized.

To summarize Meeting B, Judith demonstrates misalignment with the interactional project of diagnosis feedback throughout. She sees the meeting purpose as a discussion of her medications, does not appear to remember her assessment, suggests a different perspective of her abilities than is indicated in the testing, responds to the diagnosis with a joke, and questions the need for medication. However, this misalignment again appears to reflect a project to preserve self-identity. She highlights her deafness and vascular difficulties as sources of her problems, which, given the stigma surrounding dementia, may be more socially acceptable diagnoses. She also often laughs and jokes in serious moments, which is a common coping mechanism for Judith to maintain interactional competency in challenging situations (Saunders, 1998).

3.4.3 Meeting C

Meeting C differs from the others in that it does not start with the doctor eliciting Bill's awareness of the reason for the meeting. They instead describe their agenda (lines 1–5).

Extract 10: C1

```
01   DR:    I just want to talk with you abou:t what we' ve done
02          today:,
03   BILL:  mm:,
04   DR:    .hh what we think might be going on and how: we can
05          help you.
06          (.)
07   BILL:  .hh ↑oh.
08   DR:    is that al[ri::ght.            ]
09   BILL:            [ >>well is there<< ] more tablets,
10          [=I take eight a day] : now
11   DR:    [ahh heh heh heh    ]
12   DR:    I[know] I saw::!
13   BILL:   [ah  ]
14   BILL:  [heh! heh!]
15   DR:    [.hh so,  ] (.) in this clinic we see people with (1)
16          possible: possible mild memory problems .hh and we try
17          and deci:de (.) ↑is it due to: (.) getting olde[r,]
18   BILL:                                                 [oh] :.
19          (.)
20   DR:    or: or could it be something else li:ke a dementia.
21          (0.3)
22   BILL:  well my wife has got dementia.=I think I told
23          [the other guy]
24   DR:    [ye:s         ]
```

The doctor does not start with an expectation question as in the other examples, instead stating the meeting purpose and allowing time for a reaction, which may be a method to elicit orientation without directly threatening patient face. The statement does however forecast a potential diagnosis in stating that something 'might be going on' and that the clinic can 'help' (line 4). Bill's upward intoned, emphasized 'oh' demonstrates surprise (line 7) (Heritage, 1984). He has attended a clinic in Site A, so has just completed the cognitive testing and had a brain scan in the few hours before this meeting. Therefore, this indicates some disorientation. The doctor responds by asking for a 'go ahead' from Bill to continue (line 8). Bill's well-prefaced response in overlap again misaligns in that it does not give express permission, instead demonstrating concern regarding the need to take further medication (lines 9–10).

The doctor's response is empathic in tone, their upward intonation aligning with Bill's assessment that eight tablets a day is a lot (Heritage, 2011). Their affiliation, laughter, and indication of prior knowledge of Bill (line 12) could be performing alliance work before addressing the issue of diagnosis, which Bill's surprise suggests might be difficult. Also potentially resulting from this surprise, they give a generalized clinic description ('we see people' line 15) and minimize the symptom profile of clinic attendees ('with possible mild memory problems' line 16). They then add specificity by naming the potential diagnosis as 'something like a dementia' (line 20). It is unusual for doctors to explicitly mention dementia at this point in the meeting, with references to 'memory' being more common. This again could be in response to the fact Bill's wife has dementia: his detailed understanding of the condition in its more severe stages adds particular delicacy to breaking the diagnostic news. Bill replies with a topic shift in beginning to talk about his wife, not acknowledging the doctor's description of the meeting purpose (lines 22–24).

After some discussion of Bill's experiences leading up to the memory clinic appointment, the doctor gives a brief description of the brain scan results and a lengthy discussion of Bill's experience of the cognitive testing. Extract 11 begins with Bill accounting for his difficulties.

Extract 11: C2 – CN=companion

```
01    BILL:   yeah well you' re taken on on the spot like that' s
02            [>a bit of a job isn' t it.<]
03    DR:     [I know it' s it is        ] °er-° I appreciate it' s
04            quite[ stressful and it' s] a really hard[test.]
05    BILL:        [↓y(h)eah HH hh      ]               [I have] met
06            Margaret Thatcher >I didn' t remember< her[even]
07    DR:                                                [oh  ] but
08            you got it at the end h!
09    BILL:   yeah I know at the[e:nd h.]
10    DR:                       [ so y]ou got that point.
11    BILL:   hh[ hh ]
12    DR:       [hah] haha hah[.hh]
13    BILL:                   [and] he was at our: was it
14            Cameron?=I didn' t[know him.]
15    DR:                       [Cameron ] that' s ri:ght.=that' s
16            right.
17    BILL:   did I put him down as that[one or did I not]
18    DR:                               [    yeah no    ]
19            ((psychologist)) said he- you got both those marks cause
20            he said £just as you were about to leave you remembered
21            them both£
22    BILL:   yea::h that' s right yeah:.
23    DR:     .hh (0.3) but you scored fifty eight out of a hundred
24            on that[te:st.]
25    BILL:          [oh::  ] that' s pretty average.
26            (.)
27    DR:     and, tch (.) °uh uh° fo- for me it does show us that
```

3 (Mis)Alignment at Dementia Diagnosis

```
28                   there[probably] is a problem with your memory.
29      BILL:             [mm:.       ]
30                   (0.4)
31      DR:          tch .hh (.) now, (0.4) [with,           ]
32      BILL:                                [>what do they wa] nna do< open
33                   it up and [see: it or something? heh]
34      DR:                    [HH hehhehhehheh       .hhh] well this is the
35                   problem with making the diagno[sis of dementia,      ]
36      BILL:                                      [yeah you can' t really]
37                   can[you¿]
38      DR:             [is  ] that the on:ly way we can make an absolutely
39                   (.) definite diagnosis of dementia .hh is by taking a
40                   biopsy of the brain (0.3) and
41                   cl[early I' m not going to do tha:t.]
42      BILL:          [.hhh tch ahehh                  ]
43                   ah[heh heh .hh we don' t do] that.
44      BILL:          [praise be heh ha ha     ]
45      CN:          thank god!
```

The doctor again shows empathy within their own epistemic status as the 'tester', that they 'appreciate it's quite stressful' (lines 3–4). Bill is demonstrating awareness of and accounting for his forgetting the UK prime ministers (lines 5–17). The doctor begins to lay groundwork for the diagnosis, saying those answers were correct, 'but' Bill's score was 58/100 (lines 19–24). Bill's reception of this news and his description of the score as 'average' (line 25) indicates a lack of knowledge of what this score entails, appearing to imply that this would be in line with other people. The doctor thus follows this with an explicit diagnostic forecast in an effort to ensure understanding ('there is a problem with your memory' lines 27–28). Bill's response, similar to Judith's in Meeting B, misaligns with the forecasting of bad news by making a joke about having to open his brain up. Similar to Judith, his joking could be a method of controlling an emotional response and saving face, which is common in dementia (Hedman et al., 2014; Saunders, 1998). Similar to Doctor A, this doctor affiliates with and upgrades Bill's joke in saying that they 'clearly' won't be doing a brain biopsy and there is joint laughter.

The doctor continues by explaining how all the testing is considered to make a diagnostic decision, starting the diagnosis delivery in Extract 12.

Extract 12: C3
```
01      DR:     which I think is, (0.4) an Alzheimer' s type of prob[lem]
02      BILL:                                                       [is ]
03              it?=be da:mned >like I don' t want that I don' t want to<
04              join my: missus
05              (0.5)
06      BILL:   heh hh
07      DR:     I, I- I think you do have (0.3) a dementia¿
08              (.)
09      BILL:   ↓yeah::
```

```
10   DR:     .h u::m although as I say there's no hard and
11           [fast test that I can do but] .h but from what I can
12   BILL:   [no:: no right one yeah    ]
13   DR:     see of all the different [tests we've] done it does
14   BILL:                             [mm:.       ]
15   DR:     look like a dementia,
16           (.) ((Bill leans to look at scan result on DR computer))
17   DR:     .hh but I think it's slightly different to your wi:fe,
18           (.)
19   BILL:   is[i:t?]
20             [beca]use I think, (.) it's als- it's-
21           (.)
22   BILL:   >well it's<[ar:terial isn't it?]
23   DR:                [the com- it's- it's-] a mixed picture,=.hh
24           it's partly Alzheimer's and partly (0.5) >as you say<
25           (.) something to do with the arteries.=with the blood
26           ve[ssels]
27   BILL:     [yeah]:: what[is it?]
28   DR:                    [ vasc ]ular.
29           (0.4)
30   BILL:   vascular that's right.
31   DR:     .hh
32           (.)
33   BILL:   .HH
34   BILL:   go::sh.
35   DR:     so it's a mixed A[lzhei]mer and Vascular dementia
36   BILL:                    [mm:. ]
37   BILL:   mm m.
```

Bill has a strong negative reaction to the diagnosis, produced in overlap. Similar to Maggie, he demonstrates surprise and disappointment with a rhetorical interrogative, latched expletive, and an explicit expression of understanding in stating that he does not want to be like his wife (lines 1–3). His laughter (line 6) again could be a method of holding back further emotional reaction, particularly given that typical reactions to diagnoses tend to be stoic and restrained (Dooley et al., 2018; Maynard, 2003). He is smiling, and as the doctor reformulates the diagnosis as a 'dementia' (line 7), his smile drops. The doctor then downplays the certainty of the diagnosis, potentially in response to the strong negative reaction, saying 'there's no hard and fast test', but that it 'looks like' a dementia (lines 10–15). Bill aligns with this explanation in overlap, demonstrating knowledge ('no right one, yeah' line 12). Bill then leans forward to look at the brain scan on the doctor's computer screen (line 16).

The doctor explicitly differentiates Bill's dementia to his wife's, likely as a resource to soften the bad news in reaction to Bill's negative response (Stivers & Timmermans, 2017). Bill again aligns with this, displaying in-depth understanding of the diagnosis in reply – 'well it's arterial isn't it' (line 22) – before appearing to search for the correct term and showing recognition of the doctor's supply of 'vascular' (lines 27–30).

Bill therefore aligns with the doctor's interactional project of diagnosis, showing understanding and an emotional reaction. The doctor reassures Bill and then moves on to talk about medication.

Extract 13: C4
```
01   DR:     it might be that you'd like to consider a tablet for your
02           memory.
03           (0.5)
04   BILL:   ↑m hm hm hm heh [heh aheh heh]
05   DR:                    [.hhh          ]
06           (0.4)
07   BILL:   ↑you >want to be giving< one to (wife) actually ah
08           [(?)           hah hah]
09   DR:     [ah heh heh heh .hhh] it- (0.4) unfortunately it's not a
10           cure for memory problems.
11   BILL:   no:.
12   DR:     so it won't rever:se them,
13           (0.4)
14   BILL:   but to prescribe now you mean:.
15           (.)
16   DR:     but it- but it [should s::              ]
17   BILL:                  [but it's just going to] affect your blood
18           pressure that is.=>the thing for me was to do with the
19           blood pressure wasn't [it?<]
20   DR:                           [tch ] .hh so you're on tablets
21           for your [blood] pres [sure] but the the- one for your
22   BILL:            [khm  ]     [khm.]
23           memory isn't- wouldn't automa- wouldn't change your blood
24           pressure
25   BILL:   no:,
26   DR:     this would be about increasing one of the chemicals in
27           your brain which is called choline.
28   BILL:   ↑o[h god.    ]
29   DR:      [.hh which] helps you [make]
30   BILL:                          [↑mm ] m.
31   DR:     new memories.
32           (2)
33   DR:     you don't have to take medication,
34           (.)
35   DR:     if you fee:l that you're on enough medication and you
36           [just]
37   BILL:   [well] >I am on a [lot at the moment]
38   DR:                       [just want        ]
39   BILL:   I'm on [eight a day<]
40   DR:           [not          ] then that's fi:ne.
```

The doctor's treatment recommendation is in the form of a suggestion (Stivers et al., 2018), a recommendation format that gives Bill agency over his decision. This format is likely to be a direct response to Bill's previous resistance to taking more medication in Extract C1. There is clear misalignment here: Bill does not respond directly, instead laughing and joking that the medication should be for his wife (lines 4–7). The doctor continues with their explanation (lines 9–16), but Bill explicitly questions his need for memory tablets, entering in overlap. He formulates his diagnosis ('thing for me') as 'to do with the blood pressure', and expresses concern that the recommended medication will make this worse (lines 17–19). The doctor answers indirectly, stating that Bill is on blood pressure medication, insinuating that he need not have any concerns in that regard. They add further explanation that the tablet increases 'one of the chemicals; in the brain (lines 26–27). Similar to Maggie and Judith, Bill is demonstrating more active engagement with his physical health issues than his memory problems, and thus it may be that this is detailed, physical explanation of 'choline' is an attempt to engage Bill in discussion of the memory tablets. However, Bill's response cry ('oh god' line 28) demonstrates displeasure at this description. The doctor, likely in reaction to this strong response and continued misalignment, offers Bill the choice not to take the medication, citing Bill's previous concerns about taking too many tablets (lines 33–35). Bill aligns with this and the doctor's closing remark ('then that's fine' line 40) suggests the matter is closed.

While often providing strong and occasionally contrary reactions to what the doctor is saying, Bill does appear to align with the doctor's agenda throughout. His test results and disorientation to the meeting purpose indicate a moderate dementia, but he is engaged in and displays understanding of the diagnostic descriptions. His strong reaction to his diagnosis and his resistance to medication is embedded in a comparison between his own circumstances and those of his wife, who is in a care home with dementia. Hence, his preference to engage with the vascular description of his condition may serve to maintain his identity as the 'healthy' member of his marriage, differentiating himself from his wife's experience. Having seen first-hand what dementia is like and having been a carer of a person with dementia, receiving a dementia diagnosis is likely to be particularly emotionally challenging for Bill.

3.5   Discussion

We have presented examples of where misalignment occurs across each stage of the diagnosis feedback meeting. CA demonstrates the interactional contexts where the person receiving a dementia diagnosis chooses to align or misalign with the doctor's interactional projects of diagnosis delivery, prescribing medication, and recommending support. Examination of these instances suggests that misalignment between the assessment of symptoms may, at least in part, reflect interactional facework in the face of dementia as a challenge to self-identity.

In focus groups we conducted as part of this project, doctors said that starting the meeting by eliciting the patient's expectations about the meeting helped them decide how to approach the diagnosis delivery (Bailey et al., 2019). Two of the extracts examined in this chapter showed misalignment as to the purpose of the meeting, which reflects the wider dataset where 62 per cent of the meetings studied showed different interpretations about the meeting aim (Dooley, 2017). It is important to consider the context and how well oriented the person receiving the diagnosis may or may not be to the purpose of the meeting. Patient appointment letters in the UK do not explicitly state that memory clinics are for dementia assessment/diagnosis and General Practitioners can refer people to memory clinics without providing information on reasons for the referral or possible consequences of it (Cahill et al., 2008; Dooley, 2017). Therefore, a lack of understanding of the meeting purpose may not be due to cognitive impairment, but rather to lack of explicit information and explanation from health services. This appears to be reflected in the data. Judith (Extract 5/B1) states that the meeting is to do with her medication, which is reasonable as her appointment letter asks her to bring a list of her current medication. Bill would have seen two different clinicians in the few hours prior to the meeting, and thus his surprise that he was now in the diagnosis meeting itself may be a result of the unusual structure of the clinic, rather than his not being aware of the meeting purpose. Hence, more explicit signposting of the dementia assessment process may work to help to keep people receiving the diagnosis on board with the doctor's agenda.

Maggie, Judith, and Bill demonstrated some misalignment between their subjective view of their difficulties and the test feedback. Objective testing is a threat to self-identity, an explicit representation of change in behaviour that makes it difficult to hold on to how life has always been (Campbell et al., 2016). It is therefore unsurprising that people receiving a dementia diagnosis withhold agreement when presented with this face-threatening information. Maggie explicitly stated that her misgivings about the test feedback were because she 'thought she did things well'; Judith and Bill provided alternative accounts for their results, hearing loss and 'being put on the spot' respectively. Providing alternative accounts for their difficulties may be a coping strategy used by patients in the face of life-changing information, as previously discussed in the dementia literature (Harman & Clare, 2006).

Comparing the responses of all the people receiving the diagnosis of the results of their brain scan with their responses to cognitive test results further indicates how the stigma of dementia might lead to misalignment. All three patients in the meetings studied in this chapter were willing to accept 'physical' explanations for symptoms from the brain scans, thus showing some acknowledgment of their problems. However, they were all less engaged with the results of cognitive testing, which explores memory and cognitive abilities relevant for everyday life. All three displayed prior knowledge of their vascular conditions, which meant that the cognitive test feedback would more strongly forecast a diagnosis and be more explicit in its 'bad news' delivery. People living with dementia and their families report being 'impervious to all other information' once they receive diagnostic information (Kunneman et al., 2017:317), and withheld responses may therefore reflect processing of this bad news. Furthermore, cognitive tests fall in the realm of psychiatric assessment. While dementia awareness is increasing, this has not led to less stigma. A thematic analysis of newspaper headlines related to dementia found a prevalence of catastrophising language (e.g. 'cruel', 'dreaded'), as well as a rhetoric of blame in reporting prevention of dementia through changes in diet and lifestyle (Peel, 2014). A person receiving a dementia diagnosis may thus feel ashamed by behavioural changes and avoid talking about these to protect self-image in social contexts (Goffman, 1967; Sabat & Harre, 1992).

Previous CA studies have shown that minimal responses to a diagnosis by patients are oriented to as normal by clinicians, and diagnosis is usually followed directly by treatment recommendations (Maynard, 2003). This is even the case in other serious conditions, such as cancer. However, doctors in memory clinic diagnostic consultations pursued an extended response from the patient, making misalignment more likely. This is described in more detail in previous analyses (Dooley, 2017; Dooley et al., 2018), but is evident in Doctor A's exploration of Maggie's expectations, Doctor B's further definition of dementia types, and Doctor C's differentiation between Bill's dementia and that of his wife. This has also been demonstrated in the literature on HIV and developmental disabilities clinics, where clinicians are aiming for emotional engagement and agreement to ensure the patient will engage in long-term involvement with services (Maynard, 2003). However, doctors in memory clinics do not appear to be pursuing explicit alignment with the diagnosis. For example, in Extract 13/C4 the doctor does not disagree with Bill's view that his problems are arterial (i.e. not Alzheimer's disease). In fact, if patients withhold acceptance of diagnosis, doctors will often eschew pursuing this and instead respond with discussions of positive aspects of the diagnosis such as treatment and support (Dooley, 2017). This is evident in Extract 3/A3, where Maggie's self-assessment that she 'does things well' is immediately and enthusiastically agreed with by the doctor. This may reflect doctor understanding that misalignment stems from a person's efforts to save face in the context of being diagnosed with a stigmatized condition, and to pursue acceptance would only cause further misalignment. Additionally, following up bad news with 'good news' has been described in other settings as a method of pursuing affiliation for future projects (Stivers & Timmermans, 2017). It may therefore be that in pursuing a response from patients, doctors are laying the groundwork for recommending treatment.

Resistance to or acceptance of treatment occurred independently of whether there was misalignment in the beginning stages of the consultation. There are many factors that affect resistance to treatment recommendations, a subject that has been well explored in CA literature (Stivers & Barnes, 2018). Where Bill states that he takes too many tablets, he appears to be displaying an understandable view that he does not want to be taking so much medication, which has been shown to be a common cause for resistance, particularly in British medical settings (Bergen et al., 2018). Stigma also comes into play, with Maggie asking for medication for her symptoms, but being less engaged with discussions of support from social services. People with dementia often have stronger reactions to practical consequences of the diagnosis, such as having to stop driving or needing support in the home, than they will to the diagnostic label itself (Byszewski et al., 2007; Campbell et al., 2016). While allowing resistance to diagnosis, doctors will therefore push to put treatment and support plans in place: Maggie did eventually agree to a home visit, and although Judith and Bill explicitly questioned the need for medication, it was nonetheless prescribed. This is reflective of a pattern that occurred across the wider dataset (Dooley et al., 2019), and is unsurprising when the aim of memory clinics is to give people receiving a diagnosis of dementia and their companions access to treatment and support (Bailey et al., 2019).

3.6 Concluding Remarks

Microanalysis of misalignment in dementia diagnosis meetings sheds light on the interactional face-saving strategies of people who are faced with this life-changing news and how clinicians manage these. People with dementia are often described as showing hostility towards or disinterest in the diagnosis, with the implication that this is the result of their condition. However, this creates an assumption that people with dementia either 'have' or 'do not have' understanding of their diagnosis. This is overly simplistic, and can be damaging as it attributes further deficits to the person with dementia, instead of seeing resistance to (or misalignment with) diagnosis as a coping mechanism. Instead, strategies should be put in place to support those receiving this difficult diagnosis in maintaining their dignity and self-identity. Further information and pre-diagnostic counselling may be helpful in supporting people to prepare for a diagnostic assessment. Communication challenges in such a setting could be overcome by encouraging a safe environment where people can talk about their difficulties and addressing them in a more empathetic and therapeutic manner.

References

Albury, C. V. A.,Ziebland, S., Webb, H., Stokoe, E. and Aveyard, P. (2021) 'Discussing weight loss opportunistically and effectively in family practice: A qualitative study of clinical interactions using conversation analysis in UK family practice.' *Fam Pract*, 38: 321–328.

Bailey, C., Dooley, J. and McCabe, R. (2019) 'How do they want to know?' Doctors' perspectives on making and communicating a diagnosis of dementia.' *Dementia (London)*, 18: 3004–3022.

Bergen, C., Stivers, T., Barnes, R. K., Heritage, J., McCabe, R., Thompson, L. and Toerien, M. (2018) 'Closing the deal: A cross-cultural comparison of treatment resistance.' *Health Commun*, 33: 1377–1388.

Byszewski, A. M., Molnar, F. J., Aminzadeh, F., Eisner, M., Gardezi, F. and Bassett, R. (2007) 'Dementia diagnosis disclosure: A study of patient and caregiver perspectives.' *Alzheimer Disease & Associated Disorders*, 21: 107–114.

Cahill, S., Gibb, M., Bruce, I., Headon, M. and Drury, M. (2008) '"I was worried coming in because I don't really know why it was arranged": The subjective experience of new patients and their primary caregivers attending a memory clinic.' *Dementia*, 7: 175–189.

Campbell, S., Manthorpe, J., Samsi, K., Abley, C., Robinson, L., Watts, S., Bond, J. and Keady, J. (2016) 'Living with uncertainty: Mapping the transition from pre-diagnosis to a diagnosis of dementia.' *J Aging Stud*, 37: 40–47.

Clare, L., Whitaker, C. J., Nelis, S. M., Martyr, A., Markova, I. S., Roth, I., Woods, R. T. and Morris, R. G. (2013) 'Self-concept in early stage dementia: Profile, course, correlates, predictors and implications for quality of life.' *Int J Geriatr Psychiatry*, 28: 494–503.

Dooley, J. (2017) *Communicating a Diagnosis of Dementia*. PhD, University of Exeter.

Dooley, J., Bass, N. and McCabe, R. (2018) 'How do doctors deliver a diagnosis of dementia in memory clinics?' *Br J Psychiatry*, 212: 239–245.

Dooley, J., Bass, N., Livingston, G. and McCabe, R. (2019) 'Involving patients with dementia in decisions to initiate treatment: Effect on patient acceptance, satisfaction and medication prescription.' *Br J Psychiatry*, 214: 213–217.

Goffman, E. (1967) 'On face-work: An analysis of ritual elements in social interaction.' In Erving Goffman (ed.) *Interaction Ritual: Essays on Face-to-Face Behaviour*. Chicago: Aldine Publishing Company.

Haakana, M. (2001) 'Laughter as a patient's resource: Dealing with delicate aspects of medical interaction.' *Text & Talk*, 21: 187–219.

Harman, G. and Clare, L. (2006) 'Illness representations and lived experience in early-stage dementia.' *Qualitative Health Research*, 16: 484–502.

Hedman, R., Hellström, I., Ternestedt, B. M., Hansebo, G. and Norberg, A. (2014) 'Social positioning by people with Alzheimer's disease in a support group.' *J Aging Stud*, 28: 11–21.

Hepburn, A. and Bolden, G. B. (2013) 'The conversation analytic approach to transcription.' In A. Hepburn and G. B. Bolden (eds.) *The Handbook of Conversation Analysis*. Chichester, UK: Blackwell Publishing.

Heritage, J. (1984) 'A change of state token and aspects of its sequential placement.' In J. Atkinson and J. Heritage (eds.) *Structures of Social Action*. Cambridge: Cambridge University Press.

(2011) 'Territories of knowledge, territories of experience: Empathic moments in interaction.' In T. Stivers, L. Mondada and J. Steensig (eds.) *The Morality of Knowledge in Conversation*. Cambridge, UK: Cambridge University Press.

(2015) 'Well-prefaced turns in English conversation: A conversation analytic perspective.' *Journal of Pragmatics*, 88: 88–104.

Karnieli-Miller, O., Werner, P., Aharon-Peretz, J., Sinoff, G. and Eidelman, S. (2012) 'Expectations, experiences, and tensions in the memory clinic: The process of diagnosis disclosure of dementia within a triad.' *Int Psychogeriatr*, 24: 1756–1770.

Kunneman, M., Pel-Littel, R., Bouwman, F. H., Gillissen, F., Schoonenboom, N. S. M., Claus, J. J., Van Der Flier, W. M. and Smets, E. M. A. (2017) 'Patients' and caregivers' views on conversations and shared decision making in diagnostic testing for Alzheimer's disease: The ABIDE project.' *Alzheimers Dement (N Y)*, 3: 314–322.

Markova, I. S., Clare, L., Whitaker, C. J., Roth, I., Nelis, S. M., Martyr, A., Roberts, J. L., Woods, R. T. and Morris, R. (2014) 'Phenomena of awareness in dementia: Heterogeneity and its implications.' *Conscious Cogn*, 25: 17–26.

Maynard, D. W. (2003) *Bad News, Good News: Conversational Order in Everyday Talk and Clinical Settings*. Chicago: University of Chicago Press.

McCabe, R., Pavlickova, H., Xanthopoulou, P., Bass, N. J., Livingston, G. and Dooley, J. (2019) 'Patient and companion shared decision making and satisfaction with decisions about starting cholinesterase medication at dementia diagnosis.' *Age Ageing*, 48: 711–718.

McGlynn, S. and Schacter, D. (1989) 'Unawareness of deficits in neuropsychological syndromes.' *Journal of Clinical and Experimental Psychology*, 11: 143–205.

Milne, A. (2010) 'The 'D' word: Reflections on the relationship between stigma, discrimination and dementia.' *Journal of Mental Health*, 19: 227–233.

Mograbi, D. C., Ferri, C. P., Sosa, A. L., Stewart, R., Laks, J., Brown, R. and Morris, R. G. (2012) 'Unawareness of memory impairment in dementia: A population-based study.' *Int Psychogeriatr*, 24: 931–939.

Morgan, J. I. and Muskett, T. (2020) 'Interactional misalignment in the UK NHS 111 healthcare telephone triage service.' *International Journal of Medical Informatics*, 134: 104030.

Murdoch, J., Barnes, R., Pooler, J., Lattimer, V., Fletcher, E. and Campbell, J. L. (2015) 'The impact of using computer decision-support software in primary care nurse-led telephone triage: Interactional dilemmas and conversational consequences.' *Social Science & Medicine*, 126: 36–47.

Peel, E. (2014) '"The living death of Alzheimer's" versus "Take a walk to keep dementia at bay": Representations of dementia in print media and carer discourse.' *Sociol Health Illn*, 36: 885–901.

Quinn, C., Jones, I. R. and Clare, L. (2017) 'Illness representations in caregivers of people with dementia.' *Aging Ment Health*, 21: 553–561.

Sabat, S. and Harre, R. (1992) 'The construction and deconstruction of self in Alzheimer's disease.' *Ageing & Society*, 12: 443–461.

Saunders, P. (1998) '"You're out of your mind!": Humor as a face-saving strategy during neuropsychological examinations.' *Neurological Disorders & Brain Damage*, 10: 357–372.

Schegloff, E. A. (2007) *Sequence Organization in Interaction: A Primer in Conversation Analysis*. Cambridge, UK: Cambridge University Press.

Stivers, T. (2005) 'Parent resistance to physicians' treatment recommendations: One resource for initiating a negotiation of the treatment decision.' *Health Commun*, 18: 41–74.

Stivers, T. and Barnes, R. K. (2018) 'Treatment recommendation actions, contingencies, and responses: An introduction.' *Health Commun*, 33: 1331–1334.

Stivers, T. and Timmermans, S. (2017) 'Always look on the bright side of life: Making bad news bivalent.' *Research on Language and Social Interaction*, 50: 404–418.

Stivers, T., Heritage, J., Barnes, R. K., McCabe, R., Thompson, L. and Toerien, M. (2018) 'Treatment recommendations as actions.' *Health Commun*, 33: 1335–1344.

Voutilainen, L., Peräkylä, A. and Ruusuvuori, J. (2010) 'Misalignment as a therapeutic resource.' *Qualitative Research in Psychology*, 7: 299–315.

Wilkinson, S. and Kitzinger, C. (2006) 'Surprise as an interactional achievement: Reaction tokens in conversation.' *Social Psychology Quarterly*, 69: 150–182.

4 The Role of Applied Conversation Analysis to Enhance Equity in Care for People with Dementia from Minority Ethnic Groups

Charlotta Plejert*

4.1 Introduction

The aim of this chapter is to demonstrate how results from conversation analytical studies (CA studies) have been used in an applied way within a specific area of dementia research, that is intercultural care and support for people with dementia from minority ethnic groups[1] in Europe (see Alzheimer Europe, 2018; Gove et al., 2021). Analysis of an episode from a video-recorded, interpreter-mediated dementia assessment, and accounts from ethnographic interviews and informal conversations with stakeholders, are used as a vehicle for discussing the role of applied Conversation Analysis (CA) to intervene in the problem of inequity in care for minority ethnic persons with dementia. The chapter deals with the relationship between *micro* and *macro*, when CA is social problem-oriented and interventionist (Antaki, 2011). Even when CA studies, for example on dementia, are published and researchers present numerous important implications for relevant stakeholders, the road toward actual *application* is often long and complex. This chapter attempts to describe what such a road might look like, reporting on research conducted over a period extending for ten years, from micro-analysis to intervention.

---

* This study was conducted within the Center for Dementia Research (CEDER), which was funded by the bank of Sweden Tercentenary Foundation between the years 2011 and 2016 (Grant no. M10–0187:1) and the project Life with Dementia: Communication, Relations and Cognition, which was funded by FORTE: The Swedish Research Council for Health, Working Life and Welfare (Grant no. 2016-07207) between the years 2016 and 2022. Thanks in particular go to the patients, their relatives, interpreters, and clinicians who participated in our project on interpreter-mediated dementia assessments.

[1] Minority ethnic group denotes "a group of people who share a common cultural identity which differs in some way to that of the majority ethnic group in a particular country" (Alzheimer Europe, 2018:7). There is extensive elaboration on terms such as ethnicity, culture, identity, and intercultural care and support, etc. in Alzheimer Europe (2018), and in Gove et al. (2021), with which the author of this chapter aligns.

4.1.1 Overview of the Chapter

First, some central concepts of applied CA are presented (Sections 4.2.1 and 4.2.2). This is followed by some major challenges related to minority ethnic persons with dementia (Section 4.2.3). Analysis of an episode from an interpreter-mediated dementia assessment demonstrates micro-level circumstances that lead to macro-level problems in equity in care for the group in question (Section 4.4.2). Ethnographic accounts of clinicians and interpreters are also provided (Section 4.4.1). The chapter ends with an overview of some interventions that are connected to and were developed as a result of challenges such as those revealed in the analytical Section (Sections 4.5 and 4.6). The aim of this chapter is thus not to be only an original, empirical study. Rather, the text is organized so that the analytical section is used as a basis for discussing problems that occur every day in memory clinics for minority ethnic people, interpreters, and the medical professionals responsible for diagnosis, and how these problems can be resolved.

4.2 Background

This section provides a background on some basics of applied CA, a description of the problem to be investigated, and some prior relevant research for the chapter.

4.2.1 Prerequisites for Applied CA

Application and implementation of CA-derived findings in relation to the field of ethnicity and dementia will be described as consisting of several factors/steps,[2] in particular:

(1) Identification of a problem area, and presentation and discussion of observations and preliminary results together with relevant stakeholders;
(2) Multidisciplinary research collaborations and networks, in which results from CA are discussed alongside findings on the same topic from studies utilizing different methods and theoretical frameworks, qualitative as well as quantitative;
(3) Collaboration and dialogue with national and international interest organizations;

---

[2] A description of similar prerequisites for applied CA is presented in Antaki (2011). What is accounted for here are factors that were central for the research program to which this chapter is connected (see Section 4.2.3).

(4) Raising funds for research that is devoted to an overall problem area in need of development: for example, inequities in dementia care in relation to ethnicity, language background, and education;
(5) Presentation of results to politicians and policymakers, nationally and internationally, preferably in the shape of reports and information texts on different levels of complexity that are empirically sound, multidisciplinary, and ecologically valid, *but not too long*. This, however, is only possible if steps 1–4 have been carried out successfully.

4.2.2 Social Problem-Oriented and Interventionist CA

Antaki (2011) provides an overview of different forms of applied CA: foundational, communicational, diagnostic, institutional, social problem-oriented, and interventionist. A brief description will be given of the social problem-oriented and interventionist approaches, since they are key for the topic of this chapter. When CA is social problem-oriented, it is used to address an issue that is perceived to be challenging for a specific group or groups of people, and tied to some kind of societal context. Interventionist CA is:

> applied to a practical problem as it plays out in interaction, with the intention of bringing about some sort of change ... it is applied to an interactional problem which pre-existed the analyst's arrival; it has the strong implication that a solution will be identified via the analysis of the sequential organization of talk; and it is undertaken collaboratively, achieved with people in the local scene. (Antaki, 2011: 8)

Needless to say, an intervention cannot be meaningfully developed unless a problem has been identified. The first step is thus to explore what it is that needs intervention.

4.2.3 What Social Problem?

As part of a large program devoted to *Living with Dementia*, conducted at the Centre for Dementia Research (CEDER) at Linköping University, a subgroup of scholars formed in 2011 to investigate living with dementia in relation to ethnic and cultural diversity and multilingualism. The overall program was, by and large, concerned with the fairly culturally and linguistically homogenous setting of Sweden. As ethnicity and dementia were explored, it rapidly became clear that not only was this area surprisingly under-researched, but that the societal need (nationally as well as internationally) for increased knowledge about the impact of dementia on minority ethnic people was huge. Reviewing existing studies, several things stood out as potentially unjust in comparison to the provision of dementia care and support for majority ethnic populations in

Western societies. Some main observations could be made based on existing international research:

(1) Persons from minority ethnic groups sought help for their symptoms later than persons with a majority ethnic background, and sometimes did not seek help at all (Alzheimer Europe, 2018; Gove et al., 2021). This could be partly explained by differences in conceptions of dementia, and also cultural and religious habits, which may differ significantly from (biomedical) perspectives applied in health care in Europe and the West[3] (Alzheimer Europe, 2018).

(2) Persons from minority ethnic groups received an unspecified dementia diagnosis significantly more often in comparison to the majority ethnic population, were younger when receiving their diagnosis, had lower scores on cognitive screening tests, and were prescribed less dementia-specific medication but more anti-psychotic drugs in comparison to the majority ethnic population (Nielsen et al., 2011a, 2011b, 2011c).

(3) Tests of cognitive functioning used in memory clinics were rarely adapted to minority ethnic persons, and not available in all languages needed, neither were they adapted to people with limited education and literacy. A lack of adequately trained interpreters also made cognitive screening a particularly demanding endeavor in the overall diagnostic process (Torkpoor et al., 2022).

(4) When living in residential care and perhaps not being proficient in the language spoken by other residents and members of staff, communication was often limited, and opportunities to interact in the person's best (or only available) language were not always available (e.g., Jansson, 2014; Small et al., 2015; Söderman & Rosendahl, 2016; Alzheimer Europe, 2018, inter alia).

It should be stressed that the social problem was not the minority ethnic persons themselves, but *the unpreparedness of the majority ethnic society to be able to offer the same quality in dementia care as that provided to the majority ethnic population.*

Based on the above findings from existing research, memory clinics and residential care were identified as key environments for further scrutiny, and several studies were designed in CEDER to investigate these settings, primarily (but not only) using anthropology, ethnography, and CA (Antelius & Kiwi, 2015; Majlesi & Plejert, 2018; Jansson et al., 2019; Plejert, 2022). This chapter, however, focuses on interpreter-mediated dementia assessments in memory clinics.

---

[3] Readers interested in this aspect are referred to Alzheimer Europe, (2018), which contains references that delve deep into anthropological explanations concerning cultural conceptions of dementia.

4.2.4 Prior Work on Interaction in Dementia Assessments

Analyses of video-recorded interactions during interpreter-mediated history-taking and formal clinical dementia assessments (Van De Mieroop et al., 2012; Plejert et al., 2015; Majlesi & Plejert, 2018; Plejert, 2022) have shed further light on already documented obstacles identified by studies within related fields such as neuropsychiatry (see Nielsen et al., 2011a, 2011b, 2011c), clinical memory research (Torkpoor et al., 2022), and CA work on monolingual dementia assessments (e.g. Jones et al., 2020), as well as interpretation in other health care settings (e.g. Bolden, 2000; Raymond, 2014). Of particular interest for the present chapter is work that has investigated the lack of adequately adapted tests – linguistically, culturally, and educationally – to minority ethnic patients with limited literacy (Nielsen & Jørgensen, 2013; Gove et al., 2021; Torkpoor et al., 2022), and investigations of interaction during dementia assessment administration (Jones et al., 2020; Jones et al., Chapter 2 this volume). Prior work on interpreter-mediated dementia assessments has stressed how the interaction between participants may be characterized by lengthy sequences of repair, due to issues such as the interpreter's unfamiliarity with the test, or the patient's difficulty in understanding a task. In monolingual settings, it has also been highlighted that tests of cognitive functioning are often not carried out in standardized ways and according to formal instructions (Jones et al., 2020; Jones et al., this volume). Exactly what that means for diagnosis remains to be investigated further. However, the training of the professionals involved in the cognitive assessment appears to be a key issue, irrespective of setting or occupation (clinician or interpreter). A common denominator of monolingual and multilingual assessments is that the way a test is administered apparently has consequences for how it is understood by the patient (see Jones et al., Chapter 2 this volume for a wider discussion). This issue will be returned to in Sections 4.6 and 4.7 in this chapter.

4.3 Method

This section provides a brief account of ethical approval, setting, participants, and data.

4.3.1 Ethical Approval

The CEDER program, including the subproject on ethnicity and dementia, was ethically approved by a Swedish board for ethical vetting. The specific ethical challenges for research involving people living with dementia are elaborated on further in the introductory chapter of this volume.

4.3.2 Setting, Participants, and Data

When the project started, contact was established with a selection of memory clinics. Often, before being able to conduct any work in the field, several informal visits were made, and meetings and discussions were held with members of staff and managers, to ensure that everyone was aware of what the study was about, was able to have their say, and was willing to participate. Eventually, collaboration was established with two Swedish memory clinics, in which video recordings were made of activities such as history-taking, advice concerning daily activities, and tests of cognitive functioning, involving four patients, four interpreters, and five clinicians. Fieldwork also comprised ethnographic observations and recorded interviews with clinicians, as well as informal conversations with interpreters and clinicians. The resulting video recordings were approximately 15 hours in length, and recordings of interviews and fieldwork were approximately 20 hours in length.

The data in Section 4.4 comes from a video recording of a Turkish-speaking 80-year-old woman (PA) during the performance of a test of cognitive functioning. The woman had lived in Sweden for almost 20 years and had been able to speak some Swedish, but had successively lost parts of this ability. At the time of the assessment she could still understand some Swedish, and managed to produce Swedish words and phrases as responses to questions. The assessment took place in her home; the visit was recorded from beginning to end and consisted of three parts: history-taking, a test of cognitive functioning, and an assessment of the woman's ability to perform everyday tasks, such as making coffee. An occupational therapist (OT) responsible for the assessment had chosen to conduct the entire event in the patient's home, since OT wanted to visit PA in her everyday environment. Also present during the event was the OT, a professional interpreter (IN) speaking Turkish as her first language and Swedish as a second language, the woman's granddaughter (GD), and the granddaughter's boyfriend.

The recording lasts for an hour and a half and has been divided into eight parts: Extracts 1–8. In Section 4.4 they are transcribed verbatim in Swedish and Turkish, and an idiomatic translation into English is also provided. Transcriptions were provided by native speakers of Swedish and Turkish. Translation into idiomatic English was done by the author and is provided below each line of original language, in bold face.

The video recordings were scrutinized using CA, with multimodal notations where deemed relevant. All recordings were watched several times, and it should be noted that at the first viewing, a lot of the interaction in Turkish was not comprehensible to the researchers. This issue, was resolved once the recordings were translated and transcribed by CA-informed research assistants proficient in Turkish and Swedish, and any uncertainties were subsequently double-checked by a second native speaker of Turkish, speaking Swedish as a second language.

In contrast to Swedish and English, which are both Germanic languages with a subject–verb–object word order, Turkish ordinarily has a subject–object–verb word order, and there are also other linguistic and semantic features that may make the structure of utterances different to that found in Germanic languages. Therefore, in the extracts cited in Section 4.4, for turns that run over more than one line, the English translation is not placed below each line of the original language, but rather displayed as chunks, so that the content of what is being said is not misinterpreted as word-for-word translation. For consistency, this also applies to longer turns in Swedish as well as Turkish.

4.4   Results

This section starts with a selection of accounts provided by clinicians and interpreters working in memory clinics, as obtained by ethnographic interviews and informal conversations. This is followed by eight extracts in which the interpreter-mediated dementia assessment of the case study is analyzed using CA.

4.4.1   Ethnographic Accounts of Challenges in Interpreter-Mediated Dementia Assessments

In systematic ethnographic interviews, as well as in informal conversations, clinicians attested that interpreter-mediated assessments, and lack of adequately adapted screening materials, were great concerns. Clinicians often felt anxiety concerning assessment accuracy in relation to tests. Even if they stressed that cognitive screening was just one part of a larger assessment process, it was their viewpoint that the pathway towards certainty was more challenging and took a lot longer for minority ethnic patients in comparison to native Swedish ones. The quality of interpreting and access to proficient interpreters were worrisome: "Nuances are missing," "I sometimes have no idea what the interpreter and patient are talking about," and "I doubt everything they say is rendered to me," were frequent statements by clinicians in interviews. Some clinicians also stated that they had been taught "never to interfere or interrupt the interaction between patient and interpreter," even if they were uncertain about what was being discussed. This account also conformed to some interpreters' self-reports that they kept strictly to their professional oath of conduct (Kammarkollegiet, 2020), for example that they only rendered as exactly as possible what was said by the patient or clinician, with no omissions or additions. Readers familiar with interpreting research know that such beliefs are rarely accurate (Wadensjö, 1998; Karliner et al., 2007; Hsieh & Kramer, 2012;).

In the informal conversations with interpreters (unfortunately not recorded) during fieldwork, several other challenges were revealed, not least in terms of the interpreters' work conditions. Often, interpreters were not given the test materials in advance, and they were asked by clinicians to translate texts and test materials that were not available in the patient's language – so called *prima vista* interpreting – on the fly. This latter practice requires specific training and should be asked for in advance before an interpreter is appointed. In fact, in Sweden an interpreter not trained in *prima vista* need not do it if they feel that they cannot perform at a professional level. To support this impression from our fieldwork, it should be noted that results of a survey of 209 interpreters asking about their perspectives on mediating within logopaedic activities in Sweden showed that, despite feeling uneasy about it, they often thought that refusing a *prima vista* task would be disloyal to the patient and clinician, and they therefore often performed the task nonetheless (Aburto Maldonado & Eklind, 2021).

4.4.2 Analysis of a Video-Recorded Episode from an Interpreter-Mediated Dementia Assessment

The test material used in the episode investigated here was the Montreal Cognitive Assessment (MoCA; Nasreddine 2003–2017), which is a short screening instrument consisting of several subparts. In Extracts 1–8 the participants are engaged in a test of memory and recall, in which the patient is to repeat five words twice, try to keep them in memory, and then recall them when asked to at the end of the test. The OT had chosen to use the Swedish version of the MoCA, although a Turkish version did exist at the time. The words in Swedish were "stol" *chair*, "plånbok" *wallet*, "tång" *pliers*, "munspel" *harmonica*, and "sax" *scissors*. While the Swedish version of the test deviates in interesting ways from the English original and the Turkish version, this does not form part of the analysis considered in this chapter.[4]

At least two explanations are plausible for the OT choosing to use the Swedish version of the test. First, at the time of the recording in 2015, the Turkish version of the MoCA was in the process of being validated for different populations and diagnoses (e.g., Yildiz et al., 2014). Secondly, had the Turkish version of the test been used, the OT would have had to ask the IN to carry out the test in full, which would have given the IN a medical responsibility that was not allowed by both medical praxis and the interpreters' professional oath of conduct. However, not all clinicians take this into

---

[4] For an elaboration on this kind of translation task, see Plejert et al., 2015, in which "munspel" *harmonica* is rendered into Kurdish as *"an instrument which is played using your mouth"*: that is, one word to be remembered and recalled is transformed into a complex syntactic construction.

4 Applied Conversation Analysis

consideration when they naively treat an interpreter as an information channel (see Wadensjö, 1998): clinicians might think that they are in charge of the test when, in fact, the interpreter is performing actions well beyond their professional role (Bolden, 2000). As will also be shown, there are elements of the interpreter being assigned responsibility for the subtest, too. Administering a formal test such as the MoCA requires specific training.

Extract 1 begins at the point of transition from a picture-naming task to a memory task.

Extract 1, OT= Occupational therapist; PA= Patient; IN= Interpreter

```
01   OT:   sedan så s- går det till så här att vi ska läsa
02         upp fem ord
           then this th- will happen that we will read five words aloud
03         (0.3)
04   IN:   mm. ondan sonra beş tane kelime var orda
           mm. next there are five words
05   OT:   och kan du bara titta på de här orden och se
06         om (0.3) om de e: (.) lätta
07         *[ (å förstå)
           and can you just look at these words and tell
           if (0.3) if they are (.) easy
           *[ (to understand)
     OT:   *points with pen at test item
08   IN:   [ burda #beş beş tane kelime
09         var bu kelimeleri bir okuyun bakalım anlıycak
10         mısınız yoksa=
           [here #there are five words read these words
           we'll see if you will understand or
     IN:       #puts test sheet in front of PA
11   PA:   =stol ((said in Swedish))
           =chair
12   IN:   biliyor musunuz ne olduğunu?
           do you know what it is?
13   PA:   e: sey su sandalye
           e: it's a chair
14   IN:   tamam
           okay
15   OT:   *fast bara du ska titta   [ för att det är bara
           *but just you should look [because it's just
     OT:   *pulls paper away from PA turning it towards IN
16   IN:                             [ jaha okej
                                     [oh okay
17   OT:   *hörseln som=
           *for hearing
     OT:   *waves towards her own right ear, looks at IN
18   IN:   =hörseln okej= ben bakıp sana söyliycekmişim
19         och vad gör jag då?
           hearing okay=it's me who's to look and tell to
           you and what do I do then?
```

As already mentioned, there had been no pre-appointment briefing with the IN and she was not familiar with the MoCA. The procedure for carrying out the memory task was therefore unknown to her, and explanation-work was needed, resulting in some confusion about who was being addressed, when, and about what. The instruction provided by the OT (lines 01, 02) is initially understood by the IN as directed toward the PA, since the OT is not clearly looking straight at anyone, but rather slightly downwards toward the test sheet. The IN (line 04) thus directs her rendition towards the PA. Immediately, however, the OT addresses the IN, asking her to take a look at the words to be repeated and recalled in the test material in front of all of them (lines 05–07), pointing with her pen at them. Since the IN does not know that the PA is only to listen, repeat, and recall the words, she puts the test sheet further into the visual field of the PA and asks her to read and check if she understands the words (line 07, multimodal). Straight away there is thus a misunderstanding between the OT and the IN about how to conduct the test, where the IN in fact is doing exactly what she, in her professional role, is supposed to do, that is render what the OT is saying to the PA. She misunderstands that the question (lines 05, 06) was addressed to her, and not to the PA. The OT uses the second person singular pronoun "du" (*you*), but this is not helpful here for turn-assignment, because clinicians who are trained in how to work with an interpreter are supposed to address patients using this form, speaking to the patients directly, which is also in accordance with interpreters' professional oath of conduct. It is therefore plausible that the IN's first-hand understanding at this point is that the "you" is meant for the PA. All of this happens rapidly, and since the OT does not understand Turkish, it is the IN's non-verbal conduct of handing over the material to the PA (line 10, multimodal), who reads out "stol" (*chair*) in Swedish (line 11), that makes the OT understand that the IN mistook the question as being directed towards the PA and as a part of the test procedure. To amend this mistake, the OT initiates repair (line 15), correcting the action by the IN, adding that the PA is not to read, but just listen (lines 15, 17). This explanation is acknowledged by the IN, also addressing the patient in Turkish (line 18) before asking the OT for further information about what to do next (line 19).

Subsequently, the OT initiates a topic that indicates that she is interested in knowing whether the Swedish words to be repeated and recalled are common in Turkish (and thereby easily recognizable for the PA: see lines 05, 06 in Extract 1). The fact that confusion arises due to the language of the test material also surfaces in Extract 2. The OT acknowledges that the PA has read aloud "stol" (*chair*, Extract 1, line 11) when she saw the words in the Swedish test material.

Extract 2, OT= Occupational therapist; PA= Patient; IN= Interpreter; GD= Granddaughter

```
20   OT:   eh (0.3) stol ä lätt att säga på
21         turkiska= plånbok. (.) men tång hur ä de
22         me de? eh: vet- vet-
           eh (0.3) chair is easy to say in
           Turkish= wallet. (.) but pliers what
           about that? eh: d'you know-
23   IN:   tång ä e::=
           pliers are e::=
24   GD:   =de ä liksom=
           it's kind of-
25   PA:   =tång ağırlık değil mi?=
           isn't tång weight?=
26   IN:   =nä nä
           =no no
27   OT:   ett ver[kt- e: verktyg
           a    to[o- e: tool
28   IN:          [verktyg=ja ja[vet
                  [tool=yes I   [know
29   GD:                        [ahaa↑
```

After acknowledging the PA's reading out of "stol" (*chair*) in Swedish, the OT asks the IN about the next two words in the test, which are "plånbok" (*wallet*) and "tång" (*pliers*) (lines 20, 21). *Wallet* is mentioned in passing with falling intonation (line 21), whereas the OT asks explicitly what the situation is regarding *pliers*. The IN begins to say something about *pliers* (line 23) but is interrupted by the GD (line 24) as well as by the PA herself, who asks if "tång" means something to do with weight (line 25), which is denied by the IN (line 26). The suggestion by the PA (line 25), however, makes sense from a language-learner perspective, considering the similarity in pronunciation (as well as spelling) of the word for pliers in Swedish "tång"/tɔŋ/ and the word for heavy "tung"/tɵŋ/. It is noteworthy that the IN does not render to the OT what the PA is saying in line 25, and the episode continues as a collaborative, syntactic, co-constructed unit produced by the IN, GD, and OT (Lerner, 2004; Bockgård, 2004) about "tång" being a kind of tool (lines 23, 24, 27, 28). The IN, OT, and GD are at this point thus in agreement about the meaning of the Swedish word (see GD's acknowledgment token in line 29). The IN then checks for the Turkish translation on an online resource on her phone.

Extract 3, OT= Occupational therapist; PA= Patient; IN= Interpreter; GD=Granddaughter

```
30   IN:   vänta eh::#ja ska kolla[på en gång
           wait eh:: #I'll check  [immediately
     IN:         #lifts up her mobile phone and looks--->
31   GD:                          [de kan va
32         havstång (.) också
```

```
                                [it can be seaweed (.) also
33   OT:     ja [ja
             yea [yea
34   IN:        [nä nä inte sånt çivi falan
35              çe için=
                [no no not that like to pull a nail or so=
36   GD:     =aha:
37   IN:     aa (1.2) °jag vet° men (0.3) ah nu blev de
38           havstång kerpeten ja just de= e:: nu har
39           ja hittat de
             aa (1.2) °I know° but (0.3) ah now it became seaweed plier yes
             that's right=e:: now # I've found it
     IN: -checks phone-#
40   OT:     mm men vet hon vad det är?
             mm but does she know what it is?
41   IN:     ja ja ska k-ja ska    [fråga mm
             yea I will k- I will [ask mm
42   OT:                           [aa
((ten lines omitted))
```

The IN checks her phone at the same time as the GD suggests that "tång" may also mean "havstång," that is *seaweed* (lines 31, 32). "Tång" happens to be a homonymous word in Swedish that may refer to either a tool or a plant – it is pronounced and spelled in the exact same way. The OT acknowledges the GD's comment, but does not say anything further, and the IN overlaps (line 34), objecting to the suggestion by the GD as the non-intended meaning, supposedly since they have just reached agreement (Extract 2) about "tång" with the meaning of a tool being the target word in the test. She code-switches into Turkish, providing information about what can be done with this tool (*like to pull a nail=*) (lines 34, 35), which is accepted by the GD (line 36). The IN continues to scrutinize her mobile phone, stating, with a quiet and slightly frustrated tone of voice, that she knows (line 37), and she also happens to access the word *seaweed* on her device before, eventually, she finds the Turkish word for the tool (lines 38, 39), which is "kerpenten." For the OT, however, it is important that the PA knows what it is, so she persists in her project of making sure that the words to be tested are common in Turkish (line 40).

Ten lines have been omitted, during which the IN checks that the PA knows what pliers are. The OT checks with the IN that harmonica and scissors are also common words in Turkish, which is confirmed by the IN. After this, an attempt to restart the memory task is made.

Extract 4, OT= Occupational therapist; PA= Patient; IN= Interpreter

```
52   OT:     *för då är de så här att du- du ska
53           säga de här orden.
             *cause then it's like this that you- you are to say these words.
```

4 Applied Conversation Analysis

```
       OT:   *points at the list of words in the test form with her pen
54     IN:   på turkiska?
             in Turkish?
55     OT:   på turkiska↑ (.) å sen så ska hon säga dom (0.3) e: å då
56           markerar vi hur- vilka hon kan säga.
             in Turkish (.) and then she is to say them (0.3) e: and then we
             mark how- which ones she can say.
57     IN:   hon ska repetera alltså efter       [mig
             so she'll repeat everything after   [me
58     OT:                                       [på turkiska
                                                 [in Turkish
59     IN:   på turkiska?
             in Turkish?
60     OT:   på turkiska.
             in Turkish.
61     IN:   okej.
             okay.
```

As can be observed in Extract 4, which language to use is once more a concern for the IN (line 54) when she is given the instruction from the OT (lines 52, 53). The language is confirmed by the OT (line 55) as well as provided at the end of her instruction (line 58). It may be the case that the latter instance is not heard, since it is produced in overlap when the IN requests further information about how to carry out the task (line 57). The lack of hearing may also explain why the IN requests a confirmation of choice of language again in line 59, confirmed by the OT in line 60.

What can be observed in Extract 4 is that not only does the IN's uncertainty of what language to use need to be clarified, but more precision on how the task is to be carried out and what is expected from the PA is also required. An issue so far not addressed in detail in this analysis is the potential impact that such negotiations might have for the PA's understanding and execution of the task, since she does have some knowledge of Swedish. The PA is thus exposed to a large amount of linguistic input in two languages and visual access to the test material throughout this negotiation, which may affect her ability to remember the target words.

In the test instructions, the task is supposed to be carried out in a specific way, with the words produced at a certain pace by the test leader and then repeated by the patient; the same procedure should then be conducted a second time. After this, the patient is to receive the instruction to try to store the words in memory, and is then asked to recall them at the end of the test. As has been demonstrated, rather than providing the IN with this full explanation from the start, it is given to her bit by bit, which requires repair several times, stalling the progression of the test, as already evident from Extracts 1–4. A further example of the OT's explanation-work and the IN's requests for clarification is demonstrated in Extract 5.

**Extract 5, OT= Occupational therapist; PA= Patient;
IN= Interpreter**

```
62   OT:   å sedan så läser vi (.) du igen orden å sen
63         så ser vi då hur hon- om hon kan komma ihåg alla.
           and then we (.) you read again the words and then
           we'll see how she- if she can remember all of them.
64   IN:   mm okej (.) eh ska jag säga en och en (.) nu?=
           should I say one by one now?=
65   OT:   =ja=
           =yes=
66   IN:   eller[ska ja (xxx)
           or   [should I (xxx)
67   OT:        [ja ja men inte så fort utan att hon ska
68         hinna liksom lägga de på minnet.
           have time to put it in memory.
69   IN:   okej
           okay
70   OT:   å sen ska hon också veta att sen efter alltihopa
71         så kommer vi tillbaka (0.3) å frågar "kommer du
72         ihåg dom här orden"
           and then she should also know that then after it all
           we will come back (0.3) and ask "do you
           remember these words".
73         (.)
74   IN:   ok[ej
           ok[ay
75   OT:     [de här ä bara egentligen en repetition
             [this is in fact just a repetition
76   IN:   okej=ska jag läsa ett  [å
           okay=I should read one [and
77   OT:                          [(xx)
78   IN:   sen vänta på att hon svarar e: repeterar
           then wait for her to answer e: repeat
79   OT:   ja
           yea
80   IN:   å sen     [(xxxx)
           and then [ (xxxx)
81   OT:            [å då kan du sätta ett streck (.)
82         *så här om hon kan de=annars ingenting
           [and then you can make a mark (.)
           *like this if she knows=otherwise nothing
     OT:   *demonstrates with a pen on the sheet
```

As can be observed in lines 62–63, the IN is positioned as test administrator by the OT, by means of a repair in which the pronoun "vi" (*we*) is changed into the second person singular "du" (*you*), concerning who is to read out the list of words once more. Another salient feature in Extract 5 is the query from the IN about the way the PA is to repeat the words: if the IN is to read the words one by one (lines 64, 66, and 76), supposedly meaning that the PA should repeat each word right after it has been read out aloud. The OT responds quickly in a confirmatory way (line 67) to the first part of the question before the IN has finished her turn (line 66). The OT then provides instructions concerning the steady pace at which the reading should be conducted, and why (*not so fast cause she must kind of have time to put it in memory*) (lines 67, 68). She then returns to describing the second round of repetition (lines 70–72), although the IN once more tries to find out whether to read each item one at a time (line 76). Again, it appears that the OT assumes that the IN understands that all words should be read out at a steady pace by the IN first (as stated in the instructions) before the PA repeats them. As will be shown in Extract 6, there is still a mismatch between the participants' understanding of this procedure, since the PA repeats each word after the IN, instead of waiting, listening, and *then* repeating.

Extract 6, OT= Occupational therapist; PA= Patient; IN= Interpreter

```
83    IN:   okej şimdi ben size bazı kelimeler okuyacağım (0.3)
84          Türkçe= bu kelimeleri tekrarlayacaksınız.
85          okay now I'm going to read you some words (0.3) in
             Turkish= you are going to repeat these words.
86    PA:   mm
87    IN:   söylemeniz ile ilgili bir test bu
             this test is about you articulating
88    PA:   mm
89    IN:   e: sandalye
             e: chair
90    PA:   sandalye
             chair
91          #(1.0)
      IN:   #marks answer on test sheet
92    IN:   e:: (1.2) cüzdan
             e:: (1.2) purse
93          (0.4)
94    PA:   cüzdan
             purse
95          #(1.5)
      IN:   #marks answer on test sheet
96    IN:   eh:: kerpeten
             eh:: pliers
97          (0.3)
98    PA:   kerpeten
             pliers
99          #(1.0)
      IN:   #marks answer on test sheet
100   IN:   e: mızıka
             e: harmonica
101         (.)
102   PA:   mızıka
             harmonica
103         #(1.0)#        #(5.0)#
      IN:   #marks answer# # puts down pen, looks up from test
             sheet with a "thinking face"#
104   IN:   hi hi ((giggles)) makas
```

88   Charlotta Plejert

```
                hi hi ((giggles)) scissors
105             (0.3)
106   PA:       makas
                scissors
107   IN:       h.hhh (.) de stannar ibland hos mig också ha ha
108             så vad gör vi sen då=ska jag läsa en gång till (xx)?
                h.hhh (.) it gets stuck with me too sometimes ha ha
                so what's next=should I read once more (xx)?
((several lines omitted))
```

The pattern of the PA repeating right after the IN occurs between lines 89 and 106. The IN is still positioned as a test administrator who is responsible for marking the PA's answers on the test form. Interestingly, the IN does not object to this role, despite the fact that it goes against the interpreters' professional oath of conduct. It is hard to tell if this positioning contributes to her not rendering the PA's verbal repetitions to the OT, or if she judges her marking correctness on the test sheet as sufficient for the OT, since this action is taking place within the visual field of all participants present, and the target words are written in Swedish on the test form.

Translating text items without preparation has already resulted in negotiations about the word for "tång," when the IN had to look it up on her mobile device (Extract 3, and in talk about the other words being easily understood in Turkish). In Extract 6 the IN's mind goes blank when she is to translate the Swedish word "sax" (scissors) (line 103). Her actions of putting down the pen and looking blankly towards the right with a thinking face (Goodwin & Goodwin, 1986) are followed by a soft giggle before she turns toward the PA and produces the Turkish word for scissors (line 104). When the PA has repeated the word, the IN tries to mitigate her delay in translating by stating that she also sometimes faces memory or word-finding problems (*h.hhh it gets stuck with me too sometimes ha ha*) with laughter which, together with her facial expression, indicates embarrassment (Wilkinson, 2007; Lindholm, 2008) (line 107). Saying that she, too, faces difficulties coming up with a certain word, signals that problems with recall could happen to anyone, even an interpreter, which in a sense normalizes the PA's potential dementia condition currently being assessed. It might also be an excuse for the IN's display of a sudden lack of competence in her professional role as an interpreter.

What happens after this episode is that the OT instructs the IN to ask the PA to repeat all the words once more, which she does, and again the PA repeats straight after every word spoken by the IN. This time, the OT interrupts and provides the IN with instructions that she is to read out *all* the words first, before the PA repeats them.

The IN is ticking the boxes in the test form for each word, and does not confirm the answers in speech to the OT this round either, and the OT follows the progress and results of the PA by watching the marks being made on the sheet by the IN. At last, they manage to conduct the task in the way described in the test manual. However, this process has required a fair amount of repair work and negotiation in two languages, both of which the PA is proficient to various degrees. All participants have had a lot of visual access to the test sheet, despite the fact that this subtask on memory should be performed without visual cues.

The task is finished when the OT asks the IN to tell the PA to try to keep the words in her memory (Extract 7, line 125, 126). The PA's understanding of this instruction is displayed in line 130, as she asks for confirmation, and is positively responded to by the IN (lines 131, 133).

Extract 7, OT= Occupational therapist; PA= Patient; IN= Interpreter

```
125   OT:   de e jättebra↑(.) kan du säga nu att nu gäller
126         de för henne att hålla kvar de här sakerna
              that's great↑ (.) can you tell now that now
              she's to try to keep these things
127   IN:   şimdi bunları unutmamaya çalışın
              now try not to forget these
128   PA:   mm
129   IN:   daha sonra [dönücez
              we'll      [return to it later
130   PA:              [tekrar söyleyecek miyim bunları?
                       [am I going to say these again?
131   IN:   a: [jag ska göra (xxxx)
              a: [I'll do (xxxx)
132   OT:      [ska komma tillbaka
                [will come back
133   IN:   just det evet
              that's right yea
133   PA:   mm
```

The administration of the MoCA continues with a couple of further subtasks before it is time, as the penultimate assignment, to recall *sandalye, cüzdan, kerpeten, mızıka,* and *makas*.

Extract 8, OT= Occupational therapist; PA= Patient; IN= Interpreter

```
500   OT:   å då kommer vi tillbaka till dom här fem orden
501         som vi repeterade (.) å då ska du bara be henne
502         försöka å komma ihåg dom å för varje ord som hon
503         kommer ihåg * så sätter du ett s- en etta där.
              and then we go back to these five words
              that we repeated (.) and then you'll just ask her
              to try to remember them and for every word that
              she remembers *you mark with a s- number one there.
      OT:   *hands over test sheet to IN
```

```
504   IN:   mm (.) şimdi o denim hani bir kelimeler
505         çalışmıştık hafızanızda tutmaya çalışacağınız
506         sonra tekrar gelicez demiştim (.) o kelimelere
507         e: hatırladıklarınızı söyleyin.
            now you know we have studied some words that you are
            going to try to keep in your mind (.) then I said we
            would come back now we are returning to those words
            e: say the ones you remember.
508   PA:   en hiç hatırlatmıycek misin?
            aren't you going to remind me?
509   IN:   hayir hahaha ska ni inte påminna mig he he he
510         repetera
            no hahaha aren't you going to remind me he he he to
            repeat
511   PA:   mızıka
            harmonica
512   IN:   mm
513   PA:   eh: cüzdan
            eh: wallet
514         (0.6)
515   IN:   m:
516   PA:   sandalye
            chair
517         (14.0)
      PA:   looks straight forward. OT looking at PA, IN looking
            at test sheet
518   PA:   makas (7.0) o kadar
            scissors (7.0) that's it
519   IN:   de va #fyra stycken
            that's #four
      IN:         #hands over test sheet to OT
520   OT:   mm (.) å då ska vi se vilket ord om du frågar
521         henne (0.2) ordet hon inte tog upp (.) om ett
522         verktyg om
523         hon kan säga vilket verktyg vi pratar om
            mm (.) and then we'll see which word if you ask her
            (0.2) it was that she didn't bring up (.) about a
            tool if she can tell which tool
            we are talking about
524   IN:   mm bir de ayrıca bir böyle tamir aleti
525         [ bir kelime vardı
            mm there was also like a repair tool
            [ a word
526   PA:   [a: kerpeten
            [a: plier
527   IN:   ja tamam
            yea alright
528   OT:   mm tjusigt (0.3) jätte bra
            mm nice (0.3) well done
529   IN:   çok guzel
            very good
```

As can be observed, the IN gives the PA the instruction to try to remember the words that they had previously discussed (lines 504–507), and before the PA answers, she once more jokes about needing to be reminded herself (line 508), which is rendered by the IN with laughter (lines 509, 510). The PA is very much oriented towards the task and produces the first three target words at a fairly regular pace (lines 511–516). The PA then looks straight ahead, thinking for some time, before she comes up with the Turkish word for scissors, followed by a long silence and an account about being finished (line 518). In accordance with the test instructions, it is allowed to provide brief semantic cues at this point, which the OT instructs the IN to do (lines 520–523). When provided with this input (lines 524, 525), the PA quickly manages to remember "kerpenten," which is acknowledged as correct by the IN (line 527). The task is closed by the OT assessing the task as successful (line 528), also rendered in Turkish by the IN (line 529). Largely, the PA has completed the memory and recall task successfully. To what extent she would have scored in a similar way if conducting the test in Turkish only will never be known.

4.5 What Intervention?

In this section, findings such as those exposed in the analysis above, alongside results generated through ethnographic and informal interviews, will now be addressed in terms of how they contribute to various interventions for the target group. The impact of CA in these interventions, it should be mentioned, range on a scale: from being a main resource, to being a part of a much larger, multidisciplinary whole in accordance with the four steps for applied CA that were described in the introduction to this chapter. The interventions were primarily of three different kinds: (1) feedback to participating memory clinics; (2) presentation and discussion of research findings at training days for professionals and people from interest organizations; (3) research network outcomes in a range of forms, such as information materials and reports at different levels of difficulty and formality, policy proposals, and dialogues with policymakers.

4.5.1 Feedback to Memory Clinic Staff

During the project, the participating memory clinic teams were offered feedback using anonymous video clips and rough transcription extracts as a basis for discussion. Whereas clips like Extracts 1–8 would generate discussions about choice of test material, the role of *prima vista* interpreting, and how to better prepare interpreters for an assessment, other episodes dealt with challenges associated with patients' level of education, and cultural bias in relation to a test (see Nielsen & Jørgensen, 2013; Plejert et al., 2015). By and large, video analyses seemed to corroborate the experiences and "suspicions" that clinicians had expressed in the ethnographic interviews and informal conversations carried out before and during video-data collection. One benefit of the feedback sessions was that they appeared to be an eye-opener for many clinicians to explicitly show how challenging the situation was for interpreters, too, not just for themselves (see also Torkpoor et al., 2022).

Overall, even if clinicians were often aware of many of the issues that may influence an intercultural encounter, access to *translated* video and/or sound recordings of interpreter-mediated patient encounters made them aware of the more precise details of linguistic, cultural, and educational matters that were causing problems. Despite the small scale of this intervention with the participating teams, the sessions made clinicians consider changing certain practices, for example concerning choice of test material, to try to more systematically brief interpreters before an appointment, and to interrupt in the interpreting process when they felt uncertainty about what was going on in talk between patient and interpreter when this was not referred back to them. Based on video episodes from other activities (not considered in this chapter), there was also discussion on how different activities might be more or less challenging from the interpreter's point of view, with history-taking being a lot less demanding than being asked to translate and administer a formal test.

4.5.2   Presentations at Training Days

Analyses highlighting challenges like the ones presented in this text, published in articles as well as in more popular sources directed towards clinicians and interpreters, resulted in several invitations to speak on "training days," that is one- or two-day events for professionals involved in dementia health care. A challenge at such events was to strike a balance between criticism of existing practices and not threatening face, while at the same time suggesting easy-to-implement interventions, taking into account financial and practical constraints on the various stakeholders. Relating to the episode analyzed in this chapter that displays the struggle of the clinician and the interpreter, with several restarts of a test task before it was carried out in accordance with formal instructions and expectations, may of course be intimidating. When talking about such episodes to those concerned, it was therefore important to view and discuss them in light of circumstances at the time, that is the fact that clinicians in 2015–2017 did not have access to more suitable tests. Being an interpreter, unless as an accredited interpreter within law, is a badly paid, low-status job in most countries, including Sweden. Many interpreters in Sweden have only a very basic training. When presenting research to this group, it was therefore important to highlight differences between activities in memory clinics (e.g., history-taking being easier to interpret), and to encourage them to ask clinicians for information about tasks and materials in advance of an appointment, particularly for the more demanding tasks such as cognitive screening.

One quite straightforward intervention on these training days was to encourage implementation of the briefing–interaction–debriefing process (BID, see Langdon & Saenz, 2016). BID is a rather simple routine (and there are other ones similar to it), in which clinicians meet interpreters a little in advance of an appointment and inform them about the aims of the encounter, what materials are to be used, whether text translations might be needed, and so on. A debriefing also takes place right after the appointment, in which the interpreter and clinician discuss potential areas of confusion. The BID procedure is thus not derived from CA per se, but is an intervention that might positively affect some of the challenges revealed by CA and the problems reported in ethnographic accounts. For the session examined in this chapter, a briefing session could have prevented side-sequences during the patient encounter, for example as to whether an item to be translated was a common word in the patient's language and so on, consecutive instructions and meta-talk on how to carry out a task, or could even have provided a chance for the interpreter to say that she was not skilled in *prima vista* translation. A pre-appointment briefing in clinics, with information about tasks and materials, has proven to be high on interpreters' wish lists (Aburto Maldonado & Eklind, 2021). This was also expressed by interpreters at these training days.

It should be mentioned that staff in some memory clinics claimed to already work according to routines resembling BID, but practical issues, such as increased costs (for booking longer sessions with interpreters), and the personal needs of interpreters (for example, the need to pick up their child from nursery school, catch a bus, and so on) very often hampered the execution of a BID routine.

4.5.3 Research Network Outcomes

Substantial research funding enabled the establishment of several networks, the three most influential of which, where CA scholars had an impact, were the Research Network on Ethnicity and the Dementias, the Nordic Thematic Network on Ethnic Minorities and Dementia, and the Alzheimer Europe expert group on intercultural care and support (Gove et al., 2021). Many of the participants in these networks and groups were the same, but whereas the first network consisted exclusively of researchers conducting empirical work, the other two also comprised representatives from interest organizations, professionals from health care institutions and services, and persons assigned to report research findings to policymakers at national and international levels (Gove et al., 2021). The *research* network fed into the *thematic* network and upwards regarding everything from cultural conceptions of dementia and their consequences for help-seeking patterns, attitudes towards daycare activities, intercultural encounters, and multilingual interaction in residential care, to challenges associated with diagnostic instruments and (lack of) adequately trained interpreters, highlighting similar difficulties as those exposed in Extracts 1–8. By and large, the aim of these networks was to address the overall social problem of inequity in care for minority ethnic people with dementia, proposing recommendations and solutions on the basis of results from empirical studies using different methods and theoretical frameworks, and in dialogue with a wide range of stakeholders. Assisted by the Nordic Welfare Centre,[5] ideas and recommendations were communicated to the national boards of health and welfare of the respective Nordic countries, and to the Nordic Ministry of Health.

The Alzheimer Europe report was published in 2018 in English, French, and German, and has subsequently been modified into several shorter and more popular guides in a number of European languages, directed toward staff in residential care and health care clinics. The essence of the original report has been turned into a commentary, and also a policy proposal for improving equity in care for minority ethnic persons with dementia in Europe that was presented to the European Commission in August in 2020 (see Gove et al., 2021). In that policy proposal, factors related to analyses of language, culture, and interaction may be summarized as set out in the list below. This hopefully resonates with what can be observed in Extracts 1–8 in this chapter when it comes to the training of clinicians (Gove et al., 2021:4), who need to:

- Undergo training in cultural awareness, sensitivity, and competence so as to improve communication and build a relationship with people from minority ethnic groups, thereby helping to ensure timely, accurate, and differential diagnoses and treatment of dementia amongst members of minority ethnic groups;
- Use culturally sensitive/fair and appropriately validated screening, assessment, and diagnostic tools for people from minority ethnic groups, which are administered with the help of qualified/trained interpreters (preferably with medical accreditation) when needed – mere translations are not sufficient;
- Make every effort to enable every person to be assessed and diagnosed in their best/preferred language at no extra charge, and for people to be informed of this possibility;
- Not ask relatives and friends to act as interpreters, except for emergencies or exceptional circumstances, but to consult them during the assessment process if required and subject to the agreement of the person being assessed.

---

[5] The Nordic Welfare Centre is an institution within the Nordic Council of Ministers' social and health sector.

4.6 Summary of Findings

The aim of this chapter was to demonstrate how results from CA may be applied within a specific area identified as challenging in terms of how to provide equity in care and support for people with dementia from minority ethnic groups. In the episode with the Turkish woman analyzed above, a Swedish version of the dementia screening test MoCA was used. As can be observed, when asking the interpreter to administer the Swedish version, simultaneously translating its tasks into Turkish, the interpreter was put in charge of the procedure in (unwanted) ways that potentially affected the performance of the patient (for similar findings see Plejert et al., 2015; Torkpoor et al., 2022).

It was obvious that the interpreter had not been briefed in advance about what material was to be used and what function a certain task had, since the occupational therapist needed to supply the interpreter with instructions as the session progressed, at the same time as the interpreter turned to the patient with directions. Instructions were in this way continuously modified, as the occupational therapist realized that the task was not carried out in accordance with the Swedish manual (see Jones et al., 2020, and Chapter 2 this volume for a discussion on that issue based on monolingual data). A large amount of linguistic input in Swedish as well as in Turkish relating to the materials used in the procedures involved in the test thus occurred in repair and clarification work, which was available to the patient throughout the task.

It is of course hard to tell to what extent the metatalk in Swedish between the clinician and the interpreter affected the patient's ability to remember the words eventually, but their negotiations were, as demonstrated above, extensive. It was also noteworthy that the patient initially had visual access to the Swedish words in the test material, as the interpreter at first did not know that the words were only to be read out loud. Since the patient had some knowledge of Swedish, several linguistic cues were unintentionally available during a large part of the testing.

In sum, phenomena such as the ones examined here, which are supported by similar findings in related studies (see Torkpoor et al., 2022), compromised the progressivity of the dementia assessment in ways not observed for native Swedish patients.

4.7 Conclusion

The pathway from empirical research to intervention and practice/policy change is long and complex. To walk on such a path as a CA scholar, together with other researchers and professionals, is often extremely rewarding, but may also be frustrating at times. What perhaps causes most anxiety is the amount of funding needed in order to get from one point to the next. This does not only refer to research grants, but also to political incentives, often over a *limited period of time*, to support a service, education program, research center, and the like. Interventions are frequently like the one performed with our participating memory clinics: local, small-scale, and short-term.

A weakness of the CA study examined in this chapter is that patients were not involved in the same way and to the same extent as clinicians and interpreters, even if patients' perspectives were revealed by showing their orientations in the analyzed video-recordings. In the future, greater involvement of minority ethnic patients would allow generation of rich descriptions of a very complex social situation, and to further equity in care for these patients.

In order to end this chapter on a high note, apart from the interventions described in Section 4.5, there has been a lot of progress in the area of developing tests of cognitive functioning, such as the RUDAS and the CNTB, that are less culturally, educationally, and linguistically biased than other tests, for example the MMSE and the MoCA. This is to a great extent thanks to the work of one of the members of the networks described above, T. Rune Nielsen and his research teams that developed and trialed several test batteries, some of which are, at the time of writing in 2022, recommended by boards for health and welfare in several countries to be used in dementia assessments for minority ethnic persons (e.g., Nielsen et al., 2019). Nielsen, people at the Migrationsskolan (Migration School) in southern Sweden, and scholars at CEDER worked together for more than ten years, exchanging results, ideas, and experiences concerning dementia assessment for minority ethnic persons with dementia, combining nursing science, neuropsychiatry, clinical linguistics, anthropology, interpreting science, and CA. At the Migrationsskolan, courses were held for clinicians on how to administer the new, culturally adapted screening instruments (particularly the RUDAS), alongside providing a specific training program for interpreters, producing special "memory interpreters." An evaluation of this training program revealed that clinicians felt a lot more secure in terms of diagnostic accuracy and patient safety when they had appointed one of the memory interpreters (Migrationsskolan, 2021) in comparison to the prior situation, which had been similar to the one described in the empirical part of this chapter. All in all, even though CA results may appear as a small piece within the large puzzle of equity in care for minority ethnic people with dementia, it has hopefully been demonstrated that it is an important one.

References

Aburto Maldonado, J. and Eklind, L. (2021) *Tolksamarbete inom logopediska verksamheter. En enkätstudie ur tolkarnas perspektiv. [Interpreter Collaboration in Speech and Language Therapy Activities. A Questionnaire Study from the*

Interpreters' Perspective]. MA thesis. Linköping University. https://www.diva-portal.org/smash/get/diva2:1567407/FULLTEXT01.pdf.

Alzheimer Europe (2018) *The Development of Intercultural Care and Support for People with Dementia from Minority Ethnic Groups*. www.alzheimer-europe.org/sites/default/files/alzheimer_europe_ethics_report_2018.pdf (retrieved 19 January 2022).

Antaki, C. (2011) *Applied Conversation Analysis. Intervention and Change in Institutional Talk*. Basingstoke: Palgrave Macmillan.

Antelius, E. and Kiwi, M. (2015) 'Frankly, none of us know what dementia is: Dementia caregiving among Iranian immigrants living in Sweden'. *Care Management Journals*, 16(2): 79–94.

Bockgård, G. (2004) *Syntax som social resurs: en studie av samkonstruktionssekvensers form och funktion i svenska samtal* [*Syntax as a Social Resource: A Study of Form and Function of Co-construction Sequences in Swedish Conversation*]. Doctoral dissertation. Uppsala University.

Bolden, G. (2000) 'Toward understanding practices of medical interpreting: Interpreter's involvement in history taking. *Discourse Analysis*, 2(4): 387–419.

Goodwin, M. H. and Goodwin, C. (1986) 'Gesture and coparticipation in the activity of searching for a word.' *Semiotica*, 62: 51–75.

Gove, D., Nielsen, T. R., Smits, C., Plejert, C., Rauf, M. A., Parveen, S., Jaakson, S., Golan Shemesh, D., Lahav, D., Kaur, R., Herz, M. K., Monses, J., Thyrian, J. R. and Georges, J. (2021) 'The challenges of achieving timely diagnosis and culturally appropriate care of people with dementia from minority ethnic groups in Europe.' *International Journal of Geriatric Psychiatry*, 36: 1823–1828.

Hsieh, E. and Kramer, E. M. (2012) 'Medical interpreters as tools: Dangers and challenges in the utilitarian approach to interpreters' roles and functions.' *Patient Education & Counselling*, 89(1): 158–162.

Jansson, G. (2014) 'Bridging language barriers in multilingual care encounters.' *Multilingua*, 33(1–2): 201–232.

Jansson, G., Plejert, C. and Lindholm, C. (2019) 'The social organization of assistance in multilingual interaction in Swedish residential care.' *Discourse Studies* 21(1): 67–94.

Jones, D., Wilkinson, R., Jackson, C. and Drew, P. (2020) 'Variation and interactional non-standardization in neuropsychological tests: The case of the Addenbrooke's cognitive examination.' *Qualitative Health Research* 30(3): 458–470.

Kammarkollegiet [The Legal, Financial and Administrative Services Agency] (2020) *God tolksed* [*Good Interpreting Practice*]. www.kammarkollegiet.se/download/18.27f1fe4c168c1d817515205f/1551777027993/God_tolksed_mars2019.pdf (retrieved 19 January 2022).

Karliner, L. S., Jacobs, E. A., Chen, A. H. and Mutha, S. (2007) 'Do professional interpreters improve clinical care for patients with limited English proficiency? A systematic review of the literature.' *Health Services Research*, 42(2): 727–754.

Langdon, W. H. and Saenz, T. I. (2016) *Working with Interpreters and Translators: A Guide for Speech-Language Pathologists and Audiologists*. San Diego, CA: Plural Publishing.

Lerner, G. H. (2004) 'Collaborative turn sequences', in G. H. Lerner (ed.) *Conversation Analysis. Studies from the First Generation*. Amsterdam: John Benjamins Publishing Company, pp. 225–256.

Lindholm, C. (2008) 'Laughter, communication problems, and dementia.' *Communication & Medicine* 5(1): 3–14.

Majlesi, A. R. and Plejert, C. (2018) 'Embodiment in tests of cognitive functioning: A study of an interpreter-mediated dementia evaluation.' *Dementia – the International Journal of Social Research & Practice*, 17(2): 138–163.

Migrationsskolan (2019) *Inga om men eller varför: att främja säker och jämlik kognitiv utredning genom tolk* [*No Ifs, Buts or Whys: To Promote Safe and Equal Cognitive Screening Using an Interpreter*] Migrationsskolan report 2019:2. https://vardgivare.skane.se/kompetens-utveckling/rapporter/rapport/inga-om-men-eller-varfor/ (retrieved 19 January 2022).

Nasreddine, S. Z. (2003–2017) The Montreal Cognitive Assessment MoCA, www.mocatest.org (retrieved 19 January 2022).

Nielsen T. R. and Jørgensen, K. (2013) 'Visuoconstructional abilities in cognitively healthy illiterate Turkish immigrants: A quantitative and qualitative investigation.' *The Clinical Neuropsychologist* 27(4): 681–692.

Nielsen, T. R., Vogel, A., Phung, T. K., Gade, A. and Waldemar, G. (2011a) 'Over- and under-diagnosis of dementia in ethnic minorities: A nationwide register-based study.' *International Journal of Geriatric Psychiatry*, 26(11): 1128–1135.

Nielsen, T. R., Vogel, A., Riepe, M. W., de Mendonca, A., Rodriguez, G., Nobili, F., Fade, A. and Waldemar, G. (2011b) 'Assessment of dementia in ethnic minority patients in Europe: A European Alzheimer's disease consortium survey.' *International Psychogeriatrics*, 23(1): 89–95.

Nielsen, T. R., Andersen, B. B., Kastrup, M., Phung, T. K. T. and Waldemar, G. (2011c) 'Quality of dementia diagnostic evaluation for ethnic minority patients: A nationwide study.' *Dementia & Geriatric Cognitive Disorders*, 31: 388–396.

Nielsen, T. R., Segers, K., Vanderaspoilden, V., Beinhoff, U., Minthon, L., Pissiota, A., Bekkhus-Wetterberg, P., Hanevold Bjørkløf, G., Tsolaki, M., Gkioka, M. and Waldemar, G. (2019) 'Validation of a European cross-cultural neuropsychological test battery (CNTB) for evaluation of dementia.' *International Journal of Geriatric Psychiatry*, 34(1): 144–152.

Plejert, C. (2022) 'Challenges and remedies for interpreter-mediated dementia assessments', in L. Gavioli and C. Wadensjö (eds.) *Routledge Handbook on Public Service Interpreting*. Abingdon: Routledge.

Plejert, C., Antelius, E., Yazdanpanah, M. and Nielsen, T. R. (2015) '"There's a letter called ef." On challenges and repair in interpreter-mediated tests of cognitive functioning in dementia evaluations: A case study.' *Journal of Cross-Cultural Gerontology* 30: 163–187.

Raymond, W. C. (2014) 'Conveying information in the interpreter-mediated medical visit: The case of epistemic brokering.' *Patient Education & Counselling*, 97: 38–46.

Small, J., Chan, S. M., Drance, E., Globerman, J., Hulko, W., O'Connor, D., Perry, J., Stern, L. and Ho, L. (2015) 'Verbal and non-verbal indicators of quality of communication between care staff and residents in ethnoculturally and linguistically diverse long-term care settings.' *Journal of Cross-Cultural Gerontology*, 30: 285–304. https://doi.org/10.1007/s10823-015-9269-6.

Söderman, M. and Rosendahl, S. P. (2016) 'Caring for ethnic older people living with dementia: Experiences of nursing staff.' *Journal of Cross-Cultural Gerontology*, 31(3): 311–326.

Torkpoor, R., Fioretos, I., Essén, B. and Londos, E. (2022) 'I know hyena. Do you know hyena? Challenges in interpreter-mediated dementia assessments, focusing on the role of the interpreter.' *Journal of Cross-Cultural Gerontology*, 37: 45–67.

Van De Mieroop, D., Bevilacqua, G. and Van Hove, L. (2012) 'Negotiating discursive norms: Community interpreting in a Belgian rest home.' *Interpreting*, 14(1): 23–54.

Wadensjö, C. (1998) *Interpreting as Interaction*. London: Longman.

Wilkinson, R. (2007) 'Managing linguistic incompetence as a delicate issue in aphasic talk-in-interaction: On the use of laughter in prolonged repair sequences.' *Journal of Pragmatics*, 39(3): 542–569.

Yildiz, K., Aki, O. E., Can, U. A., Derle, E., Kibaroglu, S. and Barak, A. (2014) 'Validation of Montreal Cognitive Assessment and discriminant power of Montreal Cognitive Assessment subtests in patients with mild cognitive impairment and Alzheimer dementia in Turkish population.' *Journal of Geriatric Psychiatry and Neurology*, 27(2): 103–109.

Part 3

Dementia and Conversational Strategies

5 Using "Now What" to Discursively Compensate for Frontotemporal Dementia-related Challenges: A Longitudinal Case Study

Lisa Mikesell

5.1 Introduction

While it is accepted that individuals diagnosed with neurological impairments such as dementia have less reliable access to the same communicative and cognitive resources as individuals who are not living with dementia, it has also been recognized that "deviation from what is normal does not necessarily equate with failure or communicative ineffectiveness" (Perkins et al., 1998: 37). Accordingly, naturalistic discourse and conversation analytic studies examining the interactional achievements of individuals diagnosed with dementia have been increasingly of interest: Documenting the embodied and situated nature of collaborative human action has offered insights not only about disease-related deficits but also preserved competencies and emerging strategies individuals develop in the face of challenges they likely did not experience before disease onset (see Dooley et al., 2015; Kindell et al., 2017).

Using Conversation Analysis (CA), supplemented with ethnographic data, this chapter examines a single discourse practice – the use of the phrase "now what" – recurrently employed by an individual with the pseudonym Robert (age 63) who was diagnosed with behavioral variant frontotemporal dementia (bvFTD). As Majlesi and Ekström (2016) discuss, when a practice produced by one individual is examined in its situated context, it becomes evident that the practice is not simply produced by a single individual but also arises from the context itself. That is, one's abilities are not only "dependent on individual resources, but contingent on contextual properties" (p. 39). While "now what" is certainly not produced in a vacuum, its recurrent use helps illuminate challenges Robert is facing that are likely dementia-related (though with the data drawn upon, one cannot know this with certainty). Indeed, his use of "now what" seems to be compensatory, assisting him in navigating around particular kinds of cognitive and communicative difficulties. Moreover, the situated and sequentially sensitive examination of "now what" that CA affords allows one to more readily grasp the analytic difficulty of identifying a practice like "now what" as indicative of *either* "deficit" *or* "skill," and I will consider how Robert's use of "now what" is essentially a marker of both.

5.2 Recruiting Assistance from Others: "Atypical" Practices as Compensatory

The larger study from which these data stem followed five families, each with a member diagnosed with bvFTD. Across the data, the phrase "now what" is recurrently observed only in the interactions involving Robert and thus appears to be idiosyncratic to him. I investigated this particular usage because I was interested in discursive practices individuals systematically employed to navigate various challenges that they regularly confront. "Now what" appears to be a compensatory practice that enables Robert to actively draw on his collaborators as resources to participate appropriately in tasks and activities. As Kendrick and Drew (2016) discuss, recruiting others to help resolve troubles is ubiquitous in human interaction and interlocutors deploy both linguistic and embodied practices to achieve this, from direct requests to "subsidiary actions" that "publicly expose troubles and thereby create opportunities for others to assist" (p. 1). For Robert, such a wide array of recruitment resources may not consistently and readily be available, but "now what" effectively calls on his collaborators to identify and articulate the next step of an activity for which Robert requires clarification, and this collaborative assistance often comes in the form of directives. Thus, "now what" provides a powerful resource for Robert to navigate difficulties that likely reflect executive cognitive limitations associated with frontal lobe functioning (Alvarez & Emory, 2006; Torralva et al., 2009; see also Mikesell, 2014) so that he can more appropriately contribute to daily tasks.

A growing body of work explores how collaboration and coordination are achieved to carry out joint activities that involve individuals living with dementia (Hydén, 2014; Majlesi & Ekström, 2016; Mikesell, 2016). Collectively, this work shows the importance of collaborator-initiated instructions to direct the engagement of the individual diagnosed with dementia for the achievement of everyday activities. However, individuals living with dementia are not entirely dependent on others; they also actively draw on the sequential organization of activities and other resources to competently participate (Majlesi & Ekström, 2016). This chapter contributes to this body of work that examines coordinated engagement involving individuals living with dementia by showing how Robert strategically makes use of the phrase "now what" to solicit instruction from his collaborators.

Identifying how Robert uses "now what" to recruit assistance provides a lens with which to consider preserved competencies as well as disease-related deficits. His reliance on "now what" to do the work of recruiting assistance shows his resourcefulness in managing his participation and ability to recognize that his participation is required, while also revealing the broader sociocognitive challenges "now what" addresses, namely that he is not always able to identify the required steps to navigate multi-step activities (see Mikesell, 2014). To afford a better lens on the compensatory nature of "now what," I tracked its use over a year as Robert's dementia progressed. Initially, Robert deploys a range of recruitment practices to solicit help from others. However, over time he more regularly makes use of "now what," a presumably more readily available linguistic resource, to solicit help when facing trouble. Although over time "now what" maintains this function of recruiting others to help navigate well-defined tasks, Robert also begins to employ this same resource to navigate non-task-based activities, showing how this compensatory strategy extends in usage as he faces new challenges that he may lack resources to effectively address. Overall, as "now what" is extended to non-task-based contexts, its interactional import appears less well-suited to these moments, and it is often less effective at recruiting assistance from interlocutors who tend not to respond to "now what" when it is employed in such sequences.

In sum, this chapter details the sequential contexts in which "now what" is employed to explore the challenges that Robert works to navigate and consider how "now what" affords Robert a resource to actively participate. Additionally, a longitudinal view of this practice shows how its use varies over time as Robert's disease progresses and as his situational and activity contexts change. I show how this practice serves as a resource, assisting Robert in discursively managing evolving challenges (many of which appear to be dementia-related), and may also serve as a potential observable marker of his disease progression. This idiosyncratic use of "now what" reveals Robert's capacity to recognize when and in what ways he requires help *and* also reflects a certain level of impairment, suggesting that a dichotomous framing of atypical behavior – as *either* a deficit *or* skill, as *either* functional *or* nonsensical – may be an oversimplified approach.

5.3 Behavioral Variant Frontotemporal Dementia: Naturalistic and Longitudinal Explorations

The young onset (<65 years) neurodegenerative disorder bvFTD targets the frontal and/or temporal lobes and is characterized by changes in personality and social and emotional behavior (Mendez et al., 2014) including interpersonal and personal conduct (Kipps et al., 2007). Presenting clinical features include social disengagement, disinhibition, apathy, compulsive behaviors, and loss of social tact and social emotions for others (Desmarais et al., 2018; Roscovsky et al., 2011; Shany-Ur & Rankin, 2011). Because "loss of insight" is also common to bvFTD (O'Keefe et al., 2007), much of what is known about sociobehavioral changes associated with bvFTD stems from second-hand reports of caregivers, which may highlight especially problematic experiences and gloss behaviors at a gross level (Mikesell, 2010a), and from structured assessments in clinic settings, which "may omit, minimize, control or overlook typical bvFTD behaviors" (Mendez et al., 2014: 219). As such, "the natural course of bvFTD is less well known" than for other dementias such as Alzheimer's disease (Diehl-Schmid et al., 2011: 231). As a result, there have been efforts to explore sociobehavioral changes in bvFTD from naturalistic vantage points including ethnographic observations, real-time behavioral coding, and discourse and conversation analysis (see Barsuglia et al., 2014; Guendouzi & Müller, 2006; Mates et al., 2010; Mendez et al., 2014).

Barsuglia et al. (2014), for instance, developed a coding system of naturalistic bvFTD behaviors as observed by researchers during ordinary activities. From transcribed fieldnotes, three "social themes" were identified: (1) diminished relational interest, (2) lack of social synchrony/intersubjectivity (for establishing/maintaining relationships),[1] and (3) poor awareness and adherence to social norms. The authors concluded that these themes, which categorize deficits, correspond to caregiver reports and formalized behavioral scales, arguing that this observational work validates the diagnostic criteria of bvFTD, which have been previously questioned (Roscovsky et al., 2011). These three thematic categories, however, constitute broader abstractions of the moment-by-moment behaviors and practices that field researchers observed and thus potentially capture quite diverse sorts of social and communicative behaviors that were categorized as qualitatively similar. Coding social behaviors at such a "thematic" level may wash out the interactional achievement or function of the observed behaviors.

Complementing these efforts are video-based studies using discourse and conversation analytic approaches. Such studies provide contextualized analyses of discrete interactional practices that illustrate the difficulty of identifying a single interactional practice or behavior as *either* a deficit *or* skill (see Mikesell, 2016, 2020; Mikesell & Bromley, 2016). For instance, Mikesell (2010b) examined repetitional responses of two individuals diagnosed with bvFTD, finding that these responses were not echolalic in form (a previous diagnostic criterion; Neary et al., 1998) and were systematically employed, similar to neurotypicals (Stivers, 2005), to communicate resistance to caregivers' infantile directives concerning everyday functioning (e.g., directives to take pills with liquid). Importantly, however, these forms were also employed when diagnosed individuals were demonstrably not engaged in the normative practices for carrying out tasks (e.g., putting a pill in one's mouth without any liquid), showing that caregivers' "infantile" directives were responsive to how the individual in their care engaged in everyday tasks that they were carefully

---

[1] This included observations of abnormal social responses and impoverished verbal content.

monitoring. A CA-informed approach thus demonstrated how these forms were not random or nonsensical (which is how echolalia is defined); they were systematically employed to counter assumptions about one's lack of capacity. However, these forms simultaneously pointed to possible challenges individuals had in recognizing their own shortcomings in managing daily tasks.

There is also developing interest in longitudinal work to document disease progression. Much of this work utilizes formal assessment measures of cognitive behavior. For instance, Diehl et al. (2011) examined cognitive decline measured by the CERAD-NAB over a 13-month period and found that cognitive changes in a homogenously defined group of patients were "very heterogeneous" (p. 230) and progressed *non-linearly* over time (see Diehl et al., 2005). This heterogeneity was also demonstrated in changes in behavior. While the authors acknowledge that this might in part be due to the small sample size, they concluded that these findings likely reflect that bvFTD is "very heterogeneous regarding symptom profile and disease course" (Diehl et al., 2011: 235), another reason why case studies may be particularly useful.

Longitudinal case studies, such as the one presented here, are of course limited in scope and generalizability; nevertheless, they provide a window into the natural course of bvFTD. Such work may provide insights about how social engagement and interactional practices progress over time and how families navigate them. Additionally, using CA to carefully examine the sequentially situated, moment-by-moment production of social practices and behaviors provides a nuanced lens into the functionality of a particular practice, and thus allows us to see how it may both constitute a dementia-related challenge and simultaneously demonstrate an individual's skill and resourcefulness. Although researchers are often quick to identify behaviors as problematic, the fact that a single practice can demonstrate both deficit and skill suggests that we need to be especially careful in how we label and categorize, a process to which CA can significantly contribute.

5.4 Methods

The video data stem from an ethnographic study of five families whose length of participation ranged from between three months and two years. The data include ethnographic observations with corresponding fieldnotes from five researchers and video recordings of everyday events including mealtimes, common routines such as running errands, and a range of activities. Field researchers wrote down brief, bulleted observations during visits when feasible, which they elaborated into fieldnotes immediately after visits to share with the research team. Fieldnotes often described activities and interactions from the vantage point of the researcher, detailed the personal and emotional perspective of the researcher, identified observed challenges families and individuals faced and how they navigated these challenges, and often included references to common understandings of bvFTD as described in the literature.

As mentioned, this chapter focuses on Robert (age 63) who was diagnosed with bvFTD approximately two years prior to the collection of the data. Robert and his wife, Juliet, participated in the study for one year (November 20, 2006 until November 30, 2007) before they moved across country to be near family. The same researcher (identified as "ET" in the transcripts) regularly visited Robert and Juliet throughout the year and then again in March 2008 after their move. The study was approved by University of California, Los Angeles IRB.

This chapter draws heavily on CA to analyze Robert's *in situ* uses of "now what." CA provides a discursive lens with which to analyze both the composition of Robert's "now what", such as how its semantic meaning and turn design may contribute to its functional deployment in a particular activity or conversational turn, as well as its sequential positioning, that is, what "now what" is produced in response to and how it, in turn, is responded to. Recognizing the broader activity and sequential positioning is important for understanding what this (or any) practice achieves interactionally. Only by coming to terms with a practice's interactional achievement can we begin to understand what the recurring use of a phrase like "now what" demonstrates about Robert's interactional competencies and what it might reveal about the emerging difficulties Robert may be confronting (Erickson & Schultz, 1997). In addition to CA, I occasionally draw on ethnographic fieldnotes to complement the interactional analysis by reporting what the field researcher observed or experienced that helps contextualize Robert's challenges and how they were perceived.

5.5 Findings: The Evolving Interactional Work of "Now What"

I tracked Robert's use of "now what" from the first 62 minutes (the length of one tape) of video-recorded interactions from eight visits taking place between November 2006 and November 2007[2] (Table 5.1). The eight visits were selected to provide a window into the family's interactions in roughly equal intervals of time covering ET's second visit through her nineteenth visit. Perfect equal time intervals were not always possible; for example, there were no visits made in April, June, or July 2007.

Table 5.1 presents the larger activity contexts of those first 62 minutes of recorded interactions, which included preparing meals, a minor conflict between Juliet and Robert, purchasing items at the pharmacy, and watching television.

---

[2] I participated in this study as a field researcher and I visited Robert and Juliet on one occasion with ET.

Table 5.1 *Frequency of "now what" across eight 62-minute intervals*

Visit#	2	7	10	13[1]	14	16[3]	17	19
Date	21 Nov. 2006	17 Jan. 2007	15 Feb. 2007	15 Mar. 2007	4 May 2007	22 Aug. 2007	6 Sept. 2007	30 Nov. 2007
Uses	0	1	6	0	5	0	5	0
Activity Contexts	Rob making breakfast; seeks assistance	Running errands; Waiting in line at pharmacy to pay	Juliet reprimanding Rob; Rob making lunch with ET	Rob & ET watching TV	Setting table for dinner	Rob & ET watching TV	Making lunch	Conversation between ET and Juliet; Rob is co-present

[1]During Visits 13 and 16 Robert was not involved in any recorded activities and rarely engaged in conversation. He spent most of the hour watching television.

The table also includes the number of times Robert produced "now what" during those interactions. The data analysis that follows presents the excerpts in temporal sequence (i.e., in the time order in which they occurred).

As mentioned, Robert's practices for soliciting assistance and his use of "now what" evolve over time. During early visits, Robert seeks assistance to complete tasks, but he notably does not draw on "now what" to solicit help, as he does in later visits. Rather, he verbalizes specific requests for help or describes the problem he is facing (e.g., Extract 1, line 1). Over time his use of direct requests and problem descriptions to solicit assistance diminishes, and in later visits he employs "now what" to achieve similar interactional work. Initially, Robert employs "now what" to elicit verbal assistance from his interlocutor in the form of instructions when he is asked to accomplish specific, well-defined tasks. As an interactional resource, "now what" thus draws on a basic positional "device" of natural interaction that CA has described in some detail: the workings of adjacency pairs (Schegloff 2007; Schegloff & Sacks 1973). Paired actions are a fundamental organizational unit of natural interaction whereby an interlocutor launches an initiating action – a first-pair part (FPP) – and the receiver provides a responsive action – a second-pair part (SPP). "Now what" provides Robert a readily available and "generic" FPP that creates a sequential context that makes conditionally relevant (Schegloff 1968) an SPP that provides the subsequent required step that a current activity requires.

Over time, Robert's use of "now what" continues to evolve, as he extends its use not only to when he is facing challenges completing the next steps of an activity, but also to situations in which he faces interactional difficulty outside of well-defined tasks, such as when he is reprimanded by his wife (e.g., Extract 4). Later in the year, his productions of "now what" extend even further when they are not obviously directed to a particular interlocutor but come off as self-talk and occur in moments of seeming frustration or restlessness. Thus, throughout the year Robert consistently draws on "now what" to recruit assistance, but his later uses extend to non-task-based activities that seem less well-fitted to the interactional contexts in which they are produced.

5.5.1   Visit 2: November 21, 2006: Describing a Problem to Recruit Assistance during a Routine Activity

Extract 1 occurs early in the year and shows how Robert handles a problem he encounters when making breakfast (a routine activity) and how he recruits assistance to solve it. Here, he solicits assistance by describing the problem he is facing to his collaborator (ET) when he cannot find the colander for the blueberries. Before Extract 1, Juliet tasks Robert with making breakfast with ET's help so she can finish some work. Juliet tells him to "try to follow what

5 Using "Now What" 111

she (ET) says," displaying her understanding that Robert is likely to need guidance (not shown). Robert begins preparing fruit and quickly runs into a problem when he cannot find the colander. After searching for it, he eventually solicits help from ET by describing the problem he is facing (line 1) – "I don' see the thing for the blueberries."

Extract 1 – RO=Robert; ET=researcher
```
01   RO:   I don' see the thing for the blueberries.
02   ro    (9.1) looking in cupboards
03   ET:   No blueberries?
04   ro    (5.2) opens fridge, gets blueberries
05   RO:   .hh No(h) (I) got blueberries.
06         (2.6)
07   ET:   (But) I don't (.) see the thing for them.
08   RO:   What's the thing for them look like.
09         (0.4)
10   RO:   It's the) red thing.
11         (3.2)
12   ro    clears throat
13         (2.7)
14   RO:   (I-/W' l)
15         (0.4)
16   RO:   (I) don' see it.
17   ro    looking in cupboards; pacing kitchen
```

Although Robert's problem description contains an imprecise referent – he refers to the colander as "the thing" – his FPP makes evident that he has identified a specific obstacle to completing the activity. After observing Robert search the cupboards (line 2), ET works to clarify the problem (lines 3–10). ET's "no blueberries?" may be hearable as repair on his problem description. Robert responds by retrieving the blueberries from the refrigerator (line 4), thereby demonstrating to ET that this is not the problem he is facing. He also rejects the implication in ET's turn that there might not be blueberries (with turn-initial "no") and verbally confirms that he has them. He then repeats the description of the problem (line 7), retaining the vague referent – "thing" – for the colander that he cannot locate. ET works to clarify what "thing" means (line 8), which Robert describes a bit more precisely as "the red thing." As a newcomer to the home without shared knowledge, ET is unable to offer adequate assistance and Robert eventually seeks assistance from Juliet, which he does in much the same way, by describing to Juliet the problem he is facing ("I can't find the thing for the blueberries").

During these early visits, when Robert is tasked with a routine activity, he independently identifies the appropriate steps. That is, he does not seek assistance or need to be told what items are required or what order the steps should follow (compare Extract 3). When he does run into trouble, Robert troubleshoots first on his own, working to resolve the problem. For instance, in

Extract 1 he searches the cupboards, and when his efforts are unsuccessful, he solicits help by identifying the nature of the trouble he has run into, in this case by describing the problem to his collaborator. Although he demonstrates difficulty clarifying what the "thing" is that he cannot find, he shows resourcefulness in problem solving, recruiting assistance, and working to repair misunderstanding.

5.5.2 Visit 7: January 17, 2007: Using "Now What" to Seek Clarification about a Nonroutine Task

The following extract takes place about two months later and constitutes the first observed use of "now what" to solicit assistance. Here, "now what" seems to be employed to help orient to the purpose of a vaguely defined and nonroutinized task that Juliet has instructed him to do – "stand there" – while they are in the pharmacy picking up prescriptions.

Extract 2 – RO=Robert; JU=Juliet
```
01   JU:   Can you stand there? I'm gonna sit for a moment.
02   ju    sighs, sits down
03   ro    (0.9) standing in line; turns to look at JU
04   RO:   Now what.
05         (1.6)
06   JU:   Just wait our tu:rn.
07   ro    returns to facing front
08   JU:   We're waiting our turn.
09         (3.2)
10   RO:   (You) wan' me to use the credit card?
11   ro    (0.5) wallet is in hand
12   JU:   Yeah.
13   ro    opens wallet
14   JU:   [>Ya don' need to bring it out yet,<Rob=
```

As Robert and Juliet approach the line to pay, Juliet asks Robert to stand in line so she can sit in a nearby chair (line 1). After standing in line for nearly a second (line 3), Robert turns to Juliet and asks "now what" (line 4), an FPP that provides the sequential context for Juliet to articulate the (next) action he is to attend to. Juliet responds by directing him to "just wait our tu:rn." (line 6) and then draws on the present progressive tense to orient him to the immediate task at hand, suggesting that this is what he should be attending to for now: "we're waiting our turn" (line 8). This first observed use of "now what" thus allows Robert to point to a possible problem orienting to the current activity and also works to solicit a response from Juliet that provides clarification about the nature of the task he is engaged in.

Notably waiting in line is not an activity that Robert is often asked to perform and it is in a context outside of the home, which may be less familiar or routinized. Juliet asks him to stand, perhaps the simplest task Robert is

5 Using "Now What"

charged with in the eight hours of data examined. It is also a task without a clearly defined next step or endpoint. Robert's "now what" may thus orient, not to the complexity or multi-step nature of the task, but to its vagueness or indefiniteness. While in Extract 1 Robert's description of the trouble demonstrates his ability to independently identify the next steps required of a larger activity and solicit help in accomplishing this next step, here his use of "now what" seems to orient to a less precise understanding of the activity he is to be completing and serves as a resource to solicit specific instructions to resolve his uncertainty. Once Juliet orients him to the task he is attending to – "waiting our turn" (line 8) – he demonstrates both understanding of the larger project that standing/waiting in line is in service to and his ability to identify a likely next step to accomplish that larger project when he asks Juliet if she wants him to use the credit card (line 10) (see Mikesell, 2016).

5.5.3 Visit 10: February 15, 2007: Using "Now What" to Solicit Direct Instructions during a Routine Activity

Robert's use of "now what" becomes more commonplace over the next couple of months. In ET's fieldnotes, she first mentions Robert's use of "now what" after her eighth visit (January 24, 2007), three weeks before Extract 3 (Visit 10; February 15, 2007), when she writes: "Robert was always asking this question. He kept wanting to know what was next." During Visit 10, Robert employs "now what" six times in one hour. Both the increasing frequency of use and the sequential contexts in which "now what" is used suggest that he may be facing more difficulty independently accomplishing even routine activities. Additionally, while the first observed use of "now what" (shown in Extract 2) seemed to function as a generic request for clarification when the task was vague or unclear, in Extract 3 "now what" works to elicit specific instructions from interlocutors that precisely explicate the next steps of a multi-step activity that he seems unable to identify on his own. In other words, his use of "now what" similarly recruits others to provide assistance, but that assistance now takes the form of precisely articulating his required next actions so that he can perform them. Here, he is tasked with making sandwiches for lunch, and, after yelling to Juliet who is on the phone in another room, ET offers her help and directs him to complete the first step to make the sandwich. Following this sequence, Robert produces "now what," which prompts ET to produce a series of directives, one following the other, to guide Robert through the activity.

Extract 3 – RO=Robert; JU=Juliet; ET=researcher
((Juliet asks ET to help Robert make sandwiches))
```
01    JU:    Can you sorta guide him on it, because I often.
02           have to guide him on it
```

```
03    ju     answers phone
04    ET:    Yea yea.
05           lines omitted; JU in office
06    RO:    Ju::les!
07    ET:    W- what kinda help do you nee:d.
08    ?      ( )
09    RO:    I need- I need her help.
10    ET:    W' l she's busy right now.<Can I help?<I think (that looks)
11                 |(0.5)
12    ro     |inspecting sandwich
13    ET:    Okay, you can have one mo:re. (referring to lunch meat)
14    ro     puts lunch meat on sandwich
15    ET:    Good.
16    RO:    **Now what.**
17    ET:    How 'bout some lettuce and tomata.
18           ((lines omitted; RO gets lettuce and tomato;
19           ET and RO take sandwich to JU who asks for
20           less tomato, more lettuce, and fruit))
21    ET:    °Okay let's put that on the plate over the:re.
22    RO:    Okay.
23    et     follows RO as he walks across kitchen; leans
24           over to watch RO plate tomatoes
25    et     steps back
26    ET:    Okay. An' then- an' then what e- what else did
27           she want=did she want b- lettuce?
28    RO:    Uh (0.2) I don' know.
29    ET:    She wanted one more big piece of lettuce so
30           give her another piece of lettuce.
31    et     steps back, watches RO get more lettuce
32    ro     (9.0) puts lettuce on sandwich
33    ET:    °What 'bout for the other side?
34    ro     (gets more lettuce
35    RO:    Oh uh: ( )
36           (3.2)
37    ET:    Okay,
38    RO:    **Now what.**
39    ET:    And then she said she wanted some kind of fruit.
40           <d' you remember what kind of fruit she wanted?=
41    RO:    =Yeah, an apple.
42    ET:    An apple.
43    ro     gets an apple
44    JU:    Can you sorta guide him on it, because I often.
```

Just before Extract 3, Juliet asks Robert to make sandwiches for lunch and asks ET if she "can help him do that." She explains how she wants her sandwich (not shown) to ET (via eye gaze and bodily orientation), but RO is gazing at Juliet during her explanation and is thus an observable overhearer. At the start of making lunch, Robert calls out to Juliet (line 6). ET attempts to intervene by asking what kind of help he needs (line 7), to which Robert describes somewhat vaguely that he "need[s] her help" (line 9). In response, ET offers help (line 10) and immediately begins to assess the sandwich verbally (lines 10, 11) while visually inspecting it (line 12). After her assessment, she provides instructions to add one more slice of lunchmeat (line 13). Robert follows ET's first instruction (line 14) and, after ET's positive assessment (line 15), Robert produces "now what" (line 16), which then prompts additional step-by-step instructions from ET. She first formulates her instructions as a suggestion to add lettuce and tomato (line 17), possible next steps of sandwich construction, and later produces known-answer questions (lines 26–27, 39–40) to prompt Robert to recall Juliet's preferences as she had earlier described.

Although during ET's early visits Robert independently initiates the steps for making meals, over time he elicits instructions from interlocutors with his use of "now what." Additionally, interlocutors begin to pre-empt next steps by providing instructions even when unsolicited. For instance, in Extract 3 Robert indicates that he needs help and ET offers her own. As soon as that initial help is offered, Robert then recruits ET's assistance again with "now what." From then on, ET prompts Robert at nearly every next step, one after the other, even before Robert has an opportunity to recruit her assistance (see Majlesi & Ekström, 2016): She tells him where to put the plate on the counter to ensure there is enough counter space (line 21), monitors his cutting and plating (lines 23–24), and instructs him about what items to put on Juliet's sandwich (e.g., lines 29–30). As compared to Extract 1, Robert initiates less of the meal assembly independently, in part because his adoption of "now what" as a recruitment device is particularly effective in prompting collaborators to guide him in a step-by-step fashion.

5.5.4 Visit 10: February 15, 2007: Using "Now What" to Exit Interactionally Delicate Moments

Although Robert's uses of "now what" most frequently recruit assistance (and most often in the form of specific instructions), it is around the time of Visit 10 that its use seems to broaden in scope: In addition to task- or activity-based interactions where "now what" solicits specific instructions, he now also employs "now what" in interactions that are interactionally sensitive and emotionally charged. In Extract 4.1, Juliet animatedly reprimands Robert for several minutes, which ET describes in fieldnotes as "totally flip[ing] out," because he turned off her television recordings. Although Robert aligns with Juliet's directives to not touch the television and apologizes on several occasions, his contributions generally go unacknowledged by Juliet who continues reprimanding him. Perhaps because his acknowledgements and apologies are ineffective in closing this delicate sequence, Robert produces "now what," presumably in an attempt to shift away from the current interactional sequence by recruiting Juliet to launch a next action.

Extract 4.1 – RO=Robert; JU=Juliet

```
01   JU:    Rob. Yur- drivin me nuts, Rob.
02          I told you not to touch tha:t.
03          .hh I told you not >to touch it in any way shape
04          or fo:rm=.hh that you weren to touch it today at
05          a::ll.
06   RO:    Oka:[y.
07   JU:        [R↑o::b yu- you[ca:nt (keep)      ] touchin' it.
08   RO:                       [I'm so::rry Jules.]
09   RO:    I'm sorry I'm SOrry. I'm SORRY.
10   JU:    Rob, I have programs I've- I- I- did last nigh:-
11          that I taped last nigh:t,
12          (29 seconds omitted – Juliet continues reprimanding)
13   JU:    You are not allowed to touch this. At a:ll.
14   JU:    Anytime. Anyway.
15   JU:    You're not allowed to touch it.
16   RO:    Okay. Now what.
17   ro/ju  (3.6) looking at television
18   JU:    Gahh(d).hh
19          (0.2)
20   JU:    I'm sta- I'm supposed to be at work.
21          She thinks I'm doing something right no:w.
22   RO:    Whatur you doin'.
23   ju     (4.4) ((attending to television))
24   JU:    I'm- I'm- I'm f:- I'm putting it so that I don't mi:ss
25          all the stuff I taped last night.
26   RO:    .hh hah
27   ro     crosses legs and looks on
```

Juliet launched her reprimand about 13 seconds before line 1 in which she articulates her frustration with Robert. She then explicates the source of her frustration (lines 2–5), reminding him that he was told not to touch the television (because Juliet was recording). Although Robert acknowledges her reprimand with "okay" (line 6), Juliet continues, producing a directive to not touch the television (line 7). Robert apologizes once in overlap with her directive (line 8) and then says "I'm sorry" three more times in the clear, with each production getting louder and more forceful (line 9). Juliet does not acknowledge his apologies but continues explaining the difficulty that his actions have caused her (lines 10–11), which continues for about 29 seconds (not shown). Juliet then produces a series of emphatic directives banning Robert from touching the television (lines 13–15), which Robert accepts with "okay." He then produces "now what" (line 16). Juliet does not respond to his "now what" but remains focused on the television with remote in hand (line 17). She then continues with her reprimand by remarking on what she should be doing instead, highlighting the negative consequences of Robert's actions (lines 20–21).

The sequential context of "now what" in line 16 is notably different than the contexts previously examined: It is not produced when Robert is engaged in

5 Using "Now What" 117

accomplishing a task-based activity and needs assistance. Rather, it is used in an interactionally sensitive moment when Juliet is demonstrably upset with him. The prior task-based uses of "now what" tend to prompt his interlocutor to articulate the next step of an activity, and thus work to progress the activity-in-progress. Its use here may be an attempt to achieve the opposite, that is to *not* progress the current engagement underway, but to shift focus away from it. Whereas FPP "now what" in well-defined activity contexts works to elicit instructions that move the activity forward, here it can set up a sequential context that provides Juliet the opportunity to move away from the current interactionally sensitive sequence. Importantly, Robert does not produce "now what" immediately following Juliet's first reprimand to "not touch it." Rather, he draws on other resources to engage in this interactional moment by acknowledging/aligning with her reprimands and apologizing. Only upon not receiving any uptake does he work to shift the conversation to what might be a next, perhaps less emotionally charged direction with "now what."

Moments later, Juliet continues with her admonishment with explicit directives (Extract 4.2, lines 25–26, 29, 31–32, 35) and Robert continues to acknowledge them (lines 27–28, 31, 33–34, 37). Again, Juliet provides no recognition of his acknowledgements but continues with her reprimand, giving him further instructions to not touch the television. Following Juliet's exasperated "Gahwhd" (line 39), Robert produces "now what" (line 40), which he repeats two more times after gaps of silence (line 41 ff.) in which Juliet continues to attend to fixing Robert's error.

Extract 4.2 – RO=Robert; JU=Juliet
```
27  JU:  Rob you cannot touch this.
28  JU:  You'[re not allowed to touch this EVer.=
29  RO:      [Okay.
30  RO:  Okay.
31  JU:  EVer. For Any reason.
32  RO:  Okay =[okA:Y.          ]
33  JU:         [<if you think] you have to touch it, you have to
34       come git me.
35  RO:  O[kay.]
36  JU:   [Okay?]
37  JU:  You can't do it.
38  ju   (0.8) attending to television
39  JU:  °Gahwhd
40  RO:  Now what.
41  ju   (5.0) attending to television
42  RO:  Now what.
43  ju   (2.5) attending to television
44  RO:  Now what.
45  ju   (0.8) attending to television
46  JU:  I shouldn't even be doin' this.
47       (2.0)
```

These "extensions" in use outside of well-defined tasks may show how this practice is now not only being employed to solicit assistance to complete a multi-step activity but also works to close a current interactional sequence by attempting to shift the interactional focus away from sensitive moments that are challenging to exit. Notably, in this emotionally charged moment Juliet does not respond to Robert's "now whats" or allow them to derail her from her reprimand, just as she does not respond to his apologies. That Juliet maintains focus on her reprimand may put demands on Robert, during an already taxing situation, to figure a way out of this sequence when his brief acknowledgements and apologies fail to do so. However, he may not have a readily available repertoire of interactional resources to draw on for effectively navigating this interaction and relies on "now what" to encourage a topic shift. In this way, Juliet's lack of response contributes to his repeated uses of "now what" as a (failed) exit strategy.

5.5.5 Visit 17: September 6, 2007: "Now What" as Self-Talk

By September (seven months later) Robert is still employing "now what" to solicit assistance to navigate multi-step activities, although he is now asked to complete very few tasks and mostly routine ones. As a consequence, his use of "now what" in activity contexts is less frequent, but his use of "now what" in non-activity contexts (Extract 5), particularly when he appears distressed, anxious, or bored is more prevalent. During Visit 17, four of the five uses occurred in the context of watching television and did not appear to be directed toward an interlocutor, and as such they come off as self-talk.

Extract 5 – RO=Robert; JU=Juliet; ET=researcher
```
01    JU:     Ro:b, I'm gonna get you something-<a little something<I'll
02            get you a little dessert.
03            (0.3)
04    JU:     How's that.
05            |(   ?   )
06    ju      |leaves room
07    ET:     Have you had enough water? Toda:y?
08    RO:     Yea.
09    ro      sips from water glass in front of him
10    ro      (30.0) watching TV; shaking foot, fidgets with hands
11    RO:     |Now what. Now what ( ).
12    ro      |looking toward television
13            (0.5)
14    ro      (0.3) stands up, |starts walking out of living room
15    ET:                      |Whaddaya want.
16    RO:     I want chips.
17    ET:     She's gettin you dessert. You wanna sit do:wn? <She's
18            gonna come back with it.
```

5 Using "Now What"

```
19  ro      (29.0) sits down, resumes TV watching
20  RO:     |Now what.
21  ro      |looking toward kitchen
22  et      looks toward kitchen, resumes TV watching
23          (0.9)
24  RO:     |Now what          ( Liff  |y ).
25  ro      |looking toward kitchen |looking toward TV
26  ro/et   (32.1) watching TV
27  JU:     ET do you think you can take him for a wa:lk? ((from
28          off camera))
29  ET:     Yea: sure.
```

While watching television, Juliet gets up to get Robert dessert (lines 1–6). Following a brief exchange between Robert and ET (lines 7–8), they resume watching television. He appears visibly restless (a commonly reported bvFTD symptom), shaking his foot (line 10), and fidgeting with his fingers without any observable purpose before he produces two "now whats" (line 11), which ET does not immediately respond to. He quickly stands up and starts to head towards the kitchen (line 14), which prompts ET to ask what he wants (line 15). When he says he wants chips (line 16), ET reminds him that Juliet is bringing him dessert and directs him to sit down (lines 17). They resume watching television and he continues to fidget. Shortly after, he produces "now what" again (line 20) while redirecting his gaze from the television toward the kitchen (Juliet is off camera so it is possible that she has come into Robert's line of sight). Shortly after, Robert produces "now what" again (line 24), as he shifts his gaze from the kitchen back to the television. ET does not respond but maintains her attention toward the television and they both continue watching until Juliet returns with dessert.

Although Robert's employment of "now what" retains its function of eliciting assistance, it now is also employed during very different sorts of challenges such as when Robert displays difficulty sitting still and when there is no apparent well-defined task to attend to. Notably, ET here does not as readily respond to his "now what" FPPs. Such extended uses may provide less clear constraints on what constitutes a conditionally relevant SPP for collaborators. For instance, when watching television there is not a clearly identifiable and precise next step to direct Robert to attend to. It should also be noted that as early as February 2007, ET observed Robert's use of "now what" when he appeared restless and perseverates on a particular repetitive behavior. Following the incident when Juliet bans Robert from touching the television, ET writes:

[A]fter being banned from TV at the end of the day, he and I got in this cycle of him asking me to turn on the TV, I turning it on, and him asking me to turn it off, and I turning it off and then him asking me to turn on the TV and so on. This was REALLY annoying ... He was agitated and cursing, unable to explain why we were in a loop.

At one point, I finally said, "If I turn it off, I'm not turning it on again." And he said OK, turn it off. I asked if he was stressed out because he seemed like he was. And he kept asking me, "Now what?" As if I knew!

According to ET, following Robert's television ban, he entered into a repetitive "loop" of turning the television on and off but recruited ET's assistance to achieve these ends. Perhaps when feeling agitated or restless, "now what" similarly worked to shift focus in the absence of an immediate task to attend to.

Although Robert's use of "now what" in Extract 5 and during Juliet's reprimand are notably different (e.g., here it is not directed toward an interlocutor), for both kinds of trouble these extensions in use of "now what" may work to establish a (new) focus, demonstrating the versatility and resourcefulness of employing such a practice to recruit others when facing a variety of difficulties. Notably, in these non-task focused contexts, where precise directives may not be immediately relevant, interlocutors verbally respond less frequently to "now what" and even experience it with frustration (as evidenced in fieldnotes), perhaps because there is no obvious relevant response when the interactional outcome is unclear. Thus, these uses of "now what" seem less well-suited to achieving the topical shifts that might redirect either Robert's interlocutor's (as in the case of Juliet's reprimand) or his own attention.

By the end of the year Juliet has made plans to relocate to be near family. As she explains it to ET, she needs help because Robert is causing her extra work, which makes her feel both upset and guilty. She tells ET that Robert is no longer helping with routine activities such as meal preparation and can no longer follow simple instructions. For example, when she asks him to hand her an item, he may hand her something "not anywhere near it." During the last visit, Robert engages very little outside of responding to questions and is not asked to complete any tasks. He also never produces "now what" or seeks assistance.

5.6   Discussion

Recruiting assistance from others is not only ubiquitous in ordinary interactions (see Kendrick & Drew, 2016) but also in interactions involving individuals with dementia (see Hydén, 2014; Majlesi & Ekström, 2016). This chapter tracked Robert's uses of "now what" over the course of a year and thus provided a lens with which to view how Robert works to navigate various activity-based challenges, drawing on a single linguistic resource that works to recruit others' assistance by making conditionally relevant explicit instructions that articulate the next step of multi-step activities. Additionally, I have highlighted how, over time, Robert draws on this same resource to navigate difficulties that are observably not activity based, but nevertheless provide him a seemingly accessible strategy to recruit others' assistance to address other kinds of delicate moments that co-opt the semantic meaning of "now what" as a general strategy for sequentially organizing a potential shift in attentional focus away from the current engagement.

5.6.1 Thinking Longitudinally

Given that bvFTD is neurodegenerative, this longitudinal perspective contributes to our understanding of manifestations of the disease. As "now what" was predominantly used over the year to solicit assistance in task-based activities, the narrow focus on this one phrase provides insights into how Robert's engagement in activities evolved over time, changes which are likely due to both Robert's individually experienced difficulties participating in multi-step activities as well as his collaborators' perceptions of his difficulties. Notably, Robert's involvement in activities and responsibilities at home diminished over the year. Early on, Robert recruits assistance, but he independently initiates steps to accomplish tasks, identifies specific sources of trouble, and troubleshoots without being prompted to do so. For instance, during Visit 2 (November 21, 2006), Robert contributes to making breakfast, completing each step independently, and when he occasionally runs into trouble, he troubleshoots first on his own and eventually seeks help by describing the problem to ET.

In comparison, during Visit 17 (September 6, 2007), Juliet asks ET to help him make lunch and ET articulates each step for Robert to follow; he is not required to initiate the steps or identify points of trouble since the guidance is quite extensive and often pre-emptive. Pre-empting his needs and producing successive directives may have been an evolved strategy for Robert's familiar interlocutors. For instance, it was observed that when his interlocutors refrained from providing explicit instructions, Robert often asked "now what" to solicit instructions, sometimes even in more routinized activities.

Later in the year, many of his uses of "now what" are produced in moments of interactional difficulty (e.g., Juliet's reprimand in Extract 4) or demonstrable distress or restlessness (e.g., while watching television in Extract 5). Thus, while Robert's uses of "now what" retain some of their original functionality, they also reveal new kinds of challenges Robert seems to be facing. The analyses presented show how this resource is somewhat ill-fitted to these tasks because it is not precisely designed to address these sorts of challenges, and when Robert employs "now what" in non-task-based contexts, his interlocutors do not verbally respond to them. By the end of the year, Robert engages very little in organized activities (and did not seek others' assistance) and is given few instructions, which Juliet indicates is because he now has difficulty following even simple directives.

5.6.2 Deficit and/or Skill?

Cross-sectional studies examining coordinated work involving people with dementia typically either highlight the importance of interlocutors as resources, particularly their value in offering directives as guidance, or emphasize the skillfulness of those with dementia as they strategically draw on environmental, including human, resources. The current analysis blurs these two perspectives. The situated analysis that CA provides allows one to view Robert's use of "now what" both through the lens of deficit *and* skill, because it illuminates both the troubles Robert faces while simultaneously demonstrating his resourcefulness to navigate such troubles. Robert's use of "now what" is undoubtedly resourceful and demonstrates his ability to draw on an available resource to participate in and accomplish real-world tasks. At the same time, his reliance on this resource highlights difficulties he is facing, notably challenges with independently and incrementally progressing an activity from start to finish and handling (or exiting) delicate interactional sequences. That such compensatory practices point to both resourcefulness and difficulty suggests that a dichotomous framework – identifying a practice or behavior as either a deficit or skill – may not be the most sensitive for accurately capturing the practices of social engagement of those diagnosed with neurological disorders (see Mikesell, 2020; Mikesell & Bromley, 2016). Deficit implies a shortcoming or deficiency; skill is a developed talent or ability that brings an advantage. The previous analysis reveals how such a practice is skillful – helping an individual participate when they might have difficulties doing so – and at the same time can point to decline or incapacity, since by definition a practice that is *compensatory* functions to overcome some challenge.

The problem with identifying an atypical practice as strictly a deficit is that it overlooks what the practice provides or makes possible for the individual, and also what the practice may reveal about the resources an individual is capable of drawing on. In many cases, Robert is able to draw on rather simple language and apply it in moments of activity-centered interactions to be able to solicit assistance in a range of everyday tasks. Consequently, it allows him to participate and take part in organized activities. It also allows him to display to others his willingness to engage in these tasks. On the other hand, the problem with understanding a practice like "now what" as strictly a skill – as only what it allows an individual to accomplish – is that it de-emphasizes the significant and sometimes devastating consequences of disease or disorder and may conceal or misrepresent participants' experiences or the ensuing difficulty of a compensatory practice. In this way, third-party observations/experiences and direct, real-time observations provide unique but complementary perspectives on the sociobehavioral changes resulting from bvFTD.

Examining compensatory practices importantly helps illuminate the types of challenges individuals face. Examining "now what" highlighted Robert's challenges in navigating the sequential nature of activities that require a number of successive steps to complete. Early on, Robert demonstrated difficulties identifying a nonroutine activity (e.g., waiting in line), but once this was identified, he could identify the next step of the activity (e.g., using a credit card to pay). Later on, he demonstrated difficulty in identifying the individual steps of even routine activities, though his collaborators may have minimized his abilities to do so when pre-empting his need for step-by-step assistance. Overall, however, there seemed to be difficulties navigating the relationship between the "whole" activity and its required parts, which may reflect the executive nature of frontal lobe functioning (Mikesell, 2014, 2016). While manifesting cognitive work in observable everyday tasks is not often an explicit undertaking of conversation analytic studies, using CA to consider this delicate balance between deficit and skill contributes to the ways in which we understand the role of cognition in context (see Hutchins 1995, 2006) and provides insights into the relationship between structured clinical tasks that are *designed* to elicit 'cognition' and its real-world manifestations (see Mikesell, 2014).

5.6.3 Implications

Longitudinal case studies, such as the one presented here, are limited in scope and generalizability; however, they provide a window into the course of bvFTD from a naturalistic perspective. Such work may provide insights about how social engagement and interactional practices progress over time and how families navigate them. Employing CA, with its utilization of video recordings of real-world interactions, also provides insights into how such "atypical" practices might be categorized and coded, to avoid only capturing abstractions or gross impressions of observable behaviors that are often analyzed through the lens of deficit (see Barsuglia et al., 2014). Using CA to examine the sequentially situated, moment-by-moment production of social behaviors and interactional practices provides a nuanced lens into the functionality of a practice, and thus allows us to more easily observe how a practice can both constitute a dementia-related challenge or impairment and simultaneously demonstrate an individual's skill and resourcefulness. While Perkins et al. (1998: 37) rightly declare that "deviation from what is normal does not necessarily equate with failure or communicative ineffectiveness", such deviation may point to impairment by highlighting real-world challenges that call for workarounds.

Practices that are idiosyncratic to an individual with dementia may on the surface seem difficult to make sense of, particularly since many dementia behaviors – even those that appear common across individuals – have been framed as nonsensical and randomly produced. However, what a conversation analytic approach to examining Robert's use of "now what" reveals is that this practice, although atypical, is not nonsensical but largely systematically employed to recruit others' assistance. Notably, over time Robert's use of "now what" extends to new contexts and challenges, and in turn seems to lose some of its interactional or functional meaning for interlocutors. Thus, it may be perceived by others in those moments as randomly produced simply because these new contexts are not task-focused ones where "now what" can maintain its sequentially positioned meaning. This may account for why interlocutors responded less frequently to these uses and reported feeling frustrated by them.

As Cohen-Mansfield (2008) has argued, "disruptive" behaviors may reflect an internal state of the individual. Robert's extended uses of "now what," as his disease progressed and as his challenges extended beyond the management of discrete tasks, appeared to become more centered on his internal state of being. He increasingly displayed frustration in his tone and agitation and restlessness in his movements (often getting up and sitting down repeatedly). As such, this one practice may have the potential of serving not just as a resource for Robert, but as a resource for those who regularly interact with him and for those who are often responsible for organizing or monitoring his daily tasks. As it seems to be a "go-to" practice for navigating various challenges and uncertainties, it may, in simplistic terms, provide a marker to highlight these moments for interlocutors, giving them an opportunity to try to take Robert's perspective and identify what kind of challenge he may be currently facing when "now what" is produced.

References

Alvarez, J. A. and Emory, E. (2006) 'Executive function and the frontal lobes: A meta-analytic review.' *Neuropsychology Review*, 16:17–42. doi: https://doi.org/10.1007/s11065-006-9002-x.

Barsuglia, J. P., Nedjat-Haiem, F. R., Shapira, J. S., Valasco, C., Jimenez, E. E., Mather, M. J. and Mendez, M. F. (2014) 'Observational themes of social behavioral disturbances in frontotemporal dementia.' *International Psychogeriatrics*, 26(9): 1475–1481. doi: https://doi.org/10.1017/S104161021400091X.

Cohen-Mansfield, J. (2008) 'Agitated behavior in persons with dementia: The relationship between type of behavior, its frequency, and its disruptiveness.' *Journal of Psychiatric Research*, 43(1): 64–69. doi: https://doi.org/10.1016/j.jpsychires.2008.02.003.

Desmarais, P., Lanctot, K. L., Masellis, M., Black, S. E. and Herrmann, N. (2018) 'Social inappropriateness in neurodegenerative disorders.' *International*

Psychogeriatrics, 30(2): 197–207. doi: https://doi.org/10.1017/S1041610217001260.

Diehl-Schmid, J., Monsch, A. U., Aebi, C., Wagenpfeil, S., Krapp, S., Grimmer, T., Seeley, W., Förstl, H. and Kurz, A. (2005) 'Frontotemporal dementia, semantic dementia and Alzheimer's disease: The contribution of standard neuropsychological tests to differential diagnosis.' *Journal of Geriatric Psychiatry and Neurology*, 18: 39–44. doi: https://psycnet.apa.org/doi/10.1177/0891988704272309.

Diehl-Schmid, J., Bornschein, S., Pohl, C., Förstl, H., Jurz, A. and Jahn, T. (2011) 'Cognitive decline in the behavioral variant of frontotemporal dementia.' *International Pscyhogeriatrics*, 23(2): 230–237. doi: https://doi.org/10.1017/S104161021000164X.

Dooley, J., Bailey, C. and McCabe, R. (2015) 'Communication in healthcare interactions in dementia: A systematic review of observational studies.' *International Psychogeriatrics*, 27(8): 1277–1300. doi: https://doi.org/10.1017/S1041610214002890.

Erickson, F. and Schultz, J. (1997) 'When is a context? Some issues and methods in the analysis of social competence', in M. Cole, Y. Engeström and O. Vasquez (eds.) *Mind, Culture, and Activity*. Cambridge, UK: Cambridge University Press, pp. 22–31.

Guendouzi, J. A. and Müller, N. (2006) *Approaches to Discourse in Dementia*. Mahwah, NJ: Lawrence Erlbaum.

Hutchins E. (1995) *Cognition in the Wild*. Cambridge, MA: MIT Press.
  (2006) 'The distributed cognition perspective on human interaction', in N.J. Enfield and S. C. Levinson (eds.) *Roots of Human Sociality: Culture, Cognition and Interaction*. Oxford: Berg Publishers, pp. 375–398.

Hydén, L.-C. (2014) 'Cutting Brussels sprouts: Collaboration involving persons with dementia.' *Journal of Aging Studies*, 29: 115–123. doi: https://doi.org/10.1016/j.jaging.2014.02.004.

Kendrick, K. H. and Drew, P. (2016) 'Recruitment: Offers, requests, and the organization of assistance in interaction.' *Research on Language and Social Interaction*, 49(1): 1–19. doi: https://doi.org/10.1080/08351813.2016.1126436.

Kindell, J., Keady, J., Sage, K. and Wilkinson, R. (2017) 'Everyday conversation in dementia: A review of the literature to inform research and practice.' *International Journal of Language and Communication Disorders*, 52(4): 392–406. doi: https://doi.org/10.1111/1460-6984.12298.

Kipps, C., Knibb, J. A. and Hodges, J. R. (2007) 'Clinical presentations of frontotemporal Dementia', in J. R. Hobbs (ed.) *Frontotemporal Dementia Syndrome*. Cambridge, UK: Cambridge University Press, pp. 38–79.

Majlesi, A. R. and Ekström, A. (2016) 'Baking together – the coordination of actions in activities involving people with dementia.' *Journal of Aging Studies*, 38: 37–46. doi: https://doi.org/10.1016/j.jaging.2016.04.004.

Mates, A. W., Mikesell, L. and Smith, M. S. (eds.). (2010) *Language, Interaction and Frontotemporal Dementia: Reverse Engineering the Social Mind*. London: Equinox.

Mendez, M. F., Fong, S. S., Shapira, J. S., Jimenez, E. E., Kaiser, N. C., Kremen, S. A. and Tsai, P. (2014) 'Observation of social behavior in frontotemporal dementia.'

American Journal of Alzheimer's Disease and Other Dementias, 29(3): 215–221. doi: https://doi.org/10.1177/1533317513517035.

Mikesell, L. (2010a) 'Examining perseverative behaviors of a frontotemporal dementia patient and caregiver responses: The benefits of observing ordinary interactions and reflections on caregiver stress', in A. W. Mates, L. Mikesell and M. S. Smith (eds.) *Language, Interaction and Frontotemporal Dementia: Reverse Engineering the Social Mind*. London: Equinox, pp. 85–113.

(2010b) 'Repetitional responses in frontotemporal dementia discourse: Asserting agency or demonstrating confusion?' *Discourse Studies*, 12(4): 465–500. doi: https://doi.org/10.1177/1461445610370127.

(2014) 'Conflicting demonstrations of understanding in interactions with individuals with frontotemporal dementia: Considering cognitive resources and their implications for caring and communication', in R. Schrauf and N. Müller (eds.) *Dialogue and Dementia: Cognitive and Communicative Resources for Engagement*. New York: Psychology Press, pp. 147–180.

(2016) 'Opposing orientations in interactions with individuals with frontotemporal dementia: Blurring the boundaries between conflict and collaboration.' *Journal on Language Aggression and Conflict*, 4(1): 62–89. doi: https://doi.org/10.1075/jlac.4.1.03mik.

(2020) 'Does atypicality entail impairment? Tracing a cohesive marker in the interactions of an individual with schizophrenia', in R. Wilkinson, J. Rae and G. Rasmussen (eds.) *Atypical Interaction: Impacts of Communicative Impairments within Everyday Talk*. Cham, Switzerland: Macmillan, pp. 129–160.

Mikesell, L. and Bromley, E. (2016) 'Exploring the heterogeneity of "schizophrenic speech" outside of the clinic', in M. O'Reilly and J. Lester (eds.) *The Palgrave Handbook of Adult Mental Health: Discourse and Conversations Studies*. London: Palgrave Macmillan, pp. 329–351.

Neary, D., Snowden, J. S., Gustafson, L., Passant, U., Stuff, D., Black, S. et al. (1998) 'Frontotemporal lobar degeneration: A consensus on clinical diagnostic criteria.' *Neurology*, 51: 1546–1554.

O'Keefe, F. M., Murray, B., Coen, R. F., Dockree, P. M., Bellgrove, M. A., Garavan, H., Lynch, T. and Robertson, I. H. (2007) 'Loss of insight in frontotemporal dementia, corticobasal degeneration and progressive supranuclear palsy.' *Brain*, 130(3): 75–64. doi: https://doi.org/10.1093/brain/awl367.

Perkins, L., Whitworth, A. and Lesser, R. (1998) 'Conversing in dementia: A conversation analytic approach.' *Journal of Neurolinguistics*, 11(1–2): 33–53. doi: https://doi.org/10.1016/S0911-6044(98)00004-9.

Pomerantz, A. and Fehr, B. J. (2007) 'Conversation analysis: An approach to the study of social action as sense making practices', in T. A. van Dijk (ed.) *Discourse as Social Interaction*. Los Angeles: Sage, pp. 64–91.

Roscovsky, K., Hodges, J. R., Knopman, D. et al. (2011) 'Sensitivity of revised diagnostic criteria for the behavioural variant of frontotemporal dementia.' *Brain*,134(pt 9): 2456-77. doi: https://doi.org/10.1093/brain/awr179.

Schegloff, E. A. (1968) 'Sequencing in conversational openings.' *American Anthropologist*, 70: 1075–1095.

(2007) *Sequence Organization in Interaction: A Primer in Conversation Analysis*, vol. 1. Cambridge, UK: Cambridge University Press.

Schegloff, E. A. and Sacks, H. (1973) 'Opening up closings.' *Semiotica*, 7(4): 289–327. doi: http://dx.doi.org/10.1515/semi.1973.8.4.289.

Shany-Ur, T. and Rankin, K.P. (2011) 'Personality and social cognition in neurodegenerative disease.' *Current Opinion in Neurology*, 24(6): 550–555. doi: https://10.1097/WCO.0b013e32834cd42a.

Stivers, T. (2005) 'Modified repeats: One method for asserting primary rights from second position.' *Research on Language and Social Interaction*, 38(2): 131–158.

Torralva T., Roca, M., Gleichgerrcht, E., Bekinschtein and Manes, F. (2009) 'A neuropsychological battery to detect specific executive and social cognitive impairments in early frontotemporal dementia.' *Brain*, 132: 1299–1309. doi: https://doi.org/10.1093/brain/awp041.

6 Being Sociable
A Case Study of a Man with Vascular Dementia Singing in Conversation

Roy M. G. L. W. Foster

6.1 Introduction

This chapter is a case study of Dan, a man with vascular dementia who sings in everyday conversations with his family. Dan lives at home with his wife, Morgan, and she is his primary conversational partner. After changes in cognition, Dan began singing during conversation-based activities that did not have music as a focal point (e.g., music therapy or music as a topic of conversation). Some of Dan's singing maintains cohesion with prior talk when the song shares words with the previous turn. For example, a turn at talk that incidentally includes a song's title or lyrics might touch off his singing of that song. Dan also does something very interesting, creative, and unexpected by modifying lyrics. His modifications, which are based on prior talk and the physical environment, are the main focus of this chapter.

Dan's singing uses elements from a prior speaker's turn or objects in his immediate surroundings to modify lyrics from a small repertoire of songs. For example, Dan often changes the lyrics "Daisy, Daisy, give me your answer true. I'm half crazy over the love of you" from the song "Daisy Bell (Bicycle Built for Two)" (Dacre, 1892/1925). In Extract 1, Dan sings this song with altered lyrics during a meal with Morgan.

Extract 1 5-2014 – DA=Dan; MO=Morgan
```
01   DA:   I'm slowing down Morgan. (0.5) getting full.
02   MO:   Mmm?
03         (9.1)
04         Well you've attacked that with gusto.
05   DA:   Mm hih heh
06         (4.6)
07         ((singing modified "Bicycle Built for Two"))
08         ♫ Gusto gusto give me your answer true
09         (1.3)
10   MO:   Mmhmm
11         (5.5)
12   DA:   ♫ I'm half crazy over eating with you { looks to Morgan}
13         (1.7)
14   MO:   Well that's very kind of you
```

Dan's singing in line 8 replaces the original lyrics "Daisy Daisy" with Morgan's *gusto* (line 4). He continues with the meal theme by changing "the love of you" to *eating with you* (line 12), and Morgan treats his singing as a compliment by expressing appreciation (line 14) (see Pomerantz (1978) on compliment responses). This example is representative of how Dan creates new songs in the corpus. His singing is responsive to prior talk, accomplishes a wide range of interactional jobs (such as complimenting, complaining, and requesting) while often being humorous as well, and makes relevant a co-participant response. Furthermore, his singing is a remarkable cognitive and creative achievement. His songs maintain the original tune and some of the lyrical elements (e.g., syllabic structure and rhyme) while he simultaneously fashions novel lyrics that carry the new theme.

Musical recognition and memory may be spared in dementia despite impaired language (Cuddy & Duffin, 2005; Särkämö et al., 2012). Research into music-based interventions has rapidly grown in the hopes that capitalizing on remaining musical abilities could provide an inexpensive, easy, and enjoyable non-pharmacological treatment approach. The most robust research on dementia and singing outside of testing situations and imaging studies is on singing in the context of music therapy, recreation, and caregiving situations. The literature can roughly be divided into informal singing done by caregivers and formal singing programs led by music professionals and therapists. In a review of the studies, Chatterton et al. (2010) compared the qualifications of the singers and their goals. They concluded that music therapists and caregivers use singing to different ends. Music therapists were interested in addressing cognitive, social, and behavioral functioning. In contrast, caregivers were attempting to reduce agitation, improve quality of life, and build connections especially during specific tasks (e.g., morning routines and meals). The findings of these research areas have been thoroughly reviewed elsewhere (see e.g., Leggieri et al. (2019) for a systematic review of research on music interventions and Swall et al. (2020) for a summary of singing by caregivers). It is worth noting that while there is general agreement that music-based interventions reduce depressive and behavioral symptoms for people with dementia, it remains undetermined whether benefits extend to cognition and how they may relate to changes in the brain.

Compared to research on singing facilitated by music professionals or done by caregivers, unprompted singing by people with dementia has received less attention. Singing initiated by people with dementia has a history of being classified as noise-making and verbal disruptive behavior associated with self-stimulation (Cohen-Mansfield & Werner, 1997; Ryan et al., 1988). Although some typologies of disruptive vocalizations note that they may be goal-directed (e.g., requests for attention), this type of top-down analysis risks erasure of contextual nuances that indicate why a person vocalizes at a particular juncture in time and the role of co-participants. More recently, Hydén (2011) and Samuelsson and Hydén (2011) analyzed non-verbal vocalizations produced by people with late-stage Alzheimer's disease (e.g., screaming, repeated syllables, "singing-like" and monotonous pitch contours) to understand how co-participants orient to noise-making as meaningful communication. Their approach is in contrast to previous typologies that treat non-verbal vocalizations as an asocial expression of agitation or other inner states. Hydén also demonstrates the necessity of analyzing discursive context for understanding non-verbal vocalizations as being part of a repeated *caring practice*. This interactional approach to non-verbal vocalizations provides a model for how singing by people with dementia in everyday conversation could be analyzed. Indeed, Rasmussen (2020) analyzes the interactional environment in which a person living with frontotemporal dementia sings during the course of a conversation. The songs are positioned when the topic of talk is atrophying, and they are designed to be associated with prosodic features and words from the co-participant's earlier speaking turns.

Like the two examples described by Rasmussen, Dan's singing is more obviously directed at mutual engagement than the "loud singing" or "variety of tunes" included in classifications of disruptive vocalizations. However, Dan's frequent singing of a small set of songs could be described as an atypical, repetitive behavior using a clinical typology. This chapter shows that a bottom-up approach allows for a finer-grained description of the emergent structure and meaning of his singing. An analysis of how singing unfolds in interaction demonstrates that his songs can be quite the opposite of self-stimulation in their recipient design. Developing our understanding of how Dan uses singing as a semiotic resource for action formation and identity construction is especially important for a population in which loss of memory can be ideologically associated with incompetence and loss of self.

6.2   Data and Methodology

The data are home videos recorded by Morgan between September 2011 and December 2014. Morgan and Dan volunteered the recordings for use in my dissertation and subsequent publications. They also granted me access to Dan's cognitive-linguistic testing report and permission to summarize the results. The testing scores, along with background information provided by Morgan regarding Dan's changes in behavior, provide an important context for his singing. The University of Colorado Human Research Institutional Review Board approved the study (protocol 14-0109), and both participants provided verbal and written consent. I changed the participants' names, all names mentioned in the data, and some locations to protect the participants' privacy.

6 Being Sociable

I took a micro-level approach using Conversation Analysis to analyze Dan's singing and co-participant responses in the context of unfolding interaction. I reviewed 23.25 hours of video and transcribed 39 segments with singing. I used transcription conventions from Jefferson (2004) as a basis and added a musical note symbol (♪) to mark singing, following the notation used by Stevanovic (2012). As I am not analyzing Dan's performances for elements contained in musical notation, I have not included musical scores for each transcript. Detailed transcripts can be found in Foster (2015) as not all of the extracts from the corpus are discussed in this chapter.

6.3 Participants

Dan and Morgan live independently in their home in the USA. Morgan immigrated as an adult from the UK, and they have lived in the same house since getting married in the 1960s. At the time of the first recording, Dan was 76 years old and Morgan was 70. In 2007 Dan had an abrupt change in cognition and was later diagnosed with vascular dementia. Cognitive-linguistic testing indicates that he has severely impaired short-term memory, in the less than 1st percentile. The severity of his short-term memory loss impairs his ability to complete daily tasks despite other scores falling within normal limits (including attention, processing speed, conceptualization, auditory comprehension, expressive language, and reading comprehension). Dan's decline in cognition significantly impacts his life. He does not complete higher-level tasks (*instrumental activities of daily living* or IADLs) in any form. This means that he is wholly dependent for financial and medicine management, shopping, housework, cooking, social planning, driving, and so on. Some of Dan's basic routine activities (ADLs such as dressing) require assistance as well. Morgan provides Dan with assistance and cues to initiate and complete them, and he would not be able to live at home without her.

Dan also experienced major changes in communication. In groups and interactions outside the home, his participation is often limited to repetitive formulaic sequences, questions, and positive evaluations of objects in his surroundings (e.g., multiple productions of *those flowers are really beautiful*). Dan communicates more effectively in a dyad in a lower-stimulus and familiar environment such as his home. In these less demanding contexts, Dan still repeats topics and utterances, but he communicates with a wider range of resources (disagreeing, evaluating, inquiring, providing accounts, etc.) While this study does not go into detail about all of Dan's verbal abilities, it is important to recognize that he has resources for participation besides just singing. That is not to say that Dan's communication is unaffected by cognitive decline. It is, however, important to start an investigation into his singing by acknowledging that he has many other verbal resources for participation.

In many of the extracts, Dan appears exceptionally competent. This is in part because the extracts are removed from their larger discursive context. A five-minute clip may seem relatively "normal" when it is extracted from a two-hour recording and not viewed in the context of interactions from previous days. It is readily apparent from viewing interactions across a wider time frame that Dan's communication becomes negatively impacted by memory impairment, even in the home. While he may not have severe word-finding deficits or syntactic impairment, it is not unusual for him to repeat utterances multiple times during a single recording or across days. In many of the videos Dan repeatedly asks questions about temporal orientation or his children's life circumstances – information that has not changed in many years. He also denies that he has the memory to answer questions about his experiences in the immediate and distant past that one might expect to be in his domain of knowledge. It is clear that Dan has both deficits and remaining abilities, and this pattern of pragmatic ability and disability in the absence of other significant linguistic impairment is common in dementia. What is less typical is Dan's creative use of singing.

6.4   Background on Dan's Singing

Dan does not have professional training in music but enjoys listening to it. He started singing in conversation after changes in his cognition. Dan certainly sang before dementia, and he often sang to his children. Yet there is a difference in his earlier singing and how he uses it now as an interactional resource. His earlier singing is what one might expect from someone who sings around the house outside of primarily talking-based activities. It was only after changes in his cognition that family members noticed he would frequently repeat verses of songs in conversation, and over time he increasingly began to modify lyrics based on prior utterances. Dan's conversational use of singing was well established by the start of this study, and there is no discernible change or development in his singing patterns over the course of the recordings.

Dan has a limited repertoire and audience for his singing. He sings a fairly small set of songs that he learned in childhood and college. The nine songs that Dan sings in the data are as follows:

1. "Bicycle Built for Two" a.k.a. "Daisy Bell" (Dacre, 1892/1925)
2. "The Farmer in the Dell"
3. "The Fireman's Band" a.k.a. "The Life of a Fireman"
4. "I've Got Sixpence"
5. "Kansas City" (Rodgers & Hammerstein II, 1943)
6. "Old MacDonald"

7. "R.P.I. was R.P.I. When Union Was a Pup"
8. "She'll Be Coming Round the Mountain"
9. "There's a Meeting Here Tonight"

These songs belong to several genres: musicals, college or drinking songs, children's songs, and old popular or folk songs. The lyrics, along with musical scores and publicly available recordings, can be accessed online (www.royfoster.com). Importantly, Dan only sings with immediate family members. This means that his singing is not a form of disinhibition, perseveration, or a simple stimulus response. He is sensitive to context in terms of both conversation partner and prior discourse. The fact that Dan does not sing with some people and that he changes lyrics based on previous turns indicates sophisticated pragmatic judgment and indexes a close relationship with his conversation partners.

6.5 Analysis

Dan's singing is not random but fits systematically within the sequential organization of talk and thus emerges moment-by-moment. Recorded performances of lyrics, or *texts*, are typically produced in relatively long chunks (e.g., verses). Yet there is no guarantee that Dan will produce the whole song as it is written in a book or performed on the radio. The song's ending is arrived at jointly with his conversation partner. It can end after a single "line," or Dan can accomplish a longer, multi-unit song. The singing sequence makes relevant a response and furthers progressivity of interaction. In other words, just like talk, his singing is locally occasioned and contingent on surrounding talk and involvement of other participants.

The concepts of *preference*, *alignment*, and *affiliation* are important for understanding what Dan accomplishes with singing. Broadly, the notion of preference refers to mostly implicit principles that participants orient to when they act and respond in interaction (Pomerantz & Heritage, 2013). These principles govern multiple domains of interaction, from the design of turns to norms for responding to different types of actions (Pomerantz & Heritage, 2013; Sidnell, 2010). Most relevant to singing is the preference for a response that promotes progression of an action sequence. For example, the *action-type preference* of an invitation is an acceptance (Sidnell, 2010). Participants manage this constraint when responding in disagreement or rejection of a preceding action by designing a turn with features that project *dispreference*, such as delays, palliatives, accounts, and pro-forma agreement. Dan sometimes sings to close sequences marked by this type of dispreference. Related concepts are alignment and affiliation. Alignment refers to the current state of talk, such as participants adjusting to a change in turn-taking to accommodate storytelling – or in this case singing (Mandelbaum, 2013). Affiliation is about affective stances to events and previous talk, and participants may adopt or reject each other's interpretation of them. A recipient may exhibit conflict regarding these two orientations to talk by, for example, going along with a switch from talk to singing (alignment) but not displaying support of the singer's stance that the singing was funny (disaffiliation).

Dan performs a range of actions through singing. Humor is one of his main accomplishments, and it is an important way in which he uses singing to participate in conversation. The humor of Dan's singing is an interactional achievement, and it contributes to his situational construction of self as a funny and clever person. Humor can also contribute to the achievement of other actions, and the humorous key of his singing helps dissipate disaffiliation in sequences that are characterized by dispreference. There are further examples of Dan using singing to express appreciation and gratitude. Dan's singing in these contexts also works towards building affiliation and closeness. Yet there are contrasting examples of Dan raising a complaint by singing and also of Morgan treating his singing as making a request, which demonstrate that singing is a flexible interactional resource. In the following sections I analyze the turn-taking structure of Dan's singing. I then turn to what he accomplishes with it, first in terms of humor and then by examining specific actions including complimenting, complaining, and requesting.

6.5.1 Singing in the Turn-Taking Structure of Talk

Dan sings in a wide range of discursive locations. In terms of sections of conversation in the most general sense, Dan sings in middle and closing (or adjourning) sections. It remains inconclusive whether he sings during openings, such as greeting sequences, as those were not recorded. Sections of conversation are a relatively coarse division of interaction. In terms of fine-grained sequential structure, Dan sometimes sings modified songs to open sequences but more often as second pair parts or post-expansions. His singing is thus relatively unconstrained by position.

The length of Dan's songs spans from single, short turns to multiple turns with intervening talk. On the sparser side, 10 of Dan's 39 singing occurrences are "one liners." In Extract 2, for example, Dan produces a short singing turn, and Morgan speaks afterwards.

Extract 2 9-2011
```
01    DA:   ((modified "The Fireman's Band"))
02          ♫Oh jakey jabs oh jakey jabs
03    MO:   °Hih °hih (1.2) yeah (0.6) hhh (0.3) let's take
04          our cameras (0.6) in case there are any (1.3)
05          wildlife
```

6 Being Sociable

In an earlier sequence, Morgan informed Dan that they were going to a store she calls *Jake Jabs*. Dan uses the store name in a single line of singing, and Morgan laughs in appreciation. One could argue that she is curtailing his song by starting a new sequence about taking cameras. However, Morgan does not latch her turn onto Dan's singing turn, nor does she speak in overlap, and Dan does not continue singing during the pauses in line 3.

Dan also treats a similar single line of lyrics as complete in many other excerpts such as in Extract 3.

Extract 3 4-2014

```
01   MO:   U:m I'll get your lunch pills.
02         (0.7)
03   DA:   ((modified "The Fireman's band"))
04         ♪Oh lunchy pills oh lunchy pills
05         (0.7)
06         Boy this looks like a good lunch Morgan.
```

Here, Dan himself pauses then switches to talking after the first line of the same song seen in Extract 2. This means that a potential end to a singing turn, and thus a possible transition relevance place to next speaker, is located at the end of a relatively short turn of singing. What constitutes a "line" or turn constructional unit (TCU) is song-specific, and the data suggest that both participants treat the formulaic sequence [oh *xxx* oh *xxx*] performed with prosody from "The Fireman's Band" as a TCU (Foster, 2015).

Singing beyond the first TCU is an accomplishment that is contingent upon the actions of co-participants. Co-participants have a role in song extension through use of silences that invite more, continuers, minimal assessments, and laughter (Foster, 2015). Additionally, Dan extends songs following explicit invitation for continuation and to account for the song's relevance, as exemplified in Extract 4. Dan and Morgan have been talking about slip trailing, a technique for applying raised patterns to ceramics. Dan enjoyed making pottery as a hobby after retirement. Earlier he was complaining about his difficulty learning how to do slip trailing, and they had some disagreement over what makes it challenging. The interaction continues below with talk about his trouble. He eventually sings to the tune and general structure of "Old McDonald," a children's song in which the singer names an animal and the sound it makes on Old McDonald's farm, before ending the verse with "e–i–e–i–o."

Extract 4 3-2014

```
01   DA:   Boy I tell you I couldn't do it (.) I literally
02         couldn't do it
03   MO:   Mmm-hmm
04         (1.5)
05         With practice
06         (3.5)
07         Like everything else it's practice practice practice
```

```
08   DA:   Yeah but if: f:or a person who it's not their
09         business y' know[already] retired heh hih
10   MO:                  [Mmmhmm  ]
11   DA:   [Huh huh huh huh]
12   MO:   [Huh huh hih hih] hih hih ((sniff))
13   DA:   There aren't many years left to practice=
14   MO:   =Mmm-hmm
15         (3.8)
16   MO:   Yeah and if you're just dabbling (0.5) (to g-)
17         (0.8)
18   DA:   Yeah
19         (0.4)
20   MO:   Y- y- you can't spend that time
21         (0.6)
22   DA:   ((modified "Old MacDonald"))
23         ♫ A dabble here and a dabble there=
24         ♫ here a dabble there a dabble=
25         ♫ everywhere a dabble dabble
26         (2.5)
27   MO:   Hih hih hih ((sniff)) hih (.)
28   DA:   I won't say the rest of it
29         (0.6)
30   MO:   Oh go on huh hih hih
31   DA:   ♫ Old MacDonald had a farm
32         (0.3)
33         ♫ e-i-e-i-o
34         (3.4)
35   MO:   What did that got to- to do with pottery (.)
36         heh hih[hih
37   DA:   ♫      [With a dabble dabble here=
38         ♫ and a dabble dabble there=
39         ♫ here a dabble there a dabble=
40         ♫ everywhere a dabble dabble .hh
41         ♫ Old MacDonald had a farm
42         (2.8)
43         ♫ And on this farm he had a pottery lab
44         (.)
45         ♫ [e-i-e-i-o    ]
46   MO:     [Huh huh hih hih] hih hih hih (0.6) ((sniff)) hih
47   DA:   ((smile))
```

In line 23, Dan recontextualizes Morgan's earlier *dabble* (line 16) in his version of "Old MacDonald." Morgan volunteers laughter (line 27), and Dan comes to a possible ending of the song with *I won't say the rest of it* (line 28), which hints at the potential for more but a decision to stop. Morgan does not accept the ending and invites continuation with *oh go on* plus more laughter (line 30). Dan extends the song with the usual final verse *Old MacDonald had a farm e–i–e–i–o* (lines 31 and 33). This is another possible ending point, but Morgan again does not treat it as an acceptable one. She instead pursues an account for the song's relevance (line 35). By asking what the song had to do with pottery, Morgan's go-ahead for more singing emerges as more than a general request for additional lyrics. Singing the *rest of it* does not just mean any lyrics in this case but ones that relate to prior talk. Dan responds by singing with reference to pottery (line 43). The song again comes to a possible completion point with *e–i–e–i–o*, with Morgan laughing in overlap (lines 45–46) and Dan producing an affiliative smile. This time, the song ends. The fact that Morgan pursues more singing and Dan expands the song to account for its relevance shows that the song's ending is contingent and arrived at jointly. Dan makes decisions about appropriate stopping points, but the ending of the song is negotiable. Dan can be held accountable for how the singing relates to the ongoing action, and a lot of interactional work is done to establish progressivity by singing turns and the talk that follows.

Beyond the analytical account of how Dan's singing fits into the structure of talk, Dan's innovative songs reveal his exceptional cognitive and creative competencies. His skill at manipulating lyrics into new songs reveals strengths in at least attention, working memory, semantic memory, pattern recognition, and musical memory. These are aspects of cognition that are required to retain words and themes from previous turns and fit them into the syllabic patterns, rhyme, grammatical structures, and concepts of the original lyrics. In an exploration of the poetics of ordinary conversation, Jefferson (1996) presents a collection of talk that is produced in part by reference to previous sounds and word categories (e.g., puns, sounds repeated across turns). Dan's singing puts this type of poetics at the forefront in the way that he playfully integrates words from Morgan's turns into the formulaic structure of the song. Dan's singing positions him as someone who can astutely monitor conversation for sources of musical wordplay and as an active participant who creatively furthers interaction. In the next section I analyze how Morgan and Dan orient to his poetics as humorous and well-constructed.

6.5.2 Accomplishing Humor through Singing

Dan at times uses singing to close sequences that are characterized by dispreference and redirects the interaction toward affiliation with humor. Literature on singing in conversation by neurotypical participants is lacking with a few exceptions. In a study by Frick (2013), Finnish speakers in Estonia use singing to end extended interactional sequences that include signs of nonalignment and dispreference, such as being silent after a story and not granting requests. Frick describes how participants in one example follow singing with smiles, laughter, and other sound-making. She argues that this affiliative joint activity builds rapport and distances them from the dispreferred actions without calling for continuation of the sequence. Extract 4 illustrates a similar use of singing by Dan in English. The extended interaction has elements of dispreference and disagreement: dispreference in the blocking of progression of talk about troubles, overt disagreement about slip trailing, and conflicting characterizations of his degree of involvement in pottery. Dan's singing ends the interaction on a humorous key. Morgan laughs repeatedly during the song, and Dan's final smile solidifies affiliation as they close the sequence about his involvement with slip trailing and pottery.

Dan's singing is often treated as funny by co-participants. In many of the extracts, Morgan laughs during and after Dan's singing, sometimes even when Dan has not laughed. Jefferson (1979) compares structurally and sequentially distinct types of recipient laughter. *Volunteered laughter* is produced after a *recognition point*, which is a moment when a recipient recognizes that laughter is warranted. A recipient produces *speaker-invited laughter* after a speaker's end-of-turn or within-turn laughter. There are many examples of Dan and Morgan treating Dan's singing as humorous by using both types of laughter. The laughter may be volunteered laughter as in Extract 5.

Extract 5 9-2011
```
01    DA:   ((modified "The Fireman's Band"))
02          ♪ Oh don't you really really think
03          (2.7)
04          ♪ Vultures should stay asleep
05          (0.9)
06    MO:   Ha ha ha ha .hh heh ha ha ha hih .hh oh hh
```

After Dan sings about the vulture, which is a persistent theme throughout the interaction, Morgan produces a stretch of laughter (line 6). In Extract 5, Morgan laughs after a short gap, but she does not always wait until the end of the song to laugh. Lerner (1996: 259) writes that "a recipient need not delay affiliation until next turn" with laughter. Indeed, in other examples Morgan laughs throughout and even in overlap with Dan's singing. Her laughter in overlap demonstrates her understanding of his singing as funny, even near the onset of singing.

In addition to volunteered laughter, Morgan sometimes replies to Dan's singing with a joke of her own. Extract 6 provides an example.

Extract 6 9-2011
```
01    DA:   ((modified "The Fireman's Band"))
02          ♪ Oh don't you really really think
03          (1.1)
04    DA:   ♪ That we should see the turkey vulture
05          (0.4)
06    MO:   Huh hih ((sniff)) (.)
07    DA:   (xxx)
08    MO:   Hh (0.8) Don't go out if you're not feeling well hh
09          (2.5) ((Dan looks at Morgan and opens mouth))
10    DA:   Wh(h)at? (.)
11    MO:   Heh huh hah[ha .hh hih huh hih hih hih huh hahahahaha
```

```
12   DA:              [.Hhh HA HA .hhhhhh (H)o(h)k(h)ay .hhhh
13                    (h)I (h)w[(h)on' t .hhhhhh] uh huh uh huh .hhh
14   MO:                             [.Hh hih hih hih ]
```

In this example and on other occasions Morgan makes a humorous remark related to Dan's song immediately after he finishes singing. Morgan briefly laughs before her turn *don't go out if you're not feeling well* that teases about the possible danger of a weakened person falling prey to vultures. Dan meets her joke with astonishment – as he often does to jokes that are rude, morbid, or at his expense – by looking at Morgan with a wide-open-mouth posture and asking a question with laughter (Wilkinson & Kitzinger, 2006). In this case, Dan produces *wh(h)at* (line 10) followed by agreement (lines 12–13) and a great deal of laughter. Morgan does not treat his question as a problem with hearing or understanding but instead laughs as well. Jokes can come in tit-for-tat succession, and Morgan's laughter plus in-kind humorous responses are further evidence that some of Dan's songs are designed to be funny and are taken as such.

There is evidence that Dan and Morgan orient to wordplay within the song's original lyrical structure as constituting humor. The participants' retrospective characterization of singing in Extract 7 provides evidence of this. Morgan and Dan are finishing a meal, and Morgan invites Dan to think about a trip they have planned for the following day.

Extract 7 9-2014
```
01   DA:   I'm all outta things to say.
02         (1.6)
03   MO:   ↑Oh (0.3) okay. (0.7) well you can start thinking
04         about going to Santa Fe
05         (0.8)
06   DA:   ((modified "The Fireman's Band"))
07         ♪ .Hh oh Santa Fe old Santa Fe
08         (1.2)
09   DA:   ♪ How I love my Santa Fe=
10   MO:   =Mm ↑hmm ↑hmm
11         (0.3)
12   DA:   ♪ Oh don't you really really think
13         (0.7)
14   DA:   ♪ That we should take (0.3) a trip to Santa Fe I thin[k ]
15   MO:                                                        [hh]
16         huh hah (h)oh good[y goody heh]
17   DA:                     [Hhhh hhhh   ]
18   MO:   Hah hah
19   DA:   Heh .hh[h heh heh]
20   MO:          [.Hh heh  ] heh heh .hh
21   DA:   Oh dear[y] .
22   MO:          [O]o[oh dear.]
23   DA:              [Fool you] didn't I.=
24   MO:   =Oh y[es definitely did        ]
25   DA:        [You weren't sure what I was] gonna sa[y.]
26   MO:                                              [Y-] yeah,
```

```
27              (0.6)
28    DA:       Oh the elephant and[the (xxx)]
29    MO:                          [That was a] new variant on the
30              theme.=
31    DA:       =Yes. (.)
```

After Dan finishes singing, Morgan volunteers laughter and evaluates his song with *oh goody goody* (line 16). Dan joins in her laughter and says *fool you didn't I* (line 23). Morgan agrees, and Dan expands with *you weren't sure what I was gonna say* (line 25). Morgan again agrees and adds *that was a new variant on the theme* (lines 29–30). Both Morgan and Dan have treated the song as laughable. A laughable song can *fool you* because you won't be sure what he is *gonna say*, and part of the fun of Dan's singing is anticipating how he is going to make *a new variant on the theme* by modifying recognizable lyrics. His performances have value, in part, from the novelty and creativity in which he recontextualizes the text by changing elements based on surrounding talk. In other words, humor hinges on unpredictability within a formulaic sequence and on Dan's competent performance of clever modifications.

Morgan does not always agree with Dan's stance towards humor. This type of disaffiliation can be accomplished by withholding laughter. Morgan's absence of laughter is especially salient after Dan invites her to laugh. Jefferson (1979: 93) writes, "One technique for inviting laughter is the placement, by speaker, of a laugh just at completion of utterance, and one technique for accepting that invitation is the placement, by recipient, of a laugh just after onset of speaker's laughter." A co-participant, however, does not have to accept speaker-invited laughter. For example, in Extract 8 Morgan volunteers laughter at the start of the song but does not join Dan in laughing afterwards.

Extract 8 9-2011
```
01    MO:    O(.)kay here's some un(.)der(.)wea:r (1.5)
02           and some sockie wokies?
03           (0.5)
04    DA:    ((modified "The Fireman's Band"))
05           ♫ Oh sockie wokies oh sockie wokies
06           (0.9)
07    DA:    ♫ How I like some sockie wokies
08           (0.5)
09    MO:    Mm[hm]
10    DA:    ♫[Oh] don't [you really really] think
11    MO:              [Hh heh heh heh heh]
12           (1.3)
13    DA:    ♫ To have sockie wokies (1.0) to wear upon my feet
14    MO:    Hh
15           (0.3)
16    DA:    ↑HA HA (0.6) that song didn't wanna come out (.)
17           but it ca[me out.]
18    MO:             [Uh yeah] eh[it sort] of came out.
19    DA:                         [Heh heh]
```

Morgan is helping Dan get dressed, and after she offers him socks, Dan uses the *sockie wokies* from her turn for another version of "The Fireman's Band." Morgan volunteers laughter in the midst of Dan's singing (line 11) and takes the position that his singing is humorous in that moment. However, after Dan finishes his song, Morgan declines to laugh and even does a hard exhale (line 14) – perhaps indicating disapproval. Dan's loud laughter (line 16) makes her laughter relevant again. Morgan does not immediately laugh, and Dan continues with an assessment *that song didn't wanna come out but it came out* (lines 16–17) that puts a somewhat positive spin on his difficulty with the song. Jefferson (1979: 93) explains that one technique to decline an invitation to laugh is with recipient talk that does "serious pursuit of topic as a counter to the pursuit of laughter." Dan's *it came out* provides an alternative route for Morgan, and she declines to laugh by instead responding to Dan's assessment of the song's construction. Morgan disagrees with his stance that his rendition *came out*. She accomplishes this disaffiliation by countering with a second assessment that repeats part of his turn with the added negative qualification that *it sort of came out* (line 18).

While not made explicit, it could be that their assessments speak to how well his song's final line *to have sockie wokies to wear upon my feet* maintained the rhythmic and grammatical structure of the song's original lyrics "that we should have another drink." In any case, Morgan's stance in Extract 8 illustrates that the humor of Dan's performance is not predetermined. Whether Dan accomplishes humor or not is contingent on the unfolding structure of his lyrics, and participants may shift their stance as the song emerges. The humor of his performance is an accomplishment at every turn.

In summary, doing humor is one of the primary things that Dan accomplishes with singing. A song's ability to provoke laughter may depend on how well Dan maintains a balance between providing unique modifications while preserving the form of the original text (e.g., syllabic structure, syntactic structure, and final rhyme). Humor may also depend on how well the song reflects semantic themes of the prior discourse. Evidence that Dan and Morgan orient to these elements as constituting humor or a "good" song are found in their responses to his singing. Evaluation of the song may include reference to the song's relevance to ongoing talk (e.g., *what did that got to do with pottery* in Extract 4), the construction of the song (e.g., *that song didn't wanna come out* in Extract 8), and unpredictability of the wordplay (e.g., *fool you didn't I* in Extract 7). Although Dan and Morgan both often treat Dan's singing as laughable, Morgan does not always affiliate with Dan's stance toward his singing. The humor of Dan's singing is an interactional accomplishment that is not guaranteed by the original text, and its achievement contributes to Dan's situational construction of self as clever and funny.

6.5.3 Doing Complimenting, Complaining, and Requesting through Singing

In addition to using singing to do humor, Dan sings to accomplish a range of other actions including complimenting, complaining, and requesting. I address each of these in turn. There are multiple examples of Dan singing compliments and appreciation in the data. In the most transparent examples, Dan explicitly identifies the person or the action that he appreciates. For instance, in Extract 1 Dan is eating when he announces that he is *slowing down* with his meal and *getting full*. Morgan's *well you've attacked that with gusto* could account for why he is slowing down and getting full. Dan could simply agree with her, or he could provide an alternate account for why he ate that way (e.g., with an assessment about the meal). Dan goes down the latter path with the second part of his song *I'm half crazy over eating with you*. Morgan treats his singing as a compliment with *well that's very kind of you*. In other examples, Dan similarly does gratitude for offers of assistance (Foster, 2015).

There are also two examples in which Dan's singing turns express appreciation for his food, Extracts 9 and 10.

Extract 9 7-2014

```
01    DA:    ((modified "Bicycle Built for Two"))
02           ♫ Blueberries blueberries
03           (1.8)
04    DA:    ♫ Give me your answer true
05           (0.3)
06    MO:    M:::hm
07    DA:    ♫ I'm half crazy (0.3) for the cereal on you
08           (11.6) ((He continues eating))
09    DA:    ♫ It won't be a stylish (.) meal
10           (.)
11    DA:    ♫ I can't afford a Coors
12           (3.9)
13    DA:    ♫ But you'll taste sweet
14           (5.4)
15    DA:    ♫ On some ice cream and (0.3) cookies
16           hih hih heh heh ((He flashes gaze to Morgan))
17    MO:    Mmm[mmhmm mm hih    ]
18    DA:       [I don't know .hh] °heh °hih .hh
```

Extract 10 7-2014

```
01    DA:    ((modified "Bicycle Built for Two"))
02           ♫ Black beans black beans give me your answer true
03           (.)
04    MO:    ((in adjoining room)) Uh hhh
05    DA:    ♫ I'm half crazy over the protein in you
06           ((He eats a bite of beans.))
```

6 Being Sociable

In Extract 9, Dan starts by singing about his meal of blueberries and cereal (lines 2, 4, and 7). This portion of the song ends with *I'm half crazy for the cereal on you*. There is silence for over 11 seconds while Dan eats. He then continues singing *it won't be a stylish meal I can't afford a Coors* (beer) (lines 9 and 11) before describing an imagined meal in which the blueberries will *taste sweet on some ice cream and cookies* (lines 13 and 15). After he finishes singing, Dan laughs and looks briefly at Morgan who is preoccupied with writing an email. In the second example, Extract 10, Morgan is out of visual range but can hear Dan from the next room. In line 5, Dan does appreciation of the black beans and their protein content. In both of these extracts Morgan is within hearing distance but occupied with other activities. It could be that the main project of these singing turns is to do gratitude for the meal and/or to re-establish joint interaction with Morgan. Unfortunately, Morgan's lack of uptake means that we cannot be certain how she might treat his singing his appreciation of food. In many other examples of talk, however, Dan notices ingredients and their attributes in the food that he is eating and then thanks Morgan for taking care of him. This collocation suggests that his doing appreciation of food is part of a practice of expressing gratitude for caregiving.

Dan's singing often expresses affection by doing appreciation for companionship, gratitude for assistance, and positive evaluations of food. The songs he modifies to accomplish this is the love song "Bicycle built for two," and Dan can easily change the text to express affection that is specific to each encounter. Dan is acutely aware of the daily help that he needs, and he is quick to express thanks for assistance. He often says things such as *thank you for this meal* or *thank you for taking care of me* multiple times during a meal. Modifying songs, especially the sweet love song "Bicycle built for two," is a resource Dan uses to creatively build closeness and intimacy with Morgan.

Of course, as with talk, there is not a one-to-one correlation between singing and action. Dan at times does a complaint through singing, much in contrast to the humor and appreciation discussed earlier. In Extract 11, for example, Morgan starts a new sequence about a visual word puzzle, or "wuzzle," that was posted at her gym. Dan sometimes sings in response to Morgan's announcements of upcoming activities (see Foster (2015) for an analysis of Dan's singing in response to "mere informings" of new activities in terms of deontic congruence). In this case, Dan's singing resists the activity.

Extract 11 4-2014
```
01    MO:    Oh there was another wuzzle
02           today hh (.) one of these word puzzles
03           (2.7) ((She starts writing down the wuzzle))
04    DA:    ((modified "Old MacDonald"))
05           ♪ Wuzzle here and a wuzzle there
06           ♪ here a wuzzle there a wuzzle
```

```
07            ♪ old Mac (0.5) Donald liked his wuzzles=
08     MO:    =Mhmm?
09            (1.0)
10     DA:    ♪ e-i-e-i-o
11            (0.9)
12     DA:    ♪ And I don't like wuzzles very much
13            (0.9)
14     MO:    You're good you're pretty good at them,
15            ((She finishes writing the wuzzle))
16            (0.5)
17     DA:    We:ll,
18     MO:    ((She holds wuzzle facing Dan and walks toward him))
```

Extract 11 starts with Morgan's announcement *oh there was another wuzzle today one of these word puzzles* (lines 1–2). Her announcement projects the possibility of more than simply news of a new wuzzle. Indeed, Morgan starts writing down the wuzzle, which strengthens the possibility that her announcement is part of a larger "doing the wuzzle" project. Dan then sings a modified version of "Old MacDonald" that contrasts Old MacDonald's liking of wuzzles to his own dislike of them. The singing concludes with *I don't like wuzzles very much* (line 12) that anticipates this larger project. Morgan responds with an assessment *you're good you're pretty good at them* (line 14), and her complimenting turn could also be heard as an account for why he could do the wuzzle despite disliking them. Dan does not align with her assessment, possibly because of the problem of how to respond to compliments (see Pomerantz (1978) on the multiple constrains on compliment sequences), but an agreement might also weaken his resistance to the activity. Morgan presents him with the wuzzle in any case.

Morgan's *another wuzzle* (line 1) is relevant here as it points to a repeated activity in which Morgan brings home word puzzles for Dan. Dan struggles with comprehending and completing them. In this instance, Dan takes almost a minute to do the basic word puzzle, and Morgan provides so many clues to assist him that he complains several times *you told me* the answer. In light of this, Dan's singing can be heard as a complaint that resists the upcoming wuzzle, an activity that exposes his impaired cognition.

In addition to modifying lyrics to do an appreciation or a complaint, there are two examples in the data of either Dan or Morgan treating his singing as doing a request. Although Dan does not modify the lyrics of "The Fireman's Band" in these instances, his singing is interpreted within the framework of everyday talk and not treated as a performance of the song to be evaluated. In the first example, Extract 12, Dan sings as Morgan places a cup of coffee in front of him.

Extract 12 12-2014

```
01     DA:    (("The Fireman's band"))
02            ♪ Oh the fireman's band the fireman's band
03            ♪ here's my heart and here's my hand
```

```
04   MO:    ((Morgan puts coffee cup in front of Dan))
05   DA:    ♪ Oh don't you really really think
06          ♪ that we should have another drink
07   MO:    .Hh ha ha
08   DA:    Ha heh
09   MO:    .Hh[oka:y] there's [some coff] ee
10   DA:       [I got]          [coffee   ]
11   MO:    For y[ou .hh huh heh hih
12   DA:         [I got some coffee it worked heh
13   MO:    [It worked ok(h)]ay hih ha ha (.) ha ↘o:h dear
14   DA:    [°Hih °hih °hih ]
```

At the start of Extract 12 Morgan is walking into the room holding Dan's cup of coffee as Dan sings a drinking song. This example could be viewed as Dan matching his singing to the events occurring in the world. Retrospectively, however, Dan's turn *it worked* (line 12) positions his singing – even if jokingly – as a successful request that Morgan has fulfilled.

In the second example, Extract 13, Morgan herself responds to Dan's singing as a request that requires an account.

Extract 13 4-2014
```
01   MO:    And w:hy do you think that we should have
02          another drink. Hh
03   DA:    °I °was °just (1.9) trying to be soci[able.]
04   MO:                                         [Hh   ] hah
05   MO:    s(h)ociable.
06   DA:    Hih heh hih hah (0.3) .hh
07   MO:    Mmm
08          (0.7)
09   DA:    Hh
10   MO:    Well, you can:↑have another drink if you li:ke but
11          [it's uh root]
12   DA:    [Better be wa]ter
13   MO:    It's root beer hh[ha ha] ha .hh °hih
14   DA:                     [I see]
15   MO:    heh huh
16   MO:    Heh hhh .hhh ↓o:h ↓well. (2.1) ↓o:[ka::y    ]
17   DA:                                      [Here we are]
18          right next to Coo:rs at least close to it=
19   MO:    =Mmhmm=
20   DA:    =And I don't even get any beer.
```

Dan has sung "The Fireman's Band" just before this extract, and Morgan treats Dan's singing as an actual request for a drink. She first seeks an account for it with *and why do you think that we should have another drink* (lines 1–2) and later offers him a root beer (lines 10 and 13). Dan is aware of the fact that he has medical and pharmaceutical restrictions on how much alcohol he can drink (see *better be water* (line 12) and his lament *here we are right next to Coors at least close to it and I don't even get any beer* (lines 17–18, 20)), so it is unlikely that he meant for his singing to be taken as a sincere request for an alcoholic beverage. Indeed, Dan counters by providing an alternative version of what he was attempting to accomplish with *I was just trying to be sociable* (line 3).

In this section I have primarily focused on how Dan and Morgan give meaning to Dan's singing by how their responses – such as laughter, assessment, and pursuit of an account – treat it. Extract 13 is a rare case in which Dan uses metalanguage to describe the meaning of it. Even more, it is an example in which Morgan's treatment of Dan's singing is not in alignment with how he describes it. Enfield (2013: 101) uses the term *treating-as* to describe the response process participants usually use to characterize a speaker's actions, in contrast to a *describing-as* categorization process. For example, responding to "You look nice" with "Thank you" treats the previous turn as a compliment whereas "He gave me a compliment" explicitly describes it as one. Dan provides us with a *described-as* account for his singing that suggests a broad emic action category of *being sociable*. In this general sense, we may treat all of Dan's singing events that I have discussed as *doing being sociable*. He could simply speak instead of sing, but singing allows him to be sociable by performing entertaining songs. The texts that he sings are not neutral vehicles. They are clever and humorous variations of drinking songs, love songs, and children's songs. Dan's performances are a resource for him to position himself as funny, affectionate, and as a guy who used to enjoy a drink and who would still like to have one now.

6.6 Conclusion

Dan's account *I was just trying to be sociable* displays an orientation to singing as a form of engagement and participation. Singing is a relatively open-ended resource for Dan use to do things in interaction. There are instances in the data of him doing humor and wordplay, closing sequences to re-establish affiliation, doing appreciation and gratitude, responding to a noticing or informing turn, responding to turns that announce a new activity, and changing the trajectory of talk (Foster, 2015). Dan also uses singing to accomplish actions such as complimenting and complaining. The variety of functions does not mean that Dan's singing is random or asocial. Dan's singing is a flexible interactional resource because he astutely monitors conversation and modifies songs to the discursive context at hand.

Singing provides Dan with a route to competency despite his severe short-term memory impairment and dependence on Morgan. His technical ability to recall tunes and spontaneously alter lyrics that stay true to a conceptual theme from the prior talk while still maintaining elements of the original formulaic structure is no small feat. It manifests his cognitive strengths of attention, pattern recognition and formation, conceptualization, semantic memory, and working memory. Singing is also a medium in which he can do things that he is good at interactionally, such as being funny, affectionate, and appreciative. His singing at times provides an avenue for resisting cognitively challenging activities that expose his impairment, like the wuzzle. Morgan holds Dan accountable for the relevancy of his singing to ongoing talk, and he is also susceptible to her evaluation of his song's composition. Modified singing thus provides Dan with several avenues for displaying competence: (1) accessing musical memory to produce the tune and multiple cognitive skills to manipulate the original lyrical structure, (2) demonstrating the appropriateness of his singing by grounding texts in the immediate discursive context, and (3) showing skill in creative and clever wordplay within the structure of the lyrical text. Morgan also treats Dan as competent by responding to his singing turns as producing meaningful actions and replying with her own jokes in tit-for-tat succession. Dan and Morgan's interactions involving singing thus provide a compelling case of adaption to changes in cognition over time not only within a person but also between people.

There is a persistent notion that people with dementia lose identity along with the loss of coherence and memory, analogous even with death. Dan's singing illustrates important alternative roles that can be constructed in contrast to *person with dementia*. First, Dan's singing is a way for him to articulate creative wordplay, and each performance in which Dan accomplishes humor positions him as a funny and clever person. The stances that Dan and other participants take towards his performances position him as a particular type of singer in the moment. Those stances accumulate in a bottom-up fashion to construct Dan a more "durable" identity (such as *jokester*) than is found in his temporary participant roles (see Bucholtz and Hall (2005) on *stance accretion*, usually discussed in relation to macro identities like gender).

Second, Dan's singing is one avenue for Dan and Morgan to discursively construct their relationship as a couple. Dan's affectionate singing makes salient the intimate relationship he shares with Morgan. It points to his identity as her spouse and takes a positive affective stance towards it. Yet the relationship work they accomplish goes beyond the compliments he sings to her. His repetition of lyrical texts with situational modifications is a shared experience. Work by Goodwin (1987) and Muntigl and Choi (2010) on displays of not remembering has shown how speakers can take an epistemic orientation to talk by treating other participants as *knowing* or *unknowing* of a forgotten word or event. Depending on the type of information in question, positioning someone as having access to it can make relevant larger social identities. Talk that makes visible shared knowledge of activities may additionally provide for inferences of interpersonal relations, such as being a couple, by implying a close relationship. Both Dan and Morgan position her as a *knowing recipient* who is aware of the songs in his repertoire and his practice of modifying them. Dan's version of "The Fireman's Band" in Extract 7 could only *fool* Morgan and be recognized as a surprising *variant on the theme* if she were very familiar with his singing. Recognition of short segments of tunes and new variants of the lyrics, which could only be accomplish through repeated shared experience, thus indirectly indexes their long-term relationship.

This case study also establishes the vital importance of analyzing conversations that take place in the home in order to provide insight into interactional resources that people with dementia use in everyday life. Dan only sings in conversation with close family members, so standardized language assessment and conversation sampling in a clinical or professional care setting would not elicit his singing. In fact, his family noted that he did not sing during a short stay at a physical rehabilitation center. Since then, Dan has been able to remain at home with Morgan with assistance from professional caregivers. Morgan observed that Dan does not sing to the caregivers, even though they have been with him for over a year and a half. Without access to interactions between Dan and Morgan outside of an institutional or professional caregiving context, we would miss the interactional achievements that Dan accomplishes with his singing and also the role that his singing plays in his relationship with Morgan.

References

Bucholtz, M. and Hall, K. (2005) 'Identity and interaction: A sociocultural linguistic approach.' *Discourse Studies*, 7(4–5): 585–614.

Chatterton, W., Baker, F. and Morgan, K. (2010) 'The singer or the singing: Who sings individually to persons with dementia and what are the effects?' *American Journal of Alzheimer's Disease and Other Dementias*, 25(8): 641–649.

Cohen-Mansfield, J. and Werner, P. (1997) 'Typology of disruptive vocalizations in older persons suffering from dementia.' *International Journal of Geriatric Psychiatry*, 12(11): 1079–1091.

Cuddy, L. L. and Duffin, J. (2005) 'Music, memory, and Alzheimer's disease: Is music recognition spared in dementia, and how can it be assessed?' *Medical Hypotheses*, 64(2): 229–235.

Dacre, H. (1892/1925) *Daisy Bell (Bicycle Built for Two)*. New York: Harms, Inc.

Enfield, N. J. (2013) *Relationship Thinking: Agency, Enchrony, and Human Sociality*. Oxford: Oxford University Press.

Foster, R. M. G. L. W. (2015) *Dementia and singing: A conversation analysis case study of singing in everyday interaction*. PhD dissertation, [Online] Available at: https://scholar.colorado.edu/concern/graduate_thesis_or_dissertations/3484zg88m.

Frick, M. (2013) 'Singing and codeswitching in sequence closings.' *Pragmatics*, 23(2): 243–273.

Goodwin, C. (1987) 'Forgetfulness as an interactive resource.' *Social Psychology Quarterly*, 50(2): 115–130.

Hydén, L.-C. (2011) 'Non-verbal vocalizations, dementia and social interaction.' *Communication & Medicine*, 8(2): 135–144.

Jefferson, G. (1979) 'A technique for inviting laughter and its subsequent acceptance/declination.' In G. Psathas (ed.) *Everyday Language: Studies in Ethnomethodology*. New York: Irvington Publishers, pp. 79–96.

(1996) 'On the poetics of ordinary talk.' *Text and Performance Quarterly*, 16(1): 1–61.

(2004) 'Glossary of transcript symbols with an introduction.' In G. H. Lerner (ed.) *Conversation Analysis: Studies from the First Generation: Vol. 125 Pragmatics & Beyond New Series*. Amsterdam: John Benjamins Publishing Company, pp. 13–31.

Leggieri, M., Thaut, M. H., Fornazzari, L., Schweizer, T. A., Barfett, J., Munoz, D. G. and Fischer, C. E. (2019) 'Music intervention approaches for Alzheimer's disease: A review of the literature.' *Frontiers in Neuroscience*, 13: 132–139.

Lerner, G. H. (1996) 'On the "semi-permeable" character of grammatical units in conversation: Conditional entry into the turn space of another speaker.' In E. Ochs, E. A. Schegloff and S. A. Thompson (eds.) *Interaction and Grammar*. Cambridge: Cambridge University Press, pp. 238–276.

Mandelbaum, J. (2013) 'Storytelling in conversation'. In J. Sidnell and T. Stivers (eds.) *The Handbook of Conversation Analysis*. Chichester, UK: Wiley-Blackwell, pp. 492–507.

Muntigl, P. and Choi, K. T. (2010) 'Not remembering as a practical epistemic resource in couples therapy.' *Discourse Studies*, 12(3): 331–356.

Pomerantz, A. (1978) 'Compliment responses: Notes on the co-operation of multiple constraints.' In J. Schenkein (ed.) *Studies in the Organization of Conversational Interaction*. New York: Academic Press, pp. 79–112.

Pomerantz, A. and Heritage, J. (2013) 'Preference.' In J. Sidnell and T. Stivers (eds.) *The Handbook of Conversation Analysis*. Chichester, UK: Wiley-Blackwell, pp. 210–228.

Rasmussen, G. (2020) 'Singing as a resource in conversations involving persons with dementia.' In R. Wilkinson, J. P. Rae and G. Rasmussen (eds.) *Atypical Interaction: The Impact of Communicative Impairments within Everyday Talk*. Cham, Switzerland: Palgrave Macmillan, pp. 161–193.

Rodgers, R. and Hammerstein II, O. (1943) 'Kansas City', Act I, *Oklahoma!* New York: Williamson Music Co.

Ryan, D. P., Tainsh, S. M. M., Kolodny, V., Lendrum, B. L. and Fisher, R. H. (1988) 'Noise-making amongst the elderly in long term care.' *The Gerontologist*, 28(3): 369–371.

Samuelsson, C. and Hydén, L. C. (2011) 'Intonational patterns of nonverbal vocalizations in people with dementia.' *American Journal of Alzheimer's Disease and Other Dementias*, 26(7): 563–572.

Särkämö, T., Laitinen, S., Tervaniemi, M., Numminen, A., Kurki, M. and Rantanen, P. (2012) 'Music, emotion, and dementia: Insight from neuroscientific and clinical research.' *Music and Medicine*, 4(3): 153–162.

Sidnell, J. (2010) *Conversation Analysis: An Introduction. Language in Society*. Chichester, UK: John Wiley & Sons, Ltd.

Stevanovic, M. (2012) 'Establishing joint decisions in a dyad.' *Discourse Studies*, 14(6): 779–803.

Swall, A., Hammar, L. M. and Gransjön Craftman, Å. (2020) 'Like a bridge over troubled water – a qualitative study of professional caregiver singing and music as a way to enable person-centred care for persons with dementia.' *International Journal of Qualitative Studies on Health and Well-Being*, 15(1): 1735092.

Wilkinson, S. and Kitzinger, C. (2006) 'Surprise as an interactional achievement: Reaction tokens in conversation.' *Social Psychology Quarterly*, 69(2): 150–182.

7 On the Use of Tag Questions by Co-participants of People with Dementia
Asymmetries of Knowledge, Power and Interactional Competence

Jacqueline Kindell, John Keady and Ray Wilkinson

7.1 Introduction

In this study we use a conversation analytic approach to investigate the use of a particular type of utterance regularly deployed by the co-participants of people with dementia within conversation in our dataset, that is an utterance in the form of a tag question (Hepburn & Potter, 2010).

Grammatically, a tag question can be described as an utterance consisting of two clauses, where an interrogative clause (the 'tag', or 'interrogative tag') is added as a supplement to another clause (the 'anchor') (Huddleston & Pullum, 2002). In English, tag questions most commonly have reversed polarity, such that a positive anchor is followed by a negative tag ('he likes olives, doesn't he?'), or a negative anchor is followed by a positive tag ('he doesn't like olives, does he?').[1] Interactionally, tag questions share a number of features with other yes/no-type questions. First, via the tag at the end of a turn, a tag question can function as a means by which a current speaker selects another speaker to speak next (Sacks et al., 1974).[2] Second, that response is expected to either align or disalign with the action in the prior (tag question) turn. Third, tag questions make 'yes' or 'no' (or equivalents) relevant as the first component of the response (Heritage & Raymond, 2005). Fourth, as with other yes/no-type questions (Robinson, 2020), tag questions typically prefer responses that align with (for example, confirm or agree with) the objectives or goals of the action in the tag-formatted turn (Heritage, 2010). While utterances with a positive statement in the anchor clause followed by a negative tag (e.g., 'you're married, aren't you?') are designed to favour a 'yes' response, utterances with a negative declarative in the anchor clause followed by a positive tag (e.g., 'there's no blood in the diarrhea, is there?') are designed to favour a 'no'

---

[1] Other types of tag questions can occur in English, such as 'invariant' tags (e.g., 'right?'), but these will not be discussed further here.
[2] So-called turn-medial tags may function differently; see Hepburn and Potter (2011).

response (Heritage, 2010: 58. This feature of tag questions, whereby they display which type of response would be favoured, and thus exert some pressure on the recipient to respond in that way, has been discussed by linguists in terms of the 'conduciveness' of tag questions (Huddleston & Pullum, 2002). For example, Quirk et al. (1985: 810) talk of the 'maximum conduciveness' of tag questions compared to other types of yes/no-type questions, and Cameron et al. (1988: 87) discuss them as 'highly assertive strategies for coercing agreement'.

Our interest in the use of tag questions by co-participants of people with dementia is twofold. First, our analysis examines this type of utterance as a contribution to talk-in-interaction which is recipient-designed (Sacks et al., 1974) by the co-participant for a person with dementia and adapted to the particular cognitive and linguistic limitations (and remaining abilities) evident in the person with dementia's interactional repertoire. Second, we examine what the implications of these tag-formatted utterances are for the participation of the person with dementia within the interaction (Goodwin & Goodwin, 2004). In particular, we highlight the fact that a tag question puts interactional pressure on the person with dementia to produce an aligning response, such as an agreement (Heritage, 2010), and we examine how this property of tag questions is one that co-participants can make use of.

7.1.1 Tag Questions and the Epistemic Order, Deontic Order and Emotional Order

In outlining relevant conversation analytic research on the use of tag questions in interaction, it will be useful to discuss different types of social action (Levinson, 2013) that have been analysed in relation to their tag question turn format. It is also important to note that tag question turn formats have been shown to be one practice through which a speaker can display a particular stance concerning issues of epistemics (knowledge), deontics (power, control and agency) or emotion (or affect) in interaction (for a discussion of these three orders within interaction, see Stevanovic & Peräkylä, 2014).

In relation to *epistemic* issues, for example, a tag question displays an orientation to the knowledge status of the recipient (Ekberg et al., 2022). Designing a turn in the form of a tag question can be a means by which the speaker displays their epistemic stance (Heritage, 2013) in relation to the recipient as regards the speaker's proposition. For example, while a yes/no question such as 'are you married?' expresses that the speaker has no definite knowledge of whether the recipient is married or not, a tag question format ('you're married, aren't you?') 'conveys a strong hunch as to the likelihood of a particular response' (Heritage, 2010: 48) and indexes a smaller information gap between the speaker and the recipient compared to a yes/no interrogative

(Heritage, 2012). When a speaker produces a tag question, the epistemic status (Heritage, 2012) of the speaker relative to the recipient of the utterance will influence how that tag question will be heard and treated. When the speaker evidently has a lower epistemic status than the recipient, the tag question is hearable as requesting information from the recipient in the form of a confirmation of the tag-formatted statement proffered by the speaker (Heritage, 2012). In other cases, however, such as when a speaker and recipient have relatively equal access to the information being discussed, the tag question is hearable as a statement by the speaker that seeks agreement from the recipient (Heritage, 2012).

Tag questions have also been analysed in terms of how they are used as a turn format for a different type of action/activity, that is advice-giving (Hepburn & Potter, 2011). In their data involving child protection officers (CPOs) talking to callers on a national child protection helpline, Hepburn & Potter (2011) explore how the CPOs regularly use tags when providing advice to callers (for example, 'you need to sort it out don't you really': Hepburn & Potter, 2011: 228). Advice-giving, like directives, proposals or requests, is an activity concerned with getting others to do things, such as commit to future actions. As such, it can invoke the relative *deontic* rights of the participants (Stevanovic & Peräkylä, 2014). Hepburn and Potter (2011) explore instances where advice that has previously been resisted by the caller is presented again by the CPO, including on this latter occasion with a tag. They note that in this context when the advice-giving is produced in a tag question format, it can be seen to be 'coercive' (Hepburn & Potter, 2011: 236) in that this form of turn design prefers an affirmative response, here in the form of an agreement from the caller, even though the caller has previously resisted the advice.

A third type of action where tag questions have been discussed in relation to their tag question turn design is challenges (Keisanen, 2007). Like other actions, such as accusations, challenges can be disaffiliative (Sorjonen & Peräkylä, 2012) and, as such, can display one way in which the participants negotiate the *emotional* facets of their relationship (Stevanovic & Peräkylä, 2014). In Keisanen's data, the challenges can be produced in response to an initiating action, where the tag question turn challenges the appropriateness or relevance of that prior action. Keisanen (2007) notes that the tag question turn indexes a discrepancy in information between the participants, and this discrepancy is used as a basis for the challenge.

7.1.2 *Tag Questions in Talk-in-Interaction Involving Participants with Dementia*

Research into conversations involving people with dementia has not focused systematically on co-participants' use of tag questions, although their deployment has been noted in passing (Rasmussen et al., 2019; Svennevig & Landmark, 2019). However, one area of the literature where they regularly have been discussed is work on what has been labelled 'elderspeak'. This term is used to refer to a speech register which may be displayed by those (in the literature, particularly health and care staff) talking with older adults and people with dementia. Elderspeak is described as consisting of features including tag questions, a slower rate of speech, elevated and exaggerated pitch and volume, relatively simple grammar and vocabulary, and the use of diminutives (Williams et al., 2004). It is suggested (Williams et al., 2004) that elderspeak may be perceived by hearers as patronizing and as implying a lack of competence on the part of the recipient. The use of a tag question such as 'you want to get up now, don't you?' by a staff member to a resident with dementia has been described as 'prompt[ing] resident responses, thus suggesting the resident's inability to independently choose' (Williams et al., 2009: 12), and it has been suggested that the use of tag questions as part of elderspeak is likely to be harmful in that they 'politely push older adults' answers and behaviours in a desired direction' and 'undermine meaningful conversations and self-determined behaviours of older adults' (Schnabel et al., 2021:417).

7.2 The Current Study: Use of Tag Questions by Co-participants of People with Semantic Dementia

The data examined in the Analysis section of the chapter come from three couples where one partner has semantic dementia. We will now provide some background to semantic dementia and describe the participants and the data in this study. In the Discussion section we will revisit the use of tag questions as reported in the 'elderspeak' literature and discuss this usage in comparison to that of the spouses examined in our analysis. The chapter finishes with a discussion of what this analysis of co-participants' use of tag questions highlights about asymmetries of knowledge, power and interactional competence between persons with dementia and their co-participants, and how these asymmetries are made evident and oriented to within social interaction.

7.2.1 Semantic Dementia

Semantic dementia is a type of frontotemporal dementia (Snowden et al., 1989). It is also described as the semantic variant of primary progressive aphasia (Gorno-Tempini et al., 2011). While the presence of a progressive language disorder is required for diagnosis (Gorno-Tempini et al., 2011), it is known that with disease progression also come changes in other cognitive abilities, behaviour and personality, with symptoms often overlapping with those of behavioural variant frontotemporal dementia (Kertesz et al., 2010). Semantic dementia leads to significant challenges in communication for the person affected and their family members (Snowden et al., 2006), including difficulties for the person with dementia in understanding and in finding words when talking.

Research in semantic dementia has largely concentrated on assessing and treating underlying language (and other) impairments (e.g., Jokel et al., 2006). Less well understood is the impact of such language impairments, as well as changes in memory, behaviour and personality, on everyday conversation. To our knowledge, only two studies have specifically explored conversation in this condition. Kindell et al. (2013) used conversation analysis to analyse how Doug, a man with semantic dementia, adapted the use of his remaining linguistic and other communicative resources within conversation through regularly deploying enactment (Goodwin, 1990), that is depicting (rather than describing) an action or event using resources such as direct reported speech (Holt, 1996) and bodily behaviour such as eye gaze and gesture. Taylor-Rubin et al. (2017) used a discourse-oriented approach to explore what they termed 'trouble-indicating behaviours' (TIBs) in seven individuals with semantic dementia recorded while talking to their spouse in a clinical situation. The authors compared the number of TIBs to control subjects and found a higher presence in the turns of the people with semantic dementia. It can be seen, therefore, that both studies, while using different approaches, primarily examined the person with dementia and their communicative strengths or limitations. In this chapter, we aim to add to our knowledge of recurrent features of conversations involving people with semantic dementia by examining primarily the talk of the person with dementia's co-participants – specifically, their use of tag-formatted utterances – and in addition what the interactional implications of these tag-formatted utterances have for the participation of the person with dementia.

7.2.2   Participants and Data

In each of the three couples in this study, the person with dementia lives at home with their spouse. The couples are:

Peter (67 years old) and Joanna (64)[3]
Peter had been diagnosed with dementia five years earlier and was now experiencing significant word-finding difficulties. Peter also

---

[3] All identifying details such as person names and place names have been changed in order to preserve confidentiality.

had difficulty with understanding and retaining information in conversation.

Sarah (64) and Reg (66)
Sarah had been diagnosed with dementia four years earlier. She rarely initiated interaction at home, apart from repetitive questions about the routine of the day, and had difficulty retaining the answers Reg gave her.

Doug (71) and Karina (71)
Doug had been diagnosed with dementia five years earlier and was now experiencing significant difficulty with expressive speech, with his talking often unintelligible. Doug talked less than he used to, and when he did talk, this concerned a reduced range of topics.

In each case, therefore, the person with semantic dementia was experiencing significant difficulties with expression, comprehension and cognitive abilities, such as retaining information. This is evident in their neuropsychological test scores using the Addenbrooke's Cognitive Examination (ACE: revised version and version III) (Hodges, 2005), where Peter scored 27/100, Sarah 36/100 and Doug 18/100. Since a score below 82 on the ACE indicates likely dementia, it can be seen that each of these three people with dementia was at the more severe end of the spectrum.

Conversation was explored through analysis of video recordings of everyday conversations recorded by the couples at home. A total of 7:14 hours of conversation was recorded (couple one, 3:30 hours; couple two, 3:00 hours; couple three, 44 minutes).

An ethics committee registered with the National Health System (NHS) in the United Kingdom approved the study. The data were transcribed using the Jeffersonian transcription system (Jefferson, 2004). In the extracts in this arrows in the margins are used to direct the reader's attention to the tag questions which are the primary focus of the analysis.

7.3 Analysis

We will analyse two types of tag-formatted utterances here; there are a number of instances of each in our data set. For each type of tag question we will aim to show how its use by the co-participant is linked to the recipient's impairments associated with dementia, and how the tag question makes relevant a response, with an aligning response (the preferred option) commonly produced.

The first type of tag-formatted utterance, used particularly by the spouses Karina and Reg, involve actions, such as assertions and assessments which are largely concerned with epistemic issues (Heritage, 2012). The second type,

7 Use of Tag Questions by Co-participants

seen exclusively in the talk of the other spouse, Joanna, takes the form of challenges (Keisanen, 2007) towards Peter, the person with dementia, concerning some action or behaviour that Peter has produced. These latter actions are less concerned with epistemic issues and more with the momentary interpersonal relations between the couple, such as Joanna displaying a critical stance towards Peter's talk or conduct (i.e., they particularly concern issues within what Stevanovic & Peräkylä (2014) term the 'emotional order').

7.3.1 Tag-Formatted Assertions and Assessments

There are three features of tag-formatted assertions and assessments that we wish to highlight as regards their use by co-participants of people with dementia. The first is that they encode a certain level of access (at least to the extent of a strong hunch) on the part of the *speaker* to the information being discussed (Heritage, 2010). The second is that at the same time they acknowledge the *recipient* as having some epistemic access and authority as regards the information being talked about (Ekberg et al., 2022). The third is that they put some interactional pressure on the recipient to respond, and to do so in a way which displays alignment with the statement in the tag question.

In particular we will be showing here how co-participants can use a tag question format when they produce actions which involve providing the recipient with information that the recipient has already been told or might normally be expected to know (Stivers et al., 2011). Extract 1, involving Sarah and Reg, provides instances of this type of assertion produced by Reg both with a tag (lines 20–21) and without (e.g., lines 13, and 26–27).

Extract 1: Sar=Sarah

```
01    Reg:    Is there anything that you want now?
02    Sar:    What do you mean?
03            (0.2)
04    Reg:    To eat or drink or:
05    Sar:    °No°
06    Reg:    ((nods))
07            (1.5)
08    Reg:    So I bet you're looking forward to going to Jeans on
09            Wednesday aren't ya
10            (3.6)
11    Sar:    Wednesday?
12            (0.5)
13    Reg:    Not today, today is Monday,
14    Sar:    Yeah
15    Reg:    tomorrow Tue:sday we're [at the hospital, Wednesday you
16                                    [°Mm°
17    Reg:    go to Jea[:ns
18    Sar:             [°Mm°
19            (1.3)
```

```
20  → Reg:   You didn't go last week cos you had a bad head didnt
21  →        ya?
22    Sar:   Righ:t, oh yeah
23    Reg:   Y' know all the migraines that ya get?
24    Sar:   Yeah
25           (0.5)
26    Reg:   You had one (.) last weekend (0.7) starting on Sunday
27           [Monday
28    Sar:   [( )
29    Reg:   And Tuesday (and uh) started on the Monday
30           Tuesday (.) and the Wednesday
31           (1.3)
32    Sar:   Right
33           (0.3)
34    Reg:   So you didn't go,
35    Sar:   Right
36    Reg:   To Jeans
```

In line 08 Reg proffers a new topic (in the form of a tag question; we will return to this instance in due course). Sarah, however, does not buy into, and take forward, the proffered topic (Schegloff, 2007); it appears (from the long 3.6 second silence, and then her querying 'Wednesday?' in lines 10 and 11) that she has a problem in making sense of what Reg has just said, particularly in relation to the day that Reg has mentioned. Reg treats this as a problem relating to Sarah's dementia, that is a problem in orienting to time, including remembering which day it is that day, and proceeds to produce a series of assertions that violate the norm of not telling a recipient information they (should) already know (Stivers et al., 2011). These include what day of the week it is today (line 13), what Sarah will be doing tomorrow and the day after (lines 15 and 17), the fact that Sarah did not go to Jean's last week because she (Sarah) had a migraine (lines 20–21), and that Sarah had had migraines on a few days last week (lines 26–27 and 29–30).

One of these assertions (lines 20–21) is in the form of a tag question. As such, and unlike the other assertions here, Reg simultaneously provides information for Sarah (which, it is clear from the context, Sarah is likely to have had trouble producing herself), while treating the information being conveyed as being within Sarah's epistemic domain, and, implicitly, as something that she can remember (or at least will be able to remember after being prompted by Reg's utterance). By making expectable a response from Sarah, with a preference for an agreement, the tag question expects an affirmation by Sarah of this assertion, which in this context will be hearable as evidence that she remembers the fact being conveyed. As such, Reg's assertion is produced in a manner (i.e., tag-formatted) that treats Sarah as being able to remember the information conveyed in the assertion and affirm it. In this way, Reg bestows competence on Sarah, treating her as having these cognitive competences at this point in the interaction, whether or not she actually does remember her aborted visit to Jean the previous week.[4] With the use of this tag-formatted assertion, therefore, Reg acts to discursively construct Sarah's psychology (see Hepburn and Potter, (2011: 220) on the psychologically 'invasive' use of tag questions) as someone who will be able to remember the happening (or non-happening) that Reg is discussing.

In their talk with their spouses with dementia both Reg and Karina recurrently produce tag-formatted assertions and assessments similar to those seen in Extract 1. One use of this type of utterance for these co-participants appears to be that it allows them to produce assertions and assessments concerning issues which would be expected to be in their spouse's epistemic domain if that spouse did not have dementia, and to elicit agreement or confirmation from the person with dementia regarding what is being discussed. Of course, in these cases it may be unclear to the co-participants whether their spouse with dementia does indeed remember and have knowledge about the matters encoded in the assertion or assessment. Importantly, however, the tag-formatted utterance treats the person with dementia as if they do, bestowing competence on them and working to elicit their agreement with the matters being discussed. In addition, they engage the person with dementia in co-constructing topical talk about these issues (for example their experiences and feelings, or talk about friends, family members and acquaintances) that are within that person's lifeworld.

The three participants with dementia in our dataset initiate relatively little within these conversations and often display difficulty in contributing to the conversation due to their cognitive and linguistic impairments. As such, an ongoing issue for the co-participants is how to engage the person with dementia in topic talk and to bring into the conversation issues relating to the person's lifeworld that the person with dementia is not able to regularly bring in through their own talk.

These issues can be seen in Extract 2 involving Doug and Karina. The couple are talking about Jill (referred to in the extract as 'she' and 'her'), who is a volunteer at a social group for people with dementia which Doug attends and who gives Doug a lift home after the meetings. It is clear from the context that while Jill's main role is in relation to Doug, she also has a relationship with Karina, and the facts about Jill being discussed in this episode are treated as knowledge shared by Karina and Doug (what Labov & Fanshel (1977) refer

---

[4] As it transpires, Sarah's response of 'right, oh yeah' (line 22) is not a clear demonstration of remembering that she did not visit Jean last week due to her migraine. It neither straightforwardly affirms Reg's assertion (by starting the response with, for example, 'yes') nor marks that assertion as sparking a 'just now recollection' with, for example, 'oh, that's right' (Heritage, 1984). Reg's immediately subsequent utterances display that he is treating Sarah as still not fully remembering these details since he reiterates them (lines 23–36).

to as 'AB event' information). A notable feature of the extract is Karina's recurrent use of tag-formatted assertions (lines 01, 09–10 and 21–25) and assessments (lines 04, 12–15, and 18–21), with six produced within this 40-second episode.

Extract 2: Kar=Karina

```
01  → Kar:    And she usually brings you home anyway doesn't she.
02    Doug:   [( )-
03    Kar:    [Gives you a lift home=cos (.) not seen her for a
04  →         while be[nice to see her wouldn't it
05    Doug:           [Mm
06    Doug:   Yeah
07            (0.3)
08    Kar:    Cos she's very g- I want to ask her about her: (0.7)
09  →         breadmaking (.) cos she makes (a-) (.) all her own
10  →         bread doesn't she.
11    Doug:   Yes
12  → Kar:    I think that would be quite nice: to do (1.0) to make
13  →         bread
14            (0.4)
15  → Kar:    Don't you?
16    Doug:   Yes I °(th)-° (3.3) °ye:ah (f::::)°
17            (3.8)
18  → Kar:    (Cos) she's good at things like that in't she=bread
19  →         'n soups and=
20    Doug:   =Oh oh yeah
21  → Kar:    Things like that and she[grows ( )
22    Doug:                           [Definitely
23  → Kar:    lots of vegetables?
24            (2.2)
25  → Kar:    °Dun't she°
26            (0.5)
27    Doug:   Hhhh
28            (4.5)
29    Kar:    Which reminds me did you get your bananas yesterday?
```

Karina's tag-formatted utterances here can be seen to repeatedly make expectable responses from Doug, with a preference for Doug to produce aligning responses, agreeing with or confirming what Karina has said. In this way, Karina is able to elicit participation from Doug and to co-construct the topic talk in a particular way; while she provides the vast majority of the content, Doug's contribution can be limited to responding to – usually in the form of aligning with – that content. Here, therefore, Karina can bring into the conversation, and develop topical talk about, someone who is within Doug's lifeworld, but whom Doug himself may not have been able to topicalize within the conversation due to his impairments. At the same time, her tag-formatted utterances are hearable as an acknowledgement that this content is (or should be) within Doug's epistemic domain, and they function to elicit Doug's alignment with, and co-construction of, this content.

7 Use of Tag Questions by Co-participants

In Extracts 3 and 4 it is possible to see how a co-participant uses tag-formatted utterances to talk about what for the speaker is a 'B event' information (Labov & Fanshel, 1977), that is information that primarily is, or should be, within the recipient's epistemic domain. In each of these examples (from conversations on different days) Reg states that Sarah did not sleep well during the previous night (lines 11–12 in Extract 3; lines 11–12 in Extract 4).

Extract 3

```
01      Reg:    And Suzanne' ll (.) fetch us out n' take
02              us somewhere maybe for a meal
03              (1.3)
04      Reg     An ride round for you
05              (1.2)
06      Reg     You can say you' ve been out then.
07              (2.6)
08      Reg     Alright?
09      Sar:    °Mmm (0.3) yeah°
10              (0.5)
11  →   Reg:    Now you didn' t sleep very well last night
12  →           did ya?
13      Sar:    I don' t know. ((gaze to Reg)) °( )°
14      Reg:    You was up and down <all. night long>
15              (1.2)
16      Reg:    Saying that you couldn' t sleep.
17      Sar:    °(Right)°
```

Extract 4

```
01      Reg:    The other day there was a lot of snow in the hills,
02      Sar:    Yeah
03      Reg:    Up there.
04      Sar:    Yeah yeah w- w- its high up in' t it up there
05      Reg:    °Yeah°
06      Sar:    Mm
07              (2.2)
08      Reg:    It is.
09      Sar:    °Yeah°
10              (0.4)
11  →   Reg:    So::, you didn' t have a good night' s sleep last night
12  →           did ya
13      Sar:    I don' t know darling, didn' t I no?
14      Reg:    No no you was [awake
15      Sar:                  [(And yet) I get tired. I feel tired ↑now.
16      Reg:    Yeah.
```

Whether one has slept well or not is clearly something about which the person concerned would be expected to have primary epistemic rights. Such information concerning something experienced first-hand by the person themselves is an example of a Type 1 knowable and, as such, something that a participant has rights and obligations to know (Pomerantz, 1980). Asserting information about such issues relating to the recipient risks being heard as epistemic trespassing (Bristol & Rossano, 2020). Here this risk is mitigated to some extent by being asserted in the form of a tag question, acknowledging these issues as something which should be within the recipient's epistemic domain and eliciting a response from Sarah in regard to what is being asserted.

There is, therefore, a sense across these conversations involving a person with dementia that the co-participants are controlling the topical content of the talk through most commonly bringing into the conversation matters that they (the co-participants) already know something about, and less frequently asking the person with dementia questions to which they as questioners do not know the answer. A reason for this can be seen to be that the participants with dementia in our dataset are at a level of severity in their illness where they might not be able to provide an answer which provides the information the question is asking for. For these co-participants, tag questions are thus one alternative to producing information-seeking questions such as yes/no questions; while, like yes/no questions, they elicit a response from the person with dementia (here, typically aligning responses) and, as such, scaffold their participation in the conversation, tag questions also permit the co-participant to talk about matters about which they already have knowledge, or at least a good hunch, as to what the response might be.[5]

One area of conversation to which these issues can be seen as pertinent is topic proffers (Schegloff, 2007) by the co-participant of the person with dementia. Reg, for instance, appears to quite regularly proffer topics to Sarah in the form of tag questions. This was seen in Extract 3 (lines 11–12) and Extract 4 (lines 11–12 as well as in Extract 1 (lines 08–09). Schegloff (2007) notes that topic proffers (in conversations involving typical adult participants) are most commonly implemented by yes/no questions, and that one type of topic which is often initiated in this way is what he terms 'recipient-oriented topics' (170) where it is the recipient who is treated as the more authoritative speaker regarding the matters raised, and who is being set up to be the primary speaker in the topic. In the case of Extracts 1, 3 and 4 it is notable that Reg produces the topic proffer in the form of a tag question rather than a yes/no question. This format for doing the topic proffer means that while Reg launches a topic where he is treating Sarah as the authoritative person (regarding whether she is looking forward to visiting Jean on Wednesday, or how she slept the previous night), he does so in a way where he also has some knowledge of the matters he is proposing Sarah talks about, and thus has some control regarding how the topic might develop (compare, for example, 'did you sleep well last night?').

---

[5] As we have already suggested above, for these co-participants tag questions can also serve as an alternative to straight (non-tag formatted) assertions and assessments.

7 Use of Tag Questions by Co-participants   163

The benefits for the co-participant of having some epistemic access to the issues being discussed can be seen in Extracts 1, 3 and 4, where in each case Sarah does not take the proffered topic forward due to reasons of inability (displayed either as a statement of inability such as 'I don't know' in Extracts 3 and 4, or through her apparent disorientation in Extract 1 regarding the place in time of the issues being discussed). In such cases, Reg is then able to use his knowledge of the matters under discussion (for example, in Extracts 3 and 4 his knowledge of how well Sarah slept based on his observations of her behaviour during the night) to pick up and develop the topic.

7.3.2   Tag-Formatted Challenges

In the previous section we described the use of tag-formatted assertions and assessments by Reg and Karina, two spouses of people with semantic dementia in our dataset. In this section we describe a different type of tag-formatted utterance. This type of utterance – challenges, here in a tag-formatted form (Keisanen, 2007) – are produced by only one of the spouses, Joanna.

We discuss two episodes here. In both cases, Peter has asked Joanna a question, and following that question (either in the next turn at talk, or in a later turn) Joanna challenges it. In both Extract 5 and 6a this is done in a similar way; with 'we've just been talking about it, haven't we?' in Extract 5, and with 'we've been talking about it ... haven't we?' in Extract 6a. As such, Joanna treats the production of Peter's question at this point as inappropriate or inapposite in some manner (Heritage, 1998). That is, in requesting information, each of Peter's questions implicitly claims that he does not have access to this information, while simultaneously presupposing that Joanna does, or is likely to (Heritage, 1984). As such, Peter claims a right to ask the question, and puts some form of obligation on Joanna to answer it (Heritage & Raymond, 2012). In each case, however, Joanna produces a response which is disaligning and disaffiliative (Stivers et al., 2011); that is, rather than answering the question, she produces a challenge to Peter (see Keisanen, 2007) which disputes his implicit claim not to have had access to the information that he is requesting.

Extract 5 provides the first example.

Extract 5: Pet=Peter; Jo=Joanna
```
01      Pet:    .Hh (.) so: (.) if its clo:sed, what >what what<
02              shall I do today:?
03              (1.6)
04  →   Jo:     Ghhhh we've just been talking about it haven't we?
05      Pet:    Mm, driving range.
06              (0.3)
07      Jo:     Yup.
08      Pet:    Mm
```

The couple are chatting at breakfast. Following a lapse in the conversation Peter asks Joanna a question about what he should do that day if (due to the current cold weather) the golf course is closed (lines 01–02). In his conversations, Peter regularly asks what he or they are doing next or doing later that day, and indeed earlier in this conversation (not shown here) he has already asked a similar question ('what are we doing today?'), to which Joanna has answered that he was supposed to be playing golf with a friend but that she now has to check whether the golf course will be open or not that day. She reminds Peter they had discussed this issue earlier in the conversation and then prompts him with 'and what did I suggest?', to which Peter answers 'driving range'. So, prior to Extract 5 the couple have already discussed this issue twice in the conversation, with Joanna each time highlighting that Peter may have to go to the driving range (to practise his golf shots) rather than playing a round of golf. Peter has been able to remember this, but only after prompting.

In lines 01–02, therefore, the design of Peter's question displays that while he has remembered from earlier in the conversation that the golf course may be closed, it appears that due to his memory problems associated with dementia he has again not remembered the alternative suggested twice previously by Joanna, that is that he might go to the driving range instead. As such, Peter in lines 01–02 violates the social norm of a speaker not asking a recipient for information if the speaker has already been given that information (Stivers et al., 2011).

While an answer to the question, such as 'you could go to the driving range', would be the aligning response, Joanna does not produce this type of action. Note that such a response would ignore the inappropriateness of the question and avoid an allusion to the possible cause of that inappropriateness, that is the dementia. Instead, the delay (line 03) and laughter ('ghhhh' at the start of line 04) foreshadow a disaligning response, and when Joanna does respond (line 04), it is in the form of tag-formatted challenge to Peter's prior initiating action, with that response used to 'challenge the appropriateness or relevance of doing the action completed in the prior turn' (Keisanen, 2007: 269). Joanna's challenge in line 06 indexes Peter's question as, in effect, not justified at this juncture and, as such, can be heard as a complaint (Heinemann & Traverso, 2009). Her turn also acts as a 'counter' to Peter's question, replacing her possible answer with a question of her own (Schegloff, 2007).

The tag-formatted version of this counter-question makes two actions relevant from Peter in his response, both of which he subsequently produces (line 06): an agreement ('mm') and an answer to his own question ('driving range'). The tag format is notable since, in making relevant a response from Peter, it pushes him towards producing an aligning response, which in this case will involve him acknowledging the couple's earlier discussion of this issue. As such, Joanna's tag-formatted challenge both highlights the

7 Use of Tag Questions by Co-participants

inappropriateness of Peter's question (and, by inference, the dementia which purportedly was the cause of the inappropriate question) and pushes Peter towards acknowledging that his question was inappropriate.

Extract 6a shows a similar phenomenon. Just prior to where this extract starts, the couple have been discussing an appointment that Peter has at the hospital the following day with his cardiologist, Colin Mee. Professor Jones, a consultant who Peter sees at the same hospital concerning his dementia, has also been discussed in this conversation. As the extract starts (line 01), Joanna once again mentions Professor Jones, producing a tag-formatted assertion (which we will not further discuss here) about the hospital being the place where Peter goes to see him, with the tag eliciting an aligning response from Peter (line 02). At line 05, Peter then picks up on this mention of Professor Jones, asking 'and am I seeing ... him there?', where the 'him' refers to Professor Jones and the question clearly concerns the hospital appointment the following day. Peter has evidently forgotten, or got confused about, the earlier part of the conversation where the couple had talked about the fact that the appointment the following day was with the cardiologist, Colin Mee. As in Extract 5, Joanna treats Peter's question as an inappropriate action to have been produced at this juncture.

Extract 6a

```
01      Jo:     Its where you go to see Professor Jones (.) isn't it
02      Pet:    ⌈Mm
03      Jo:     ⌊At the hospital.
04              (3.8)
05      Pet:    And am I seeing (1.3) him there?
06      Jo:     ((head shake)) No::,
07              (2.1)
08      Jo:     No we've just discussed wh- why you're going
09              (3.8)
10      Jo:     Why are you going tomorrow?
11              (3.1)
12      Jo:     Who are you going to see?
13              (3.7)
14      Pet:    I don't know.
15      Jo:     (('disappointed' look)) Owwhh (.) you do know.
16      Pet:    ((turns head away; sighs))
17   →  Jo:     ↑We've been talking about it
18              (0.7)
19   →  Jo:     Haven't we?
20      Pet:    Mm.
21              (4.0)
22      Jo:     Going to see the <cardiologist.>
23      Pet:    ↑Oh:::: god!
```

In response to Peter's question, Joanna produces a disaffirmation (line 06). Since Joanna clearly knows who Peter is seeing at the hospital the next day, her turn consisting of a head shake and 'no' is hearable as purposefully withholding the other information that would fully answer Peter's question, that is the identity of the relevant doctor. With this turn and the several turns that follow (i.e., lines 06, 08, 10, 12, 15 and 17–19) Joanna is clearly acting in a pedagogic manner, attempting (unsuccessfully) to elicit from Peter the identity of the doctor. The last of these turns (lines 17–19) is a tag-formatted challenge which, like that in Extract 5, pushes Peter towards acknowledging (line 20) that the couple had indeed been talking earlier in the conversation about which doctor they will be seeing the following day (who is not Professor Jones), and that his question was therefore inappropriate.

In Extracts 5 and 6a the tag-formatted nature of Joanna's turns can be seen to add an element of coercion (see Hepburn & Potter, 2011) to the challenges by putting interactional pressure on Peter to acknowledge that the matters he has asked about had been discussed earlier in that conversation.[6] This element of coercion is evident when these two tag-formatted challenges (Extract 5, line 06; Extract 6a, lines 17–19) are compared with another challenge in Extract 6a by Joanna in response to Peter's question: 'no we've just discussed wh- why you're going' in line 08. While this utterance is still hearable as challenging Peter's question and implying criticism of it, the lack of an interrogative tag means that Peter is not under interactional pressure to confirm this previous discussion and thus to acknowledge any 'fault' or 'blame' on his part. Indeed, he does not produce an agreement (nor any other talk) in the next available slot (line 09), and it is Joanna who speaks next (line 10).

This coercive feature of tag-formatted challenges is seen particularly clearly in a final instance, Extract 6b, which is a continuation of Extract 6a. After his confirmation in line 20, Peter still displays an inability to identify the doctor (line 21), and at this point Joanna produces part of the answer to her own test (or 'known-answer' (Schegloff, 2007)) question in line 12, in effect reminding Peter that he is going to see the cardiologist (line 22). Joanna's production of this action is produced with a tag (line 25).

Extract 6b
```
19  → Jo:    Haven't we?
20    Pet:   Mm.
21           (4.0)
22  → Jo:    Going to see the <cardiologist.>
23    Pet:   ↑Oh::::: god!
24           (0.3)
```

---

[6] Somewhat similarly to the situation discussed above in relation to Extract 1, the tag-formatted utterances in Extracts 5 and 6a bestow competence on Peter by treating him (in a context where he has been displaying forgetfulness) as being able to remember and affirm the information being presented to him. In the case of these latter extracts, however, this bestowing of competence is done by the co-participant as part of a larger activity of complaining about the person with dementia's forgetting and not knowing (see also in this regard lines 14–15 in Extract 6a).

```
25  → Jo:    Aren't you?
26    Pet:   Yeah.
27    Jo:    The hear:t man.
28           (1.4)
29    Jo:    Colin Mee.
30           (0.4)
31    Pet:   ↑Oh: go::d! ↑yeah!
32           (3.1)
33    Pet:   Yeah yeah
34    Jo:    (('disappointed' look, breaking into small smile))
35    Pet:   I'm sorry lovey.
36    Jo:    ((reaches over and touches his hand)) no you don't
37           Have to say sorry=I know you can't help it. (0.4) Pete
38           (0.3) but-but we have y' know we've just talked about it
39    Pet:   Mm, (.) mm,
40    Jo:    Literally two minutes ago.
```

Like the tag-formatted challenges in Extracts 5 and 6a, this tag functions to elicit agreement from Peter that he had previously had access to the information requested, and indeed he then produces an agreement in line 26. A notable feature of the tag in this case, however, is that it is delayed. Not only is it separated in time from the action (line 22) that is attached to, it is also produced after a response cry (Goffman, 1978) of 'oh god' from Peter, which is hearable as claiming some form of realization that the cardiologist had indeed been discussed earlier in the conversation. In this context, therefore, Joanna's subsequent addition of the tag in line 25 acts to elicit a *further* agreement from Peter, acknowledging that he had been provided with this information earlier.

Cameron et al. (1988) discuss a somewhat similar coercive function of tag-formatted actions where the action is also indexing some action or activity of the recipient as blame-worthy. In their study, the tag-formatted utterance discussed is produced by a magistrate to a defendant and takes the form of 'you're not making much effort to pay off these arrears, are you?' Cameron et al. observe that designing this accusation with an interrogative tag is hearable 'as a way of increasing the addressee's humiliation. Not only is the defendant ... being accused of bad faith and idleness, he is also being invited (in an extremely conducive manner) to agree with the magistrate's assessment of his behaviour' (p. 88). As with Cameron et al.'s example, Joanna's tag-formatted utterances in Extracts 5, 6a and 6b work not only to critically challenge Peter and put him on the spot regarding not remembering something that (as Joanna treats it) he should have remembered, they also put interactional pressure on him to respond in a manner which will publicly acknowledge this 'blameworthy' forgetting.

As noted above, Joanna is the only spouse of the three who engages in such challenges which act to highlight some aspect of the person with dementia's conduct as inappropriate. Evidence from persons with other types of communicative impairments suggests that one motivation for the conversation partner to highlight the incompetence of the person with the impairment within conversation may be to improve that person's talk/conduct in the future (Wilkinson, 2014). Whatever Joanna's motivation, it is clear that at these points in the conversation she is choosing to display a critical stance towards the consequences of Peter's memory impairments that have resulted from his dementia and to highlight his incompetence in this regard. One consequence of this critical stance that is evident in Extracts 6a and 6b is that Peter subsequently apologizes for forgetting who the couple have been talking about (line 35). In effect, Peter has been brought to a position of apologizing for the consequences of his dementia, and Joanna's tag-formatted utterances have been a feature of her talk that have pushed him towards acknowledging, and then later apologizing for, this forgetting.

7.4 Discussion

In the Analysis section, we examined two different forms of tag-formatted utterances used by the co-participants of people with dementia in domestic conversations, that is tag-formatted assertions and assessments (Extracts 1–4) and tag-formatted challenges (Extracts 5 and 6). In the introductory section we also noted that tag questions have been discussed in the literature as a recurrent feature of 'elderspeak' talk. We will now briefly examine some tag-formatted utterances from that literature before drawing together some general features concerning tag question use by co-participants of people with dementia.

Three examples from the elderspeak literature are set out below:

> Extract 7: 'you want to get up now, don't you?' (Williams et al., 2009: 12)
> Extract 8: 'you want to take your medicine now, don't you?' (Williams et al., 2004: 6)
> Extract 9: 'you would rather wear the blue socks, wouldn't you?' (Williams et al., 2004: 7)

We should note straightaway that these three examples have limitations in terms of standard conversation analytic investigation. While the papers the examples come from are based on observational studies of nursing care for people with dementia, the examples seen in Extracts 7–9 are presented there as isolated utterances, with no talk prior to, or following, the tag-formatted utterance provided. As such, we have little information about the sequential context within which each of these utterances was produced, or how each was responded to. Nevertheless, it is possible to see from the extracts and from the discussion in the papers from which they come that in each case the care staff member is attempting to get the recipient to do something (to get up, to take their medicine, to choose a certain item of clothing). They do this using a particular turn design whereby they provide an assertion concerning what the person with dementia wants or would like (compare, for example, 'I think you should get up now' or 'it's time to take your medicine now') with a tag question appended. The tag in each case increases the deontic force of the staff member's utterance by putting interactional pressure on the person with dementia to align with what is being asserted that the person with dementia wants.[7] An aligning response by the person with dementia will be heard here as acquiescence to the suggested course of action put forward by the staff member. By analysing how the turns are designed in these ways, it is possible to see the linguistic and interactional practices through which the utterances seen in Extracts 7–9 might 'politely push older adults' answers and behaviours in a desired direction' (Schnabel et al., 2021:417).

At the start of this chapter we highlighted two reasons for analysing these tag-formatted utterances produced by co-participants of persons with dementia. One concerned how this type of utterance could be seen to be recipient-designed for a person with dementia. We have aimed to show here how the tag-formatted assertions and assessments seen in Extracts 1–4, the tag-formatted challenges seen in Extracts 5, 6a and 6b and the tag-formatted utterances by care staff suggesting what the person with dementia wants (Extracts 7–9) can each be seen to be designed in ways which take into account the fact that the recipient has dementia. As such, we suggest, such uses of tag-question-formatted turns are one way in which these co-participants have systematically adapted aspects of the way they talk, in particular in relation to turn design (Drew, 2013), when interacting with the person with dementia (see Wilkinson et al. (2011) for a discussion of adaptation, including by the co-participants of people with communicative impairments).

The second reason concerned one consequence of this adapted form of talk, that is how the tag-formatted utterances by the co-participants might influence (and, in particular, constrain) the contributions of the persons with dementia. We have noted that the tag questions produced by the co-participant put interactional pressure on the person with dementia to produce an aligning response. In the case of some types of tag-formatted utterances this aspect of tag questions appeared particularly coercive (Hepburn & Potter, 2011). For example, in Extracts 5, 6a and 6b the tags pushed Peter, the person with dementia, to confirm that questions he had asked were inappropriate due to the fact that earlier in the conversation he had been provided with information that he was now asking about. In Extracts 7–9 the person with dementia

---

[7] These utterances thus display both the coercive and psychologically invasive use of tag questions that Hepburn and Potter (2011) discuss.

appeared to be being pushed to acquiesce with a particular line of action (e.g., taking medicine now) that was suggested as being what the person with dementia themselves wanted.

It is therefore possible to see how tag questions use by co-participants of persons with dementia might be viewed negatively, as is the case in much of the elderspeak literature. However, examples such as those seen in Extracts 1 to 4 highlight a more facilitative use of this form of adapted talk, that is encouraging the participation of the person with dementia in topic talk concerning matters within that person's lifeworld. As such, an implication of the findings presented here is that tag questions per se should not be viewed as necessarily a negative or problematic feature of the talk of those interacting with people with dementia; rather, the tag-formatted utterance needs to be analysed as a whole (including in relation to the action produced in the anchor clause) within its interactive context.

Finally, and more broadly, the analysis of co-participants' use of tag questions in these extracts has highlighted how dementia can impact particular 'orders' (Stevanovic & Peräkylä, 2014) or 'territories' (Heritage, 2012) involved in human social relations, that is what Stevanovic & Peräkylä, 2014 term the epistemic order, the deontic order and the emotional order. As has been noted here, the effects of dementia can impact the affected person's control of these territories and the maintenance of their own agency in this regard.

Concerning the epistemic domain, or what Heritage (2012:4) terms 'territories of information', the impairments associated with dementia can regularly result in the person with dementia not being able to remember, and therefore not currently knowing about, features of their life which would normally be assumed as being central to an adult's epistemic domain. As seen in the extracts above, this includes personal information such as what they did recently, whether they slept well last night and other forms of Type 1 knowables (Pomerantz, 1980). As was evident in Extracts 1–4, co-participants' tag-formatted assertions and assessments can function to allow the co-participant to produce utterances which would normally be seen as epistemically trespassing (Bristol & Rossano, 2020) into the recipient's territory of information while at the same time mitigating this to some extent through the use of those tags.

Concerning the deontic order, the impairments associated with dementia may make it harder for the person with dementia to carry out everyday activities, either independently or with another person's assistance. In such circumstances, a co-participant, such as a care worker, may talk in ways (Extracts 7–9) which can be heard as encroaching on the recipient's deontic territory and, through the use of tags, putting interactional pressure on the person with dementia to acquiesce with the co-participant's suggestion as to what the person with dementia wants to do and should do.

Finally, concerning the emotional order, the impairments associated with dementia can result in the person with dementia displaying interactional incompetence in the form of, for example, producing inappropriate actions (such as asking a question concerning information which they have already been given) while being apparently unaware of this inappropriacy. In this situation, the co-participant might take it upon themselves to display a critical stance towards this presentation of interactional incompetence. Again, tags can play a role in this through eliciting agreement from the person with dementia in acknowledging the inappropriacy.

As such, it can be seen that dementia can impact on the affected person's ability to preserve their 'negative face', that is 'the basic claim to territories, personal preserves, rights to non-distraction – i.e. to freedom of action and freedom from imposition' which 'all competent members of a society have' (Brown & Levinson, 1987: 61). In the case of dementia, as seen in the extracts presented here, the co-participant of a person with dementia can orient to knowledge, power or interactional competence as being asymmetrically shared between the dyad and can produce talk which is hearable as encroaching upon the person with dementia's epistemic, deontic or emotional territory. A warrant for this can be that the person with dementia is judged by the co-participant to be not sufficiently competent (Brown & Levinson, 1987) to act independently as regards, for example, remembering what they did in the previous week (Extract 1), recognizing their inappropriate question (Extracts 5, 6a and 6b) or deciding which socks they would prefer to wear (Extract 9). In this situation, the co-participant can produce talk which, while hearably trespassing into one or more domains of the person with dementia, can act – so the co-participant could argue – to achieve something (e.g., scaffold the participation of the person with dementia in the conversation in Extracts 1–4, make the person with dementia aware of their inappropriacy in Extracts 5, 6a and 6b, or in Extracts 7–9 get a task done, such as getting the person with dementia to take their medicine). While these ways of talking can be reasonably argued as having negative consequences for the person with dementia, at least in some cases (e.g., Williams et al., 2009; Schnabel et al., 2021), they also highlight some of the difficult interactional dilemmas that co-participants of people with dementia can face in regard to how they design their talk when interacting with the affected person (see also Elsey, 2020).

References

Bristol, R. and Rossano, F. (2020) 'Epistemic trespassing and disagreement.' *Journal of Memory and Language*, 110: 104067.

Brown, P. and Levinson, S. C. (1987) *Politeness: Some Universals in Language Usage.* Cambridge: Cambridge University Press.

Cameron, D., McAlinden, F. and O'Leary, K. (1988) 'Lakoff in context: The social and linguistic functions of tag questions.' In J. Coates and D. Cameron (eds.) *Women in Their Speech Communities: New Perspectives on Language and Sex.* New York: Longman, pp. 74–93.

Drew, P. (2013) 'Turn design.' In J. Sidnell and T. Stivers (eds.) *Handbook of Conversation Analysis.* Oxford: Blackwell-Wiley, pp. 131–149.

Ekberg, K., Ekberg, S., Weinglass, L., Rendl-Short, J., Bluebond-Langner, M., Yates, P., Bradford, N. and Danby, S. (2022) 'Attending to child agency in paediatric palliative care consultations: Adult's use of tag questions directed to the child.' *Sociology of Health & Illness,* 44(3): 566–585.

Elsey, C. (2020) 'Dementia in conversation: Observations from triadic memory clinic interactions.' In R. Wilkinson, J. P. Rae and G. Rasmussen (eds.) *Atypical Interaction: The Impact of Communicative Impairments within Everyday Talk.* London: Palgrave Macmillan, pp. 195–221.

Goffman, E. (1978) 'Response cries.' *Language* 54(4): 787–815.

Goodwin, C. and Goodwin, M. H. (2004) 'Participation.' In A. Duranti (ed.) *A Companion to Linguistic Anthropology.* Malden, MA: Blackwell, pp. 222–244.

Goodwin, M. H. (1990) *He-Said-She-Said: Talk as Social Organization among Black Children.* Bloomington: Indiana University Press.

Gorno-Tempini, M. L., Hillis, A. E., Weintraub, S., Kertesz, A., Mendez, M., Cappa, S. F., Ogar, J. M., Rohrer, J. D., Black, S., Boeve, B. F., Manes, F., Dronkers, N. F., Vandenberghe, R. M. D., Rascovsky, K., Patterson, K., Miller, B. L., Knopman, D. S., Hodges, J. R., Mesulam, M. M. and Grossman, M. (2011) 'Classification of primary progressive aphasia and its variants'. *Neurology,* 76(11): 1006–1014.

Heinemann, T. and Traverso, V. (2009) 'Complaining in interaction.' *Journal of Pragmatics,* 41: 2381–2384.

Hepburn, A. and Potter, J. (2010). 'Interrogating tears: Some uses of tag questions in a child protection helpline.' In A. F. Freed and S. Ehrlich (eds.) *'Why Do You Ask?': The Function of Questions in Institutional Discourse.* New York: Oxford University Press, pp. 69–86.

(2011) 'Designing the recipient: Managing advice resistance in institutional settings.' *Social Psychology Quarterly,* 74(2): 216–241.

Heritage, J. (1984) *Garfinkel and Ethnomethodology.* Cambridge: Polity Press.

(1998) 'Oh-prefaced responses to inquiry.' *Language in Society,* 27(3): 291–334.

(2010) 'Questioning in medicine.' In A. F. Freed, and S. Ehrlich (eds.) *'Why Do You Ask?': The Function of Questions in Institutional Discourse.* New York: Oxford University Press, pp. 42–68.

(2012) 'Epistemics in action: Action formation and territories of knowledge.' *Research on Language and Social Interaction,* 45(1):1–29.

(2013) 'Epistemics in conversation.' In J. Sidnell and T. Stivers (eds.) *Handbook of Conversation Analysis.* Boston, MA: Wiley-Blackwell, pp. 370–394.

Heritage, J. and Raymond, G. (2005) 'The terms of agreement: Indexing epistemic authority and subordination in talk-in-interaction.' *Social Psychology Quarterly,* 68(1): 15–38.

(2012) 'Navigating epistemic landscapes: Acquiescence, agency and resistance in responses to polar questions.' In J.-P. De Ruiter (ed.) *Questions: Formal,*

Functional and Interactional Perspectives. Cambridge: Cambridge University Press, pp. 179–192.

Hodges, J. R. (2005) *Addenbrook's cognitive examination* [Online]. www.neurovascularmedicine.com/ace.pdf.

Holt, E. (1996) 'Reporting on talk: The use of direct reported speech in conversation.' *Research on Language and Social Interaction,* 29(3): 219–245.

Huddleston, R. and Pullum, G. K. (2002) *The Cambridge Grammar of English Language.* Cambridge: Cambridge University Press.

Jefferson, G. (2004) 'Glossary of transcript symbols with an introduction.' In G. Lerner (ed) *Conversation Analysis: Studies from the First Generation.* Amsterdam: John Benjamins, pp. 13–31.

Jokel, R., Rochon, E. and Leonard, C. (2006) 'Treating anomia in semantic dementia: Improvement, maintenance, or both?' *Neuropsychological Rehabilitation,* 16(3):241–256.

Keisanen, T. (2007). 'Stancetaking as an interactional activity: Challenging the prior speaker.' In R. Englebretson (ed.) *Stancetaking in Discourse: Subjectivity, Evaluation, Interaction,* Amsterdam: Benjamins, pp. 253–281.

Kertesz, A., Jesso, S., Harciarek, M., Blair, M. and McMonagle, P. (2010) 'What is semantic dementia? A cohort study of diagnostic and clinical boundaries.' *Archives of Neurology,* 67(4): 483–489.

Kindell, J., Sage, K., Keady, J. and Wilkinson, R. (2013) 'Adapting to conversation with semantic dementia: Using enactment as a compensatory strategy in everyday social interaction.' *International Journal of Language and Communication Disorders,* 48(5): 497–507.

Labov, W. and Fanshel, D. (1977) *Therapeutic Discourse: Psychotherapy as Conversation.* New York: Academic Press.

Levinson, S. C. (2013) 'Action formation and ascription.' In J. Sidnell and T. Stivers (eds.) *Handbook of Conversation Analysis.* Boston, MA: Blackwell-Wiley, pp. 103–130.

Pomerantz, A. (1980) '"Telling my side": "Limited access" as a "fishing" device.' *Sociological Inquiry,* 50(3–4): 186–198.

Quirk, R., Greenbaum, S., Leech, G. and Svartvik, J. (1985) *A Comprehensive Grammar of the English Language.* London: Longman.

Rasmussen, G., Dalby, K. E. and Muth, E. (2019) 'Working out availability, unavailability and awayness in social face-to-face encounters: The case of dementia.' *Discourse Studies,* 21(3): 258–279.

Robinson, J. D. (2020) 'One type of polar, information-seeking question and its stance of probability: Implications for the preference for agreement.' *Research on Language and Social Interaction,* 53(4): 425–442.

Sacks, H., Schegloff, E. A. and Jefferson, G. (1974) 'A simplest systematics for the organization of turn-taking in conversation.' *Language,* 50(4): 696–735.

Schegloff, E. A. (2007) *Sequence Organization in Interaction.* Cambridge: Cambridge University Press.

Schnabel, E. L., Wahl, H. W., Streib, C. and Schmidt, T. (2021) 'Elderspeak in acute hospitals? The role of context, cognitive and functional impairment.' *Research on Aging,* 43(9–10): 416–427.

Snowden, J., Goulding, P. J. and Neary, D. (1989) 'Semantic dementia: A form of circumscribed cerebral atrophy.' *Behavioural Neurology,* 2(3): 167–182.

Snowden, J., Kindell, J. and Neary, D. (2006) 'Diagnosing semantic dementia and managing communication difficulties.' In K. Bryan and J. Maxim (eds.) *Communication Disability in the Dementias*. London: Whurr, pp. 125–146.

Sorjonen, M.-L. and Peräkylä, A. (2012) 'Introduction.' In A. Peräkylä and M.-L. Sorjonen (eds.) *Emotion in Interaction*. Oxford: Oxford University Press, pp. 3–15.

Stevanovic, M. and Peräkylä, A. (2014) 'Three orders in the organization of human action: On the interface between knowledge, power, and emotion in interaction and social relations.' *Language in Society*, 43(2): 185–207.

Stivers, T., Mondada, L. and Steensig, J. (eds.) (2011) *The Morality of Knowledge in Conversation*. Cambridge: Cambridge University Press.

Svennevig, J. and Landmark, A. M. D. (2019) 'Accounting for forgetfulness in dementia interaction.' *Linguistics Vanguard*, 5(s2).

Taylor-Rubin, C., Croot, K., Power, E., Savage, S. A., Hodges, J. R. and Togher, L. (2017) 'Communication behaviors associated with successful conversation in semantic variant primary progressive aphasia.' *International Psychogeriatrics*, 29(10): 1619–1632.

Wilkinson, R. (2014) 'Intervening with Conversation Analysis in speech and language therapy: Improving aphasic conversation.' *Research on Language and Social Interaction*, 47(3): 219–238.

Wilkinson, R., Lock, S., Bryan, K. and Sage, K., 2011. 'Interaction-focused intervention for acquired language disorders: Facilitating mutual adaptation in couples where one partner has aphasia.' *International Journal of Speech-Language Pathology*, 13(1): 74–87.

Williams, K., Kemper, S. and Hummert, M. L. (2004) 'Enhancing communication with older adults overcoming elderspeak.' *Journal of Gerontological Nursing*, 30(10): 17–25.

Williams, K. N., Herman, R., Gajewski, B. and Wilson, K. (2009). 'Elderspeak communication: Impact on dementia care.' *American Journal of Alzheimer's Disease & Other Dementias*, 24(1): 11–20.

8 Initiating and Pursuing a Topical Agenda with Limited Communicative Resources

Anne Marie Dalby Landmark and Jan Svennevig*

8.1 Introduction

The capacity to take the initiative in conversation and influence the development and outcome of the talk may be reduced for persons living with dementia. Limited communicative resources and loss of episodic and working memory can be consequential for the opportunities of persons with dementia to voice their opinions and initiate and pursue communicative projects in interaction. In conversation, persons with dementia often take (and are given) a passive role, restricted to providing responses and answers to initiatives taken by others (Backhaus, 2018). Moreover, the epistemic authority of persons with dementia may be reduced in situations where their knowledge claims are treated by conversational partners as uncertain or unreliable (Lindholm, 2015). Also, their deontic authority may be at risk, affecting their influence on everyday matters (Lindholm & Stevanovic, 2022). As a dementia condition progresses, a person living with dementia will usually need support from formal or informal caregivers in order to meet basic needs and handle everyday tasks. People in need of institutional care may lose autonomy by caregivers imposing on their right to decide for themselves (Heinemann, 2011).

In this chapter we present a case study of an extended negotiation between a person with a dementia diagnosis and his homecare nurse, illustrating how a speaker with limited communicative resources influences the course of action and interactional outcome by taking topical initiative and persistently pursuing it across a series of sequences. The analysis focuses on how the person with dementia pursues his communicative project in two interrelated domains: first, how he argues for a specific understanding of the world, thus

---

* The authors are grateful for valuable comments by the editors, and to members of the Dementia, Language, Interaction, and Cognition Network and the research group Conversation analysis and Interactional linguistics at the University of Oslo for comments on previous versions. We also want to acknowledge the Norwegian registry of persons assessed for cognitive symptoms (NorCog) for providing access to patient data. We are indebted to the participants in the MultiLing Dementia study for taking part. This work was partly supported by the Research Council of Norway through its Centers of Excellence funding scheme, project number 223265, as well as through project number 250093.

pursuing an epistemic project of deciding 'how the world is'; second, how he promotes and pursues a decision about how to handle a practical problem, and thus seeks to accomplish a deontic project of deciding how the world 'ought to be' (Stevanovic, 2013: 298). The case is special in that it shows how a person with dementia manages to overcome interactional challenges, gain acceptance of his knowledge claims and recruit assistance with a practical task.

8.1.1   Epistemics and Dementia

In conversation, social actors regularly present and argue for specific versions of events or states in the world. As described in the field of social epistemics, knowledge is socially organized and implies normative rights and obligations concerning who is expected to know and be able to report what (Stivers et al., 2011). In typical interaction, social actors are expected to have privileged access to certain domains of knowledge, especially personal experiences (Pomerantz, 1980). Furthermore, they have epistemic authority and primary rights to report and evaluate events and states-of-affairs within these domains (Heritage & Raymond, 2005).

A central problem in atypical interaction involving persons with dementia (and other cognitive impairments) is that these fundamental expectations and rights may not always be taken for granted. Several studies have investigated how problems with episodic memory may lead to communicative problems, such as being unable to answer questions about personal history (Nilsson, 2017; Hamilton, 2019; Svennevig & Landmark, 2019; Schrauf, 2020) or making factual statements that are (more or less obviously) incorrect (Lindholm, 2015; Hydén & Samuelsson, 2019; Landmark et al., 2021). Consequently, persons living with dementia have an epistemic status that makes their knowledge claims vulnerable to doubts concerning their epistemic value (Lindholm & Stevanovic, 2022).

Such reduced expectations of epistemic access are manifested in several characteristic patterns of interaction involving persons with dementia. For instance, interlocutors may format their questions in a way that displays lowered expectations of epistemic access, such as 'do you remember...' (e.g., Williams et al., 2019) or by suggesting candidate answers in the question itself (Svennevig & Landmark, 2019). They may also perform blunt other-corrections of statements rather than inviting the persons with dementia to self-correct, thus displaying lowered expectations that they are able to access the correct information themselves (Landmark et al., 2021). When talking to third parties, spouses and other accompanying persons may answer on their behalf instead of letting the person with dementia speak for themselves (Österholm & Samuelsson, 2015; Nilsson, Ekström & Majlesi, 2018; Hamilton, 2019).

8.1.2 Deontics, Elderly Care and Agency

In conversation, social actors also negotiate rights to determine future actions (Stevanovic & Peräkylä, 2014; Rossi & Zinken, 2017). The field of social deontics studies how participants seek to define and get acceptance for what is necessary and desirable, and what should, or should not, be done in the immediate or remote future. It also investigates how they negotiate who has the right to tell others what to do and the obligation to do what others tell them to (Stevanovic & Peräkylä, 2012). The manifestations of deontic rights in conversation may vary in explicitness and degree of imposition. As shown by Kendrick and Drew (2016), ways of recruiting assistance vary along a continuum involving at least three forms. At one end we find explicit requests, in the middle we find reports or embodied displays of trouble, giving the interlocutor an opportunity to offer assistance, and at the other end of the continuum we find projectable trouble, in which the interlocutor offers assistance pre-emptively in the face of a projectable (or anticipated) trouble.

Studies from elderly care have shown that care recipients' opportunities to exert agency and influence their everyday life may sometimes be at risk. The notion of agency can be described as 'the fundamental conditions and constraints under which we pursue our goals, from the simplest everyday actions to the greatest uses and abuses of power in society' (Enfield & Kockelman, 2017: xv). In this study, agency is understood as the interactional realization of interlocutors' communicative projects, and their opportunity to exert influence over how the world *is* (epistemic rights) and how the world *ought to be* (deontic rights) (Stevanovic & Peräkylä, 2014; Antaki & Crompton, 2015). Providing help and assistance with everyday needs and tasks (e.g., health-related, social, and practical) are often given much weight in formal care settings. In later life, and especially for those living with dementia, the need for assistance, and thus reliance on others, may be pressing (Lindström, 2005; Persson & Wästerfors, 2009; Ryvicker, 2009; Brooker & Kitwood, 2019). In such cases, agency may be distributed, that is 'divided up and shared out among multiple people in relation to a single course of action' (Enfield, 2017: 9).

Elderly people in need of formal care have been shown to gradually lose autonomy and agency through the communicative practices that evolve in interaction with their caregivers. Heinemann (2011) shows how various routine activities in homecare develop over time with the effect that the roles become increasingly institutional and asymmetric, and the care recipients are gradually ascribed less autonomy. For instance, in the case of giving advice, she notes that 'advice is delivered in a way that clearly positions the caregiver as the expert with the appropriate competence to say what is, or is not, good for the care recipient, while the care recipient is treated almost like a child who is unable to determine for herself what is necessary' (Heinemann, 2011: 105).

A few studies have investigated how care recipients manage to accomplish practical tasks or resolve trouble in close collaboration with their care providers. Lindström (2005) describes a variety of syntactic structures care recipients deploy for requesting assistance in the Swedish home help service. Jansson et al. (2019) show the range of multimodal resources elderly multilinguals draw on when seeking assistance in Swedish residential care. The study describes 'the fine interplay among talk, prosody, gesture and the manipulation of an object' (p. 23) utilized for recruiting assistance from the care provider, in concert with the extensive efforts made by care providers in figuring out what kind of assistance is being sought. As pointed out by the authors, these sequences of seeking and achieving assistance 'involve great interactional efforts on the parts of both caregiver and resident' (p. 3).

Related to the question of deciding on remote actions in the future is the issue of deciding on actions in the present situation, more specifically, the development of the talk and the course of the interaction. People engage in conversation in order to accomplish communicative projects (Linell, 2009) and engage in social activities (Levinson, 1979; Mazeland, 2019). Participants may establish a joint project by agreeing on a task (such as making an appointment to go to the movies) to be carried out in collaboration through their conversational contributions. Deontic authority is manifested in the ways the participants launch such projects and influence their development. One way this may be done is by producing 'first actions' in adjacency pairs (Schegloff, 1968). First actions, such as questions and requests, set *topical agendas* and *action agendas* that enable and constrain second actions by creating expectations of alignment with the proposed topical content and the projected responsive action type (e.g., an acceptance of a request) (Heritage & Clayman, 2011). Another way deontic authority may be manifested is by pursuing an action agenda in the face of resistance or other forms of misalignment from the interlocutor (Pomerantz, 1984).

In a study of resident–staff interaction in a Japanese eldercare facility, Backhaus (2018) found a general pattern that care providers shaped the interactional flow and course of action by producing first pair parts (FPP) of adjacency pairs. Consequently, 'the residents' common lack of access to FPP turns severely curtails their agency, assigning them a largely passive role that calls for reaction rather than action' (p. 215). Of particular interest for the present study, a few deviant cases showed examples of residents going first. Backhaus noted that this 'reversed turn structure thus allows the resident to more substantially influence the course of the actions' (p. 214). The present study contributes to this line of inquiry by investigating how a person with a dementia diagnosis and limited verbal resources may successfully influence the course of action by taking topical initiatives and persistently pursuing them in the face of resistance across a series of sequences.

8.2 Data and Method

The data investigated in this chapter were collected within a larger research project on multilingual speakers with dementia in Norway (Svennevig et al., 2019). The data include audio and video recordings of seven elderly multilingual speakers with dementia collected in three different settings: psycholinguistic language testing, research interviews about their language background, and naturally occurring conversations with family, friends, and health care professionals. The data for this case study were drawn from the latter part and consists of a 38-minute-long video recording of a homecare visit. The participants were recruited from a memory clinic and from day care centres for elderly people. Informed consent was secured both in writing and orally from all participants in the study. Identifiable information such as names of persons and places are anonymized. The study has been approved by the Regional Committee for Medical and Health Research Ethics in Southeast Norway (2016/597).

The participants in the study are 'Koki' (aged 85) and his homecare nurse 'Amina'. Koki is diagnosed with amnestic Alzheimer's disease, which means that memory problems constitute the primary symptom (McKhann et al., 2011). At the time of recording, he was at a moderate stage of his dementia and lived alone in his home with support from health care professionals (nurses and home help providers) visiting three times a day for assistance in meal preparation. Amina is his primary responsible nurse, visiting Koki almost daily. Both participants are second language (L2) speakers of Norwegian. Amina has an East African background. Koki has a Northeast Asian background, and he has lived and worked in Norway since early adulthood. As L2 speakers, some of their utterances include unidiomatic constructions and non-standard pronunciation and intonation patterns, which in some cases may influence their mutual understanding. Unidiomatic constructions in the original language are marked with asterisks in the transcription, although these constructions are not always visible in the English translation (for instance when the speakers employ a word order consistent with English rather than Norwegian syntax). The data have been transcribed following the conventions developed by Gail Jefferson (2004) and are presented with a two-line transcription, where the first line represents the original talk. The second line represents an idiomatic English translation, as Norwegian and English are closely related languages, and the analysis does not focus on grammar specifically (Hepburn & Bolden, 2013).

The case is selected because it provides an illustrative example of a person with dementia managing to accomplish both epistemic and deontic goals despite limited communicative resources and a misalignment with a healthy interlocutor. By describing the communicative resources available to the person with dementia in managing a disagreement about factual states of affairs and recruiting assistance in accomplishing a practical task, it illustrates the communicative opportunities rather than the limitations of persons with cognitive and communicative challenges due to dementia. As such, it may provide important knowledge to those supporting persons with dementia in mobilizing and supporting their remaining communicative resources.

Conversation analysis (CA) is used for analysing the establishment and development of a negotiation concerning both a factual disagreement (within an epistemic domain) and a related negotiation of a practical problem (within a deontic domain). The analysis thus identifies the epistemic and deontic claims made by the participants related to these issues and investigates to what degree they are accepted or challenged by the interlocutor. Five extracts are selected for close analysis, representing the main parts of this extended, coherent negotiation about a tube of dental adhesive that Koki uses for fastening his dental prosthesis. The extracts represent the key events in the establishment of a disagreement about the origin of the tube and the resolution of it. Furthermore, they show how the participants agree on a practical task, namely to acquire a new and different type of adhesive. As such, they are chosen because they illustrate Koki's active role in furthering his epistemic and deontic goals.

8.3   Analysis

This section presents five extracts of an extended negotiation between Koki (K) and his homecare nurse Amina (A) during a dinner visit in Koki's home. The analysis focuses on how Koki initiates and pursues two (interrelated) communicative projects within an epistemic and deontic domain respectively, and what resources the interlocutors mobilize for realizing these projects.

8.3.1   The Disagreement Emerges

The first extract shows how Koki initiates a topic and thereby sets both the topic and the action agenda of the ensuing talk. Furthermore, it shows how he contradicts the nurse, thereby initiating a disagreement.

Prior to Extract 1, Amina has asked about whether he is using the dental prosthesis today. She finds out that the (pink) tube of dental adhesive he normally uses for fastening the prosthesis is empty and promises to buy a new one the next day (data not shown). Around five minutes later, while Koki and Amina are sitting by the kitchen table waiting for the soup to be ready, Koki picks up a different tube of dental adhesive standing on the table in front of him and starts inspecting it. Amina notices the embodied action, and provides a topic proffer that develops into (more) talk about the adhesive:

Extract 1 (10:57–11:29): A=Amina; K=Koki

```
01         (8.0) ((K grabs tube and inspects it))
02    A:   Er det li:m? (.) til tannprotesen?
```
Is it adhe:sive? (.) for the dental prosthesis?
```
03         (1.5)
04    K:   Har jeg fått ny:lig?
```
Have I got re:cently?
```
05         (.) ((K gazes towards A))
06    A:   .H ne:i.
```
.H no:.
```
07         (.)
08    A:   Den e' kke ny, ((head shake))
```
It isn't new,
```
09         (1.0) ((K looks down again))
10    A:   Den er gammel,= men den er ikke like god som den andre,
```
It is old,= but it is not as good as the other,
```
11    K:   Nei det e::r ny tror jeg.=
```
No it i::s new I think.=
```
           ((K takes tube out of the box))
12    A:   =Ja:.
```
=Ye:s.
```
13         (1.0) ((K holds tube up in front of him))
14    K:   Den er ny:.=
```
It is ne:w.=
```
15    A:   =Den er ny. ((small nods))
```
=It is new.
```
16         (1.0)
17    A:   Du kan br↑uke den hvis du vil altså
```
You can ↑use it if you want (you know)
```
18    A:   Så lenge- ((A points towards her teeth))
```
For now-
```
19         (0.5)
20    K:   [Je- (br)    ]
           [I-          ]
21    A:   [Jeg skal kjø]pe den andre,
```
[I will bu]y the other,

Amina topicalizes Koki's inspection of the tube by asking him whether it is adhesive that he is holding (line 02). Koki, in response does not answer the question, but directs and narrows down the topic by launching a new FPP, asking whether he has got it 'recently' (line 04). Koki's prolonged inspection of the tube and his subsequent inquiry about its origin indicate puzzlement about some state of affairs. As will become clear later in the extract, the source of this puzzlement seems to be that the tube has a different colour than the one he usually uses, as it is a weaker type of adhesive. Amina disconfirms that he got it 'recently' with an unmitigated negation, thus taking a strong epistemic stance on the matter (line 06). As Koki does not produce any receipt of information, she increments her answer twice. First, she merely explicates the import of her negation ('it isn't new', line 08, 'it is old', line 10), but subsequently she provides some additional information addressing a potential underlying concern of Koki's question (line 10). By comparing the tube to 'the other' (type), she treats his question as being concerned with the unusual appearance of the tube.

At this point, Koki initiates disagreement by producing an explicit rejection ('no') and an opposing claim ('it is new') in line 11. His epistemic position is thus upgraded from a question expressing an assumption to a declarative taking a knowing stance on the matter. The disagreeing turn is produced without delay but is somewhat mitigated by a turn final epistemic hedge ('I think').

Amina's response in line 12 is somewhat puzzling. She merely confirms his opposing claim, without any account of her change of position (such as for instance a token of 'realization'; see Emmertsen & Heinemann, 2010). The unusual character of such a response seems to be reflected in Koki's repetition of the claim, this time without any hedging (line 14). Amina again confirms (line 15), this time with an upgraded agreement, an 'echo answer' (Ferrara, 1994; Svennevig, 2003), but still without providing any account for her shift in position.

There may be several possible explanations for this unusual response. One may be that she interprets Koki's statement as not being in opposition to her own, for instance in that it invokes a different meaning of the word 'new'. The tube may not be 'new' in the apartment (that is, newly bought) but 'new' in the sense of a new type of adhesive. Another may be that she merely 'goes along' with Koki, renouncing her position on the question in the service of avoiding further disagreement (Lindholm, 2015). Both interpretations are in line with her subsequent elaboration (lines 17–18, 21), where she changes the focus from the 'newness' of the tube to its practical usefulness for Koki. There, she reorients the discussion from an *epistemic problem* related to the origin of the tube to a potential *deontic problem*, instructing him to use the current tube for now, while promising to get a new and different one. Amina thus seems to orient to Koki's original question about the tube as indicating a potential trouble with it by pre-emptively offering to buy one of the other type (Kendrick & Drew, 2016). Given that procuring food and supplies is typically a responsibility of the homecare service, she offers assistance by explicitly committing to buying a new tube.

8.3.2 Pursuing the Disagreement by Upgrading Epistemic Stance

At this point, it may seem that they have solved the epistemic problem (about the origin of the adhesive) and the deontic problem (about the usage and replacement of the adhesive). Nevertheless, in Extract 2 (following immediately after Extract 1), Koki pursues the matter further and maintains his opposing claim about the newness of the tube.

Extract (2) (11:29–12:00)

```
22   K:   Fr- fra hvem*jeg har fått den?
          Fr- from whom *I have got that?
          ((K holds tube up in the air))
23   A:   Fra o:ss, for lenge siden= ((hand over her shoulder))
          From u:s, a long time ago=
24   A:   =Den var her, ((points at the table))
          =It was here,
25        (0.7)
26   K:   ↑lE:nge siden?= ((leans forward))
          ↑Lo:ng ago?=
27   A:   =J(h)A::.(HHhh)
          =Ye(h)::s.(HHhh)
28        (1.0)
29   A:   Du har ikke sett den men den blir stående bare:
          You have not seen it but it just stays there:
30        på kjøkkenet,
          in the kitchen,
          ((A points at the table))
31        (3.5) ((K looks down, still holding the tube))
32   A:   Du kan bruke tannprotesen altså.=
          You can use the dental prosthesis (you know).=
33   K:   =Ne:i, det*komme ny:lig, ((lifts tube in the air))
          =No:, it *come re:cently,
34        (3.5) ((A wrinkles eyebrows and gazes at tube, K twists the lid
          off the tube))
35   A:   Den ↑var her i går.
          It ↑was here yesterday.
36        (1.5) ((K gaze into the tube opening))
37   K:   Ja kanskje, me:n- ((nod))
          Yes maybe, bu:t-
38        (0.5)
39   A:   ↑Ja, ((nod, glances at K, then back to the tube))
          ↑Yes,
40        (1.0)
41   K:   °M°- det*komme ny:lig. ((puts the lid back on, gazes at A))
          °M°- it *come re:cently.
42   A:   ↓Ja:. det kan hende. ((small nods, wrinkles nose))
          ↓Ye:s. that might be.
```

Koki's information-seeking question in line 22 redirects the topical agenda back to the origin of the adhesive, asking about who procured the tube. He thereby maintains control of the topical agenda. In her answer (line 23), Amina also volunteers information about the 'newness' of it, thereby relating it to the previous discussion and reverting to her original claim (in lines 08–10) that the tube came there 'a long time ago' (line 23). Koki treats this information as new and surprising by repeating the temporal expression with emphatic stress and rising intonation (line 26) (Selting, 1996). As a 'questioning repeat' (Jefferson, 1972) it merely requests confirmation, but the emphatic prosody displays a problem beyond hearing and thus makes an elaboration relevant, addressing a problem of understanding or acceptance. Amina attends to this problem indication by providing an account (lines 29–30), in which she claims that the tube has been standing in the kitchen without him noticing it. Interestingly, although she here makes a strong claim about Koki's personal experiences (what he has seen) and his personal 'territory' (his kitchen, where he spends most of his time when awake), she does not mitigate her claim of epistemic access. A long pause ensues (line 31), during which Koki withholds any expression of acceptance or rejection. Amina then self-selects and seems to move towards closure of the topic (line 32). This is done in a similar way as in Extract 1, repeating the conclusion to the practical problem about the use of the prosthesis (and the adhesive).

Koki does not respond to the closing-implicative move, but instead pursues the negotiation about the adhesive by rejecting Amina's claim with an explicit negation ('no') and an opposing claim ('it come recently') in line 33. By using falling intonation, he upgrades his epistemic stance and invites her to agree with him. Amina does not respond verbally for the next 3.5 seconds, but instead looks at the tube with an expression of concentration (wrinkled eyebrows) (line 34). By doing so, she seems to be seeking information and thus to be investigating the possibility that she might have been wrong. In conclusion to this activity, she produces a new statement ('it was here yesterday', line 35), which bolsters her position by providing evidence for her claim. Koki, in line 37, concedes to this claim, but projects further opposition by initiating a contrastive clause ('but'), which is subsequently aborted and left hanging in the air. Amina pursues a stronger expression of agreement by producing a prompt, an acknowledgement token with high pitch and rising intonation, accompanied by a nod (line 39). Koki does not accept her claim and instead repeats his own claim, upgrading his epistemic stance by producing it with falling intonation (line 41). At this point, Amina once again (cf. lines 12, 15 in extract 1) concedes to his claim by stating 'that might be' (line 42), thus backing down from her initial position. The disagreement is thereby potentially resolved by Koki gaining at least partial acceptance for his repeated claim that the tube is new. Yet, by not displaying full agreement, Amina takes an agnostic stance that does not concede full epistemic authority to Koki on the matter (Lindholm, 2015; Lindholm & Stevanovic, 2022).

8.3.3 Indicating a Practical Problem

Extract 3 shows how Koki takes a new topical initiative in the conversation, this time seemingly related to his practical concerns with the use of the adhesive.

Extract 3 (12:00–12:09)

```
43            (0.4)
44    K:      Jeg trengte den men e::,   ((lifts the tube up))
              I needed it but e::,
45    A:      Men du trenger ↑nå: eller,   ((A points to her teeth))
              But you need   ↑no:w or,
46            (0.5)
47    A:      Sk[ al du ta-     ]
              Ar[e you taking-]
48    K:         [Ikke nå:       ]
                 [ Not no:w   ]
49    K:      Ikke nå: [men e:]
              Not no:w [but e:]
50    A:               [Nei.   ] er den fast- godt nok fast?
                       [No.   ] is it tight- tight enough?
```

By pointing to a previous (unmet) need related to the adhesive, Koki redirects the topical agenda over to the deontic domain (line 44). As he runs into trouble formulating his utterance to completion, Amina seeks to help him by producing a collaborative completion (line 45). She treats the (incomplete) report as a problem alert by inquiring about his needs here and now, thereby projecting an offer of assistance (Kendrick & Drew, 2016). Koki denies having any problems at present (line 48) but proceeds by reissuing the incomplete disjunctive turn initiation ('but' from line 44) in line 49, thus projecting some other potential problem. Once again, Amina curtails his attempt to formulate his concern. Instead of giving him time to continue the turn initiation, she asks a new question about the current state of the prosthesis. In this way, Koki's two attempts to formulate his problem with the adhesive or prosthesis are both met by pre-emptive questions that orient to his needs but do not seem to contribute to clarifying his underlying concern.

8.3.4   Settling the Disagreement

Extract 4 shows how Amina settles the disagreement by further conceding to Koki's claim and providing an account for how the tube might have been brought there during the day.

Extract 4 (12:18–12:43)

```
58    K:      Men-
              But-
59            (1.5)
60    A:      Vi pleier å kjøpe til deg fordi ho: (.) som har
              We usually buy for you because she: (.) who has
61            vært før meg, hon handlet for deg=sikkert kanskje
              been before me, she shopped for you=probably maybe
62            hun har kjøpt for deg,
              she has bought for you,
```

```
63          (1.0)
64   K:     Hm?
65   A:     Du hadde handledag også i ↑dag,
            You had shopping day also ↑today,
66   K:     [ Å, ]
            [Oh,]
67   A:     [ Og ] *sikkert de har kjøpt for deg i ↑dag,
            [And] *probably they have bought for you ↑today,
68          (1.2)
69   K:     Jeg hu:sker ikke.
            I do:n't remember.
70   A:     N#e:i, det er ikke så viktig men du hadde
            N#o:, it is not so important but you had
71          handledag i dag. vi kjøpte*deg litt      [ ma::t? ]
            shopping day today. we bought *you some [foo::d?]
72   K:                                              [ Me:n-  ]
                                                     [ Bu:t-  ]
```

After yet another but-initiation by Koki, which is left incomplete (lines 58–59), Amina returns to the topic of the origin of the adhesive. This time she presents a hypothetical scenario as a potential explanation for how the tube may have been brought there during the day, thus supporting Koki's position that it has 'come recently' (lines 60–62). The downgraded epistemic stance ('probably maybe' [sic]) marks it as a tentative account. In response to Koki's open class repair initiator (Drew, 1997) (line 64), possibly orienting to the abrupt topic shift, Amina restates the alternative account, this time with an upgraded epistemic stance ('probably' line 67). Although these events are potentially accessible to Koki, having spent the day there, she treats the information as new to him and informs him about her conjectures rather than asking him about what he knows. So, despite claiming superior epistemic rights to events within Koki's epistemic domain, this seems appropriate in this situation, as Koki responds with a news receipt in the form of a change-of-state token (Heritage, 1984) (line 66), and a subsequent statement claiming lack of access to any memories of the events (line 69).

8.3.5 Resolving the Practical Problem

In Extracts 3 and 4 we saw that Koki repeatedly tried to initiate a topical shift by producing the contrastive conjunction *men* ('but'), and that he hinted at a practical problem. Extract 5 shows how Koki finally manages to formulate his practical concern, his wish to get a different tube of adhesive, and gets Amina to commit to providing him with one.

Extract 5 (12:42–13:22)
```
72   K:     [ Me:n-]
            [ Bu:t-]
```

```
73        (0.4)
74   K:   Får jeg flere*sånn?
          Will I get more (of) *these?
75   A:   Jeg kan godt gjør det slik atte det*blir ikke
          I     can very well do so    that it    *isn't
76        så tomt,
          so empty,
77        (1.5)
78   A:   Vil  du  ha  flere?
          Would you like more?
79   K:   Ja::? fordi:
          Ye::s? beca:use
80        (1.0) ((K coughs))
81   A:   Liker du bedre den rosa kanskje.
          Do you like better the pink maybe.
82   K:   Hm?
83   A:   Du liker bedre den rosa*form?
          You like better the pink *form?
84        (.) ((K leans forward))
85   A:   <Den som er ro:sa?> du liker den.
          <The one that is pi:nk?> you like that one.
86        (.) ((K gaze to the left))
87   A:   Den er hvit farge.
          That one is white color.
88   K:   Åja ro:sa ja.
          Oh yes pi:nk yes.
89   A:   Ja,
          Yes,
90   K:   Ja den*jeg liker.
          Yes that *I like.
91   A:   Ikke sant? da kan jeg kjøpe*deg i morgen.
          Right?  then I can buy *you tomorrow.
92   K:   Takk   takk   takk   takk.
          Thanks thanks thanks thanks.
93   A:   Hh i li:ge måde, Hh hh hh.
          Hh the sa:me (to you), Hh hh hh.
94   A:   Jeg ve:t du liker det.
          I kno:w you like it.
```

Koki's initiative is formulated as a request for information about the future (line 74), which Amina treats as indicating a wish to have more adhesive, which she offers to get 'so that it isn't so empty' (lines 75–76). In the face of no uptake from Koki (line 77), she pursues a response by inquiring whether he wants more (line 78). Koki immediately confirms this and initiates an account, which is, however, aborted (lines 79–80). Here Koki contributes to changing the topical agenda from the epistemic puzzle about the origin of the tube to the deontic question about what to do about the state of affairs. This also has consequences for the action agenda. By offering to procure another tube of adhesive, Amina treats Koki's question as indicating a problem with the current situation and invokes a potential solution to it. In terms of Kendrick and Drew's (2016) recruitment continuum, there is a report of a need which occasions an offer of assistance. This creates a rather equal distribution of agency in establishing the communicative project of deciding to get a new tube of adhesive.

In line 81 Amina starts making practical arrangements for the accomplishment of the service by offering a candidate guess about which colour Koki prefers. This question simultaneously provides a potential account for why he wants additional tubes of adhesive, namely that he wants a different type. After an extended repair sequence clarifying the right type ('the pink') (lines 82–90), Amina affirms her commitment to buying the adhesive (line 91), as is normatively required in granting remote action requests (Lindström, 1999). Koki responds to this by thanking her, a post-expansion that serves to ratify Amina's interpretation of line 74 as a request, his acceptance of the offer and his proposed closure of the sequence (Lindström, 2005). In addition, the fourfold reduplication of it adds an expressive and affective dimension to it, displaying (and co-constructing) the importance of the concern to him and his satisfaction with the solution (line 92). Amina reciprocates the thanking and further expands the sequence by reaffirming that she knows his preferences, thus expressing affiliation with him (lines 93–94). These affiliative contributions seem oriented towards redressing and reaffirming the social relationship between them after this prolonged negotiation.

As an epilogue, it may be noted that Koki brings up the topic of the tube twice more, approximately 10 and 22 minutes later in the visit. Both times, Koki requests confirmation of the fact that the tube is new and who brought it. In response, Amina sticks to the story that her colleague has bought the tube earlier that day. Without any epistemic hedges, she responds with 'it is new. we shop- we shopped (*you) today,'. And in response to whether he got it from her, stating 'no from my colleague who been before me here today' (data not shown). In that way, even though Koki may have forgotten their previous agreement on the state of affairs, or at least seeks confirmation of it, Amina goes along with and confirms that the tube 'came there recently'.

8.4 Discussion

This study illustrates how a person with dementia can influence the course of action and interactional outcome of a collaboratively negotiated communicative project in a naturally occurring institutional setting. By taking a topical initiative and persistently pursuing it across a series of sequences in a routine homecare visit, the person with dementia succeeds in achieving two interrelated projects in collaboration with the homecare nurse, one being within an epistemic domain (clarifying the origin of the adhesive) and the other within a deontic domain (getting the right type of adhesive). Multiple interactional resources are used for accomplishing this. First, a persistent use of first actions contributes to maintaining control over the topical agenda and establishing talk about the adhesive as a joint communicative project. The topic of the origin of the adhesive is kept on the agenda until the factual disagreement is resolved, despite the interlocutor's attempts to change the topic to related practical concerns. Second, the person with dementia's repeated knowledge claims and the interlocutor's concessions and exploration of alternative explanations contribute to moving the distribution of epistemic rights in a more symmetrical direction. Finally, the verbal and embodied displays of problems with the tube contribute to influencing the action agenda. By indicating a need for a different type of adhesive, Koki manages to recruit assistance in resolving the problem and obtaining an explicit commitment by Amina to buying a different tube.

As noted, previous studies have largely documented how the epistemic authority of persons with dementia is reduced in interaction with healthy interlocutors (e.g., Nilsson, 2017; Hamilton, 2019; Svennevig & Landmark, 2019; Lindholm & Stevanovic, 2022; see also Jones, Chapter 12 this volume; Muntigl & Hödl Chapter 9 this volume). The current study partly supports these findings, in that Amina initially treats Koki as having reduced epistemic access by taking a strong epistemic stance on a matter within the domain of Koki's personal experiences, possibly interpreting his understanding of the matters as somewhat confused. She contradicts his claims that the tube is new without accounting for her claim of epistemic authority, and she informs him about events occurring earlier that day (her colleagues shopping for him) of which she has only indirect and inferential evidence, as compared to his direct personal experience. She even claims explicitly that he has not seen the tube standing on the table, thus taking a strong epistemic stance on his perceptual experiences. In this way, she risks missing information by not exploring what he knows and instead taking for granted that he does not have access to it. However, when Koki insists on his factual claims, she changes her line of action by making concessions to his point of view and exploring alternative explanations. In this way, the case study also shows that persons with dementia may succeed in having their knowledge claims accepted and be able to engage the interlocutor in establishing a likely account of what happened, despite manifest cognitive and communicative limitations and differences in initial understandings. As stated by Antaki and Webb (2019: 1564), 'people with cognitive impairments' low epistemic status, and dubious deontic authority, always put them at risk of exclusion'. In such cases, healthy interlocutors may profit from taking time to explore the epistemic grounds for differences of opinion.

Within the deontic domain, previous research has shown that persons in elderly care may have reduced influence on decisions concerning practical courses of action in their daily life (Heinemann, 2011; Backhaus, 2018). The current study corroborates and elaborates on previous findings (e.g., Jansson et al., 2019), illustrating how persons with dementia, and with limited verbal resources, may nevertheless assert deontic authority in interaction through collaboratively recruiting assistance with practical tasks. As such, the study may contribute to our understanding of how persons with dementia may mobilize their remaining communicative resources for taking and pursuing initiatives in interaction, and how family and caregivers may recognize and support such initiatives (Svennevig & Hamilton, 2022). These findings may also be relevant beyond the case of dementia, in the support of persons with complex communicative needs caused by conditions other than dementia.

The study points to a subtle resource for recruiting assistance, namely to rely on shared knowledge. By merely drawing attention to and topicalizing the origin of the adhesive, Koki relies on the interlocutor's specific knowledge about his usage and preferences regarding this remedy for figuring out that there is a problem with it and volunteering a solution. The embodied resources used in this case thus move beyond that of 'searching' as an indicator of trouble (Drew & Kendrick, 2018), in that merely 'scrutinizing' an object in his hand is treated as a potential trouble indicator by the interlocutor. This highlights the inherent reliance on shared epistemic access as a prerequisite for identifying potential trouble alerts. Unlike the general knowledge being drawn upon for recognizing a trouble in Kendrick & Drew's (2016) and Drew and Kendrick's (2018) examples (e.g., a lighter is needed for lighting a cigarette), here, the knowledge being drawn upon for recognizing a problem is quite specific, and in this case only shared between these two persons.

This remark on shared epistemic access leads us to another implication for practice for those caring for persons with dementia. This case study exemplifies empirically the importance and benefits of continuity of dementia care, increasing the opportunity for shared epistemic access: Koki draws on the homecare nurse's specific knowledge about his preferences and care routines as a resource for solving a practical trouble. It is reasonable to assume that the road to accomplishing the same thing would have been longer if the health care professional did not know the person with dementia that well.

Our study also supports Jansson et al.'s (2019) related finding, that health care professionals are attentive to, and go to great lengths in solving everyday practical, or 'deontic needs' of the person with dementia. In addition, the present study adds that 'epistemic needs', understood as the need to sort out how the world 'is' may be given less attention by the health care professional. But in the face of Koki's topical insistence, the health care professional revises her initial position and collaborates in also resolving his 'epistemic need'. This may indicate that the 'epistemic needs' of persons with dementia (e.g., due to memory problems) may be easily overlooked in the face of multiple 'deontic needs' that must be worked out in order to provide good care (e.g., Brooker & Kitwood, 2019).

Moreover, this case study also alerts us to the danger that healthy interlocutors, in trying to assist persons with limited communicative resources in formulating their concerns, may risk derailing their project. Koki repeatedly tries to introduce a new (deontic) concern by initiating a new utterance with the contrastive conjunction 'but'. However, instead of giving him time to formulate this concern by himself, the nurse on two occasions curtails the continuation of his utterance by proposing candidate formulations of his potential concerns (Extract 3, lines 45 and 50). These suggestions turn out not to be in line with Koki's actual concern and instead end up making it more difficult for him to formulate his concern. This may alert us to the difficult balance between assisting persons with dementia in formulating their utterances and 'putting words in their mouths', a dilemma that has also been observed for conversations with L2 speakers (Svennevig, 2013). Sometimes, giving time may be more effective than making suggestions.

Finally, in the field of dementia, repetitive first actions have mainly been ascribed to the cognitive deficits caused by dementia. Examples of repeated formula (Lindholm, 2016), repeated tellings (Hydén & Örulv, 2009), and repeated assertions, narratives and questions (Hamilton, 2019) have been documented in previous studies. Hamilton describes how a person with dementia repeats assertions despite the interlocutor's attempts to close the topic. Furthermore, Hamilton (2019: 112) describes how (quite general) questions, that can be asked to anyone, are used by a person with dementia 'to move the conversation forward', although repeating the same question several times across the same interaction may also counteract the progressivity of the interaction and put the interlocutor in a challenging situation of how to respond and orient to the norm of not asking about things they (should) already know (Stivers et al., 2011). This case study tells a different story, in that Koki's repetitive actions contribute to pursuing and realizing a communicative project despite his limited cognitive and communicative resources. By repeating his first actions, he pursues a topical and action agenda in which he claims both epistemic and deontic rights. And, instead of dismissing these repeated initiatives as repetitive 'hang-ups', the care provider gradually starts exploring them and contributes to co-constructing his statement of opinion and request for action. In this way, the success of the communicative project launched by Koki is to a large extent a result of collaboration and distributed agency.

References

Antaki, C. and Crompton, R. J. (2015) 'Conversational practices promoting a discourse of agency for adults with intellectual disabilities.' *Discourse & Society*, 26(6): 645–661.

Antaki, C. and Webb, J. (2019) 'When the larger objective matters more: Support workers' epistemic and deontic authority over adult service-users.' *Sociology of Health & Illness*, 41(8): 1549–1567.

Backhaus, P. (2018) 'Reclaiming agency in resident–staff interaction: A case study from a Japanese eldercare facility.' *Discourse Studies*, 20(2): 205–220.

Brooker, D. and Kitwood, T. (2019) *Dementia Reconsidered, Revisited: The Person Still Comes First*. London: Open University Press.

Drew, P. (1997) ''Open' class repair initiators in response to sequential sources of troubles in conversation.' *Journal of Pragmatics*, 28(1): 69–101.

Drew, P. and Kendrick, K. H. (2018) 'Searching for trouble: Recruiting assistance through embodied action.' *Social Interaction. Video-Based Studies of Human Sociality*, 1(1): 1–15.

Emmertsen, S. and Heinemann, T. (2010) 'Realization as a device for remedying problems of affiliation in interaction.' *Research on Language and Social Interaction*, 43(2): 109–132.

Enfield, N. (2017) 'Distribution of agency.' In N.J. Enfield and P. Kockelman (eds.) *Distributed Agency*. New York: Oxford University Press, pp. 9–14.

Enfield, N. J. and Kockelman, P. (2017) 'Editors' Preface.' In N.J. Enfield and P. Kockelman (eds.) *Distributed Agency*. New York: Oxford University Press, pp. xi–xv.

Ferrara, K. (1994) 'Repetition as rejoinder in therapeutic discourse: Echoing and mirroring.' In B. Johnstone (ed.) *Repetition in Discourse: Interdisciplinary Perspectives* (2 vols.). Norwood, NJ: Ablex, pp. 66–84.

Hamilton, H. E. (2019) *Language, Dementia and Meaning Making*. Cham: Palgrave Macmillan.

Heinemann, T. (2011) 'From home to institution: Roles, relations and the loss of autonomy in the care of old people in Denmark.' In P. Backhaus (ed.) *Communication in Elderly Care: Crosscultural Perspectives*. London: Bloomsbury, pp. 90–111.

Hepburn, A. and Bolden, G.B. (2013) 'The conversation analytic approach to transcription.' In J. Sidnell and T. Stivers (eds.) *The Handbook of Conversation Analysis*. Chichester: John Wiley & Sons, pp. 57–76.

Heritage, J. (1984) 'A change-of-state token and aspects of its sequential placement.' In J.M. Atkinson and J. Heritage (eds.) *Structures of Social Action: Studies in Conversation Analysis*, pp. 299–345.

Heritage, J. and Clayman, S. (2011) *Talk in Action: Interactions, Identities, and Institutions* (Vol. 44). Oxford: John Wiley & Sons.

Heritage, J. and Raymond, G. (2005) 'The terms of agreement: Indexing epistemic authority and subordination in talk-in-interaction.' *Social Psychology Quarterly*, 68(1): 15–38.

Hydén, L. C. and Örulv, L. (2009) 'Narrative and identity in Alzheimer's disease: A case study.' *Journal of Aging Studies*, 23(4): 205–214.

Hydén, L. C. and Samuelsson, C. (2019) '"So they are not alive?": Dementia, reality disjunctions and conversational strategies.' *Dementia*, 18(7–8): 2662–2678.

Jansson, G., Plejert, C. and Lindholm, C. (2019) 'The social organization of assistance in multilingual interaction in Swedish residential care.' *Discourse Studies*, 21(1): 67–94.

Jefferson, G. (1972) 'Side sequences.' In D. Sudnow (ed.) *Studies in Social Interaction.* New York: The Free Press, pp. 295–331.

(2004) 'Glossary of transcript symbols.' *Conversation Analysis: Studies from the First Generation*, Amsterdam: John Benjamins, pp. 24–31.

Kendrick, K. H. and Drew, P. (2016) 'Recruitment: Offers, requests, and the organization of assistance in interaction.' *Research on Language and Social Interaction*, 49(1): 1–19.

Landmark, A. M. D., Nilsson, E., Ekström, A. and Svennevig, J. (2021) 'Couples living with dementia managing conflicting knowledge claims.' *Discourse Studies*, 23(2): 191–212.

Levinson, S. C. (1979) 'Activity types and language.' *Linguistics*, 17(5–6): 365–399.

Lindholm, C. (2015) 'Parallel realities: the interactional management of confabulation in dementia care encounters.' *Research on Language and Social Interaction*, 48(2): 176–199.

(2016) 'Boundaries of participation in care home settings: Use of the Swedish token *jaså* by a person with dementia.' *Clinical Linguistics & Phonetics*, 30(10): 832–848.

Lindholm, C. and Stevanovic, M. (2022) 'Challenges of trust in atypical interaction.' *Pragmatics & Society*, 13(1): 109–127.

Lindström, A. (1999) 'Language as social action: Grammar, prosody, and interaction in Swedish conversation (Grammatik, prosodi och interaktion i svenska samtal)', Doctoral dissertation, Acta Universitatis Upsaliensis.

(2005) 'Language as social action: A study of how senior citizens request assistance.' In A. Hakulinen and M. Selting (eds.) *Syntax and Lexis in Conversation: Studies on the Use of Linguistic Resources in Talk-in-Interaction.* Amsterdam: John Benjamins Publishing, pp. 209–233.

Linell, P. (2009) *Rethinking Language, Mind, and World Dialogically: Interactional and Contextual Theories of Human Sense-Making.* Charlotte, NC: Information Age.

Mazeland, H. (2019) 'Activities as discrete organizational domains.' In E. Reber and C. Gerhardt (eds.) *Embodied Activities in Face-to-Face and Mediated Settings: Social Encounters in Time and Space.* Cham: Palgrave Macmillan, pp. 29–61.

McKhann, G. M., Knopman, D. S., Chertkow, H. et al. (2011) 'The diagnosis of dementia due to Alzheimer's disease: Recommendations from the National Institute on Aging-Alzheimer's Association workgroups on diagnostic guidelines for Alzheimer's disease.' *Alzheimer's & Dementia*, 7(3): 263–269.

Nilsson, E. (2017) 'Fishing for answers: Couples living with dementia managing trouble with recollection.' *Educational Gerontology*, 43(2): 73–88.

Nilsson, E., Ekström, A. and Majlesi, A. R. (2018) 'Speaking for and about a spouse with dementia: A matter of inclusion or exclusion?' *Discourse Studies*, 20(6): 770–791.

Österholm, J. H. and Samuelsson, C. (2015) 'Orally positioning persons with dementia in assessment meetings.' *Ageing & Society*, 35(2): 367–388.

Persson, T. and Wästerfors, D. (2009) '"Such trivial matters": How staff account for restrictions of residents' influence in nursing homes.' *Journal of Aging Studies*, 23(1): 1–11.

Pomerantz, A. (1980) 'Telling my side: "Limited access" as a "fishing" device.' *Sociological Inquiry*, 50(3–4): 186–198.

(1984) 'Pursuing a response.' In J. M. Atkinson and J. Heritage (eds.) *Structures of Social Action*. Cambridge: Cambridge University Press, pp. 152–164.

Rossi, G. and Zinken, J. (2017) 'Social agency and grammar.' In N. J. Enfield and P. Kockelman (eds.) *Distributed Agency*. New York: Oxford University Press, pp. 79–86.

Ryvicker, M. (2009) 'Preservation of self in the nursing home: Contradictory practices within two models of care.' *Journal of Aging Studies*, 23(1): 12–23.

Schegloff, E. A. (1968) 'Sequencing in conversational openings 1.' *American Anthropologist*, 70(6): 1075–1095.

Schrauf, R. W. (2020) 'Epistemic responsibility – Labored, loosened, and lost: Staging Alzheimer's disease.' *Journal of Pragmatics*, 168: 56–68.

Selting, M. (1996) 'Prosody as an activity-type distinctive cue in conversation: The case of so-called "astonished" questions in repair initiation.' In E. Couper-Kuhlen and M. Selting (eds.) *Prosody in Conversation: Interactional Studies*. Cambridge: Cambridge University Press, pp. 231–270.

Stevanovic, M. (2013) 'Deontic rights in interaction: A conversation analytic study on authority and cooperation'. Doctoral dissertation, University of Helsinki, Helsinki.

Stevanovic, M. and Peräkylä, A. (2012) 'Deontic authority in interaction: The right to announce, propose, and decide.' *Research on Language & Social Interaction*, 45(3): 297–321.

(2014) 'Three orders in the organization of human action: On the interface between knowledge, power, and emotion in interaction and social relations.' *Language in Society*, 43(2): 185–207.

Stivers, T., Mondada, L. and Steensig, J. (eds.) (2011) *The Morality of Knowledge in Conversation* (Vol. 29). Cambridge: Cambridge University Press.

Svennevig, J. (2003) 'Echo answers in native/non-native interaction.' *Pragmatics. Quarterly Publication of the International Pragmatics Association (IPrA)*, 13(2): 285–309.

(2013) 'Reformulation of questions with candidate answers.' *International Journal of Bilingualism*, 17(2): 189–204.

Svennevig, J. and Hamilton, H. (2022) 'Fostering storytelling by persons with dementia in multiparty conversation.' In U. Røyneland and R. Blackwood (eds.) *Multilingualism across the Lifespan*. London: Routledge, pp. 169–188.

Svennevig, J. and Landmark, A. M. (2019) 'Accounting for forgetfulness in dementia interaction.' *Linguistics Vanguard*, 5(s2): 1–12.

Svennevig, J., Hansen, P., Simonsen, H. G. and Landmark, A. M. D. (2019) 'Code-switching in multilinguals with dementia: Patterns across speech contexts.' *Clinical Linguistics & Phonetics*, 33(10–11): 1009–1030.

Williams, V., Webb, J., Dowling, S. and Gall, M. (2019) 'Direct and indirect ways of managing epistemic asymmetries when eliciting memories.' *Discourse Studies*, 21(2): 199–215.

Part 4

Dementia and Epistemics

9 Identifying Family Members in Photographs
Practical Epistemic and Deontic Challenges for a Person with Frontotemporal Dementia

Peter Muntigl and Stephanie Hödl

9.1 Introduction

The behavioural variant of frontotemporal dementia (bvFTD), unlike Alzheimer type dementia, is not typically characterized by a decline in cognitive ability or memory, but rather by a marked decline in social and emotional functioning (Neary et al., 1998). Although memory impairment may not be prevalent in bvFTD, especially in the early stages of the illness, difficulties in accessing personal domains of knowledge may become present and noticeable. Many people with bvFTD, for example, are largely ignorant of any changes in their behaviour, displaying a 'lack of insight' concerning the effects that bvFTD is having on them and their family members (O'Keeffe et al., 2007). Persons with bvFTD are also considered to be unable to construe an appropriate *theory of mind* (ToM), which generally refers to the ability to take the perspective of another person in terms of their beliefs and intentions (Kipps & Hodges, 2006). Some persons also have difficulty in recognizing familiar faces (i.e., friends and relatives), as for example on photographs (*prosopagnosia*). Although much research has focused on studying these aspects of knowledge from a medical standpoint, much less work has been done to uncover the interactional processes by which a person with bvFTD's knowledge displays are realized and managed in dialogue.

For this chapter, we use the methods of conversation analysis (CA) to examine the practical epistemic and deontic organization of viewing family photos. In particular, the focus is placed on sequences that involve difficulties in identifying persons in photos and how talk and conduct is managed to facilitate person identification. Our data are taken from a case study that involves one individual, Trudy, who was diagnosed with bvFTD and who lived at home and was regularly attended to by a caregiver and a nurse. To explore the interactional organization of identifying persons in photos in this context, we examine the following questions: (1) how is person identification organized as an activity and which interaction formats are used in its accomplishment?; (2) how does this activity shed light on the person with bvFTD's epistemic domain vis-à-vis the other conversational participants?;

(3) which sequences index a 'reduced' epistemic domain (e.g., through uncertainty or not knowing) and which maintain Trudy's epistemic status of being the primary knower of her own biography? Advantages and pitfalls of this activity for persons with bvFTD are also discussed.

9.2 Epistemics and Deontics

Conversation analytic research has shown that *epistemic* and/or *deontic* features tend to permeate social actions in sequence (Drew, 2018; Heritage, 2013; Stevanovic & Peräkylä, 2014; Stevanovic & Svennevig, 2015). Whereas the term 'epistemics' generally refers to how *knowledge* is displayed and organized in talk and conduct, 'deontics' refers to how actions around *goods and services* are negotiated.

Epistemics can be considered along three different vantage points: *domain, status* and *stance* (Heritage, 2013). For the first, it is recognized that people have knowledge about different kinds of experiential domains. A similar view has been put forward by Labov and Fanshel (1977), who make the distinction between *A-events* and *B-events*. A-events may refer to knowledge derived from first-hand experience, whereas B-events refer to knowledge that is indirectly acquired through reports or inference (see also Pomerantz, 1980). Further, experiential domains or *territories of knowledge* may transcend 'everyday' knowledge and be unequally distributed amongst different persons and/or groups (Heritage, 2013). For example, through socialization and training, doctors acquire direct access and rights to so-called medical knowledge, whereas patients generally retain access to 'lifeworld knowledge' (Mishler, 1984). Differential access and rights to a given epistemic domain (e.g., someone's personal life-world experiences or specialized medical knowledge) will give rise to differences in epistemic status pertaining to a given domain. In this way, persons are generally considered to have greater authority and entitlement to know about their own biographies – what happened to them, past events in their own lives – as do specialists working in a given field (e.g., medicine, law, engineering, restaurant cuisine, construction, fashion, etc.).

Epistemic stance, on the other hand, is looked upon as a more transient construct, and is gauged by a speaker's momentary use of a vast array of discursive/interactional resources to convey degree of rights and access to knowledge – including grammatical mood (i.e., interrogative, declarative), modality, prosody, facial expressions and others (Heritage, 2013). Each instance of stance-taking occurs in a sequentially unfolding context and thus creates ongoing (and sometimes changing) points of reference to speakers' statuses as related to various epistemic domains. In CA, stances that index an upgraded epistemic position is represented as [K⁺], whereas a downgraded position is represented as [K⁻] (Heritage, 2013).

Deontics is a relevant concept for actions that get others to do things, such as requests, commands, proposals or suggestions (Couper-Kuhlen, 2014; Landmark et al., 2015; Stevanovic & Svennevig, 2015). These actions, which generally fall under the rubric of *directives*, involve some future event or task to be accomplished, orient to speakers' rights and responsibilities, and make relevant some form of acceptance or compliance by the recipient or commitment to carry out the task (Couper-Kuhlen, 2014). It has been shown that the discursive make-up of directives (e.g., the expressions and words used to design the directive) orient to various general principles that involve the degree of *entitlement* to direct another's actions, *contingencies* associated with the potential for refusal (e.g., ability or willingness to comply), sensitivities to the speakers' role relationships with respect to agency and who will benefit from the action, the amount of work or 'cost' needed to recruit another into action and the degree of immediacy or urgency for directing another (Clayman & Heritage, 2014; Drew & Couper-Kuhlen, 2014; Kendrick & Drew, 2016; Mikesell, Chapter 5 this volume; Rossi, 2012; Sorjonen et al., 2017).

Recent research on persons with Alzheimer's dementia (AD) has been examining epistemics and especially A-events (or *Type 1 knowables* involving the person's biographical knowledge: Pomerantz (1980)). The focus has been on forgetfulness and the kinds of *fishing devices* used to either get persons with AD to 'remember' (Nilsson, 2017) or the kinds of practices that persons with dementia use to account for their lack of knowledge or ability to remember (Jones 2015, Chapter 12 this volume; Svennevig & Landmark, 2019). Epistemic research on bvFTD has examined how persons with bvFTD display degrees of insight or understanding (or a lack thereof) when asked about personal life events (Avineri, 2010; Mikesell, 2014; Muntigl et al., 2014). By examining the practical epistemic and deontic organization of viewing family photos, this chapter extends understanding of how a person with bvFTD may navigate everyday contexts in which displaying and/or accessing her own biographical knowledge may prove difficult.

9.3 Data/Method

The data are taken from a study that was undertaken in Austria to investigate the talk and conduct of persons with bvFTD (see Muntigl et al., 2014). One component of this study involved participants taking part in an activity that involved looking at family photographs and discussing aspects of the photos (e.g., who the people in the photo are, where the photograph was taken, what happened on that day, etc.). From a total of seven persons who had been diagnosed with bvFTD, a female participant, Trudy, was selected for this chapter. It was initially observed that she had difficulty in identifying persons in photos and thus we thought that interactions with Trudy would shed important light on how knowledge is organized in contexts involving a larger social epistemic network. Trudy was seventy at the time, living in a house in a rural area. She had three grown-up children, grandchildren and a great-grandchild. A caregiver who was responsible for taking care of Trudy's everyday needs lived with her and she also received regular visits from a nurse. The following people participated in these conversations: Trudy = Tr/ the person with bvFTD; a researcher = R; Trudy's daughter, Joanna = D; a caregiver = CA; a nurse = N. All conversations did not follow a pre-determined script and unfolded in a spontaneous manner.

The conversation was videotaped and transcribed using the transcription conventions from Hepburn & Bolden (2013). Transcriptions of bodily comportment and multimodality were further informed by Mondada (2018); for example, simultaneous or concurring vocal and non-vocal conduct was indicated using special symbols (e.g., '+', '#') – see the key at the beginning of the book. All examples used in this chapter contain English translations from the original Austrian German. Identifying information was removed from the transcriptions and all persons involved were given pseudonyms. The method used to analyse the conversations was CA (Sidnell, 2013) and the analytic concepts *epistemics* and *deontics* were taken from Heritage (2013) and Stevanovic & Svennevig (2015). The analytic focus was placed on sequences in which Trudy was asked to identify a family member in a photograph. Attention was given to the initiating action (e.g., what type of action was it? what were the design features?), Trudy's response (or lack of response) and the ensuing talk that attended to getting Trudy to identify the person in the photo.

9.4   Analysis

Examination of the videotaped conversation revealed that the activity of identifying family members was accomplished via several sequence types. In general, these involved sequences that contained initiating actions with *wh*-interrogative or imperative formats. Differences were found in the epistemic stances taken up by participants and in the sequence organization when 'correct' vs. 'incorrect' answers were produced. Further, although Trudy did tend to regularly display uncertainty when asked to identify a family member in a photo, she was able to display certainty and knowledge about aspects of her own (Type 1) biography in 'face-to-face' contexts with a family member.

9 Identifying Family Members in Photographs

These various epistemic/deontic aspects pertaining to identifying family members will be reviewed in subsequent sections.

9.4.1 Practices to Request Information

Three different kinds of request formats were used to get Trudy to identify persons in the photographs. The first two were most often produced in *wh*-interrogative format: *Who are they?* and *Who is that?* The third practice, *Find X*, used a directive format to initiate a 'seek and find' activity. From the perspective of deontics, the other family members use these request formats to exercise control of the conversation, deciding on the topic (identifying a person) and speaker selection (Trudy is directed to answer).

9.4.1.1 Wh-interrogative: 'Who Are They?'

One type of action used to request identification of persons from Trudy is the *wh*-interrogative '*Who are they?*' This format creates some 'openness' with respect to Trudy's options for answering: that is, she has some choice in deciding whom to identify and thus in displaying what she knows. For example, if she cannot recall any specific names, she has the option of choosing a descriptor – such as 'my grandchildren', 'my daughter's children' and so on. Thus, by asking 'who', the researcher is generating options in terms of descriptor response – Trudy could answer with a name or a more general descriptor. Extract 1 provides an example of this interrogative format by the researcher, whose epistemic domain regarding Trudy's family relations is negligible (the *wh*-interrogative is in bold).

Extract 1: R=researcher; Tr=Trudy; D=daughter; CA=caregiver

```
01    R:      +Wer sind die+
              +Who are they+
      R       +points to 3 different persons in photo, her grandchildren+
      Tr      looks at photo

02            (5.7)
      Tr      looks away from photo and towards her daughter

03    D:      Na schau das genau an wer dort auf'm bühdl is.
              Well look at that carefully who there is on the picture.

04            (0.8)

05    Tr:     Ja we::r.
              Yeah who::.
      Tr      looks at photo

06    CA:     Du kennst zicher zehr gut.
              You know certainly very well.

07            (0.5)
```

08	Tr:	Bist es d̲u.
Is it y̲ou.
	Tr	looks over at others
09	D:	Na schau' s ↓an und dann sagst unsers.
Well look ↓at it and then tell us.
10	CA:	Noch e̲inmal.
Once a̲gain.
	Tr	looks again at photo
11	D:	Ganz genau anschauen
Look at it ve̲ry carefully
12		(1.0)
13	Tr:	Is des S̲usi.
Is that S̲usi.
	Tr	points at photo, repeatedly tapping it with her finger
14	D:	[↓Na::
[↓*No::*
15	CA:	[Hm hm. des is-
[*Hm hm. it is-*
16		(3.4)

At the beginning of this extract, the researcher seeks information by posing a *wh*-interrogative question ('who are they'), while simultaneously pointing to and drawing mutual gaze/attention towards the various people on the photo (i.e., Trudy's grandchildren, who are not present in the room). The pronoun 'they' offers the addressee some flexibility in responding because she has some authority in deciding whom she will identify; for example, she could name the people she knows or she could simply name one person, thus satisfying the requirements of the question, at least in part. This *wh*-format also creates a certain epistemic scene by presupposing that Trudy *can* identify the people in the picture – compare an alternative design such as 'do you know who they are?', which would leave open the possibility that Trudy does not possess this knowledge. In line 2, rather than orient to the researcher, Trudy looks at – and thus possibly seeks help from – the others in the room with whom she is more familiar (possibly also trying to form a connection between the person in the photo and the people in the room). Thus, although the long silence does imply some difficulty in knowing the answer, her gaze may suggest some incipient knowledge of who can help her and who might know the answer. The daughter, in line 3, then directs Trudy to focus on the picture using an imperative format ('well look at that carefully who there is on the picture'), thus reinforcing Trudy's epistemic position as K⁺. Trudy then responds in line 5 by requesting help, implying that she does not know and is thus unable to take up this knowledge position ('yeah who::'). In the next turn, the caregiver then provides encouragement by explicitly ratifying Trudy's epistemic status of knowing the identity of the persons in the photo ('you know certainly very well'). Trudy responds with a guess and by looking over at her daughter ('is it you'), signalling out one of the persons. However, in line 9 the daughter resists providing confirmation and again places the burden of answering back onto Trudy by using an imperative format to direct her to focus on the picture and to identify the person ('well look ↓at it and then tell us'). Thus, by not confirming (or disconfirming), the daughter treats Trudy's utterance as merely a guess and, further, implies that her guess was incorrect. In sum, what began as a *wh*-interrogative produced by someone who has low epistemic status (i.e., who does not know the identities of the people in the photo and is 'genuinely' seeking this information) is transformed into imperative-initiated sequences produced by persons with high epistemic status (i.e., they know the identities of the people in the photo), who now direct Trudy into providing an answer by focusing on the photo – the subsequent unfolding of this interaction is shown in Extract 8.

9.4.1.2 Wh-interrogative: 'Who Is That?'

Another type of initiating *wh*-interrogative format, '*Who is that?*', provides a more constrained set of identifying response options because the relevant next action is to name the individual being referred to (either with a proper name or even a person category reference such as 'my daughter'), rather than choosing freely to name some or all of the persons. This kind of format appears in Extract 2 and occurs about a minute after Extract 1.

Extract 2: R=researcher; Tr=Trudy; D=daughter; CA=caregiver

```
25    R:    Probier ma anders- anders foto.
            Let's try a different- different photo.
      Tr    looks directly at photo ———————>

26          (               4.1                  )
      Tr    ———> looks away towards others in room

27    CA:   ↓Ja::
            ↓Yes::

28    Tr:   [H(h)ah hah hah hah hah hah.

29    R:    [+Wer is des. wer is des.+
            [+Who is that. who is that.+
      R     +points at a specific person with a tapping motion+
```

30	CA:	Wer is #das. du kennst zicher. Trudy. **Who is #that.** *you know for certain. Trudy.*
	Tr	#looks again at photo
31		(1.2)
32	Tr:	Jo<u>a</u>nna. bist des <u>du</u>. *Jo<u>a</u>nna. is that <u>you</u>.*
	Tr	taps finger on photo
	Tr	looks towards D, towards the photo, then towards D
33	D:	<u>G</u>enau. =des bin <u>i</u>:. *<u>Ex</u>actly. =that's <u>me</u>:.*
34	CA:	Super. perfekt. ja:? *Super. perfect. yes:?*
35	Tr:	i hab ma's hoit a so d(h)e(h)nkt. *I just kinda th(h)ou(h)t so.*
	Tr	looks at the photo

The researcher begins this extract by suggesting that they move on to a different photograph. The *wh*-interrogative in line 29 this time targets a specific person ('who is that. who is that'), making it relevant to name the individual and thus constraining the options for producing a next action. Here, as in Extract 1, the *wh*-format presupposes that Trudy possesses the requisite knowledge needed to answer correctly. The researcher simultaneously points at the individual and so may be attempting to draw mutual gaze/attention back towards this person. Trudy's looking away from the photo and towards the others may not only be conveying a lack of engagement with the activity but also a request for others to help by providing an answer. The caregiver immediately responds in line 30 by first redoing the request ('who is that') and then by offering 'encouragement', ratifying Trudy's higher epistemic status ('you know for certain. Trudy'). Again, as in Extract 1 the change of speaker doing the initiating actions – from researcher to caregiver – marks a shift in the epistemic alignment, or *footing* (Goffman 1981), between requester and requestee. Whereas the researcher does not know who is in the picture, the caregiver does, and thus has certain entitlements to make claims about Trudy's epistemic status. Trudy then answers by providing the name of her daughter ('<u>Joanna</u>'), but then downgrades her epistemic stance by requesting confirmation from her daughter ('is that <u>you</u>'). The daughter provides confirmation in line 33 and the caregiver provides strong positive assessment in line 34 ('super. perfect. yes:?').

To summarize, this extract marks a change in activity from the researcher *seeking information* from Trudy from a K⁻ position (i.e., the researcher does not know the identity of the person in the picture) to an *exam question* in which a 'social network member' (SNM) such as the daughter or caregiver knows the

Table 9.1 *Epistemic positions compared for seeking information vs. exam questions*

	Seeking Information		Exam Question	
Position	Speaker	Epistemic position	Speaker	Epistemic position
1. Question	Researcher	K^-	SNM	K^+
2. Response	Trudy	K^+	Trudy	$K^{+/-}$
3. Response	Researcher	K^-	SNM	K^+

person's identify and thus tests Trudy's knowledge from a K^+ position. The initial epistemic position in sequence is important because it sets the stage for what is to come. In seeking information, respondents are placed in a K^+ position and, because the questioner does not know the answer, a relevant third position action is to claim information receipt as K^- (Heritage, 1984). It should be emphasized that, for information-seeking questions, respondents are positioned as K^+ regardless of whether or not they know the answer. It is most likely for this reason that respondents generally provide accounts to explain why they cannot take up the assumed K^+ position. Exam questions, which are claimed to follow a *question–answer–comment* sequence (Mchoul, 1978; Mehan, 1979), have a different epistemic organization. Because questioners already possess knowledge, they take up a K^+ position. Further, the epistemic status of the respondent is 'undetermined' and dependent on the third position feedback of the questioner. Thus the questioner remains as K^+ in this sequence and respondents will be positioned as K^+ if they are correct, or as K^- if they are not – see Table 9.1 for an overview of the epistemic organization of these sequences.

Relating these observations to conversations involving persons with dementia, Drew (2018) makes the point that, drawing from Jones (2015), this reversal in epistemic status in exam questions may be used as a way of monitoring the person with dementia's declining mental state and, further, may cause anxiety because the person with dementia is expected to know but may not be able to demonstrate this knowledge. Thus these exam questions may yield face-threatening situations, leading to disaffiliation between SNMs and the person with dementia (see also Jones, Chapter 12 this volume, and Webb, Chapter 15 this volume, for similar arguments).

9.4.1.3 Directives: Find 'X' [=Specific Person]

The third format, shown in Extract 3, is a directive that is initiated by members of Trudy's close social network. Although this directive format may presuppose that Trudy can take up a K^+ position by identifying the person, it also appears as a 'test' and thus may be more similar to exam questions in which the person giving the directive knows and the person being directed has a 'yet-to-be-determined' knowledge state – the researcher does not have this expert knowledge and therefore this directive format is not available for him to use. The directive also indexes a certain deontic alignment, with the daughter/caregiver leading the trajectory of talk and Trudy following their lead.

Extract 3: R=researcher; Tr=Trudy; D=daughter; CA=caregiver

```
01   D:    Na +wo is dein sohn.
           Well where is your son.
     Tr     +looks towards D

02         (1.8)
     Tr    maintains gaze @ D ->

03   D:    Tsoarg uns.
           Show us.
     Tr    ————————>

04   CA:   Wo is dein #drittes kind Trude. [dein drittes kind.
           Where is your third child Trude. [your third child.

05   D:                                    [Da fesche bua
                                           [The handsome boy.
     Tr    ————————>
     Tr             #looks back at photo ————————>

06         (2.0)

07   CA:   Dein brave bub. mm?
           Your good boy. mm?

08   Tr:   Da maxi?
           Maxi?

09   CA:   Na::.
           No::.

10   D:    Dein so:hn.
           Your so:n.

11         (7.3)
     Tr    towards end of the silence briefly glances up then back at photo

12   Tr:   (1.2)
     Tr    points at and rests finger on a person in photo

13   CA:   Su:::per.

14         (0.7)

15   D:    Genau. des is a.
           Exactly. that's him.
```

The extract begins with the daughter issuing a directive to Trudy, telling her to locate her son in the photo ('<u>where</u> is your son'). This represents Type 1 autobiographical knowledge and so the assumption is that Trudy should be able to take up a K$^+$ position by identifying her son. Rather than looking at the picture and engaging in the activity of finding the person, she instead continues to look at her daughter. This leads the daughter to issue a directive in imperative format ('show us'), which orients to Trudy as not looking at the photo and thus not properly engaging with the activity. In line 4 the caregiver latches onto this turn by adding more *granularity* (i.e., detail) to the directive (Schegloff, 2000), specifying that Trudy should search for her third child, and the daughter, as an overlapping turn, deepens granularity by adding another attribute ('the handsome boy'). Trudy shifts her gaze to the photo, but does not respond, which results in a 2-second silence, leaving the caregiver to provide another attribute ('your good boy') and a turn-final expression that seeks elicitation ('mm?') in line 7. What then follows is a conversational practice that has been termed *try-marking* (Sacks & Schegloff, 1979; Schegloff, 2007). This generally involves the use of a 'first name recognitional' with an upward intonational contour. Thus, Trudy makes a try or guess as to whom she is supposed to be looking for, but this is immediately rejected by the caregiver in line 9 and also countered by the daughter (line 10), by which it can be inferred that Maxi is not her son. Trudy continues to focus her attention on the photograph for some time and then, in line 12, she identifies an individual by pointing at and resting her finger on a person in the photo. Her response then receives upgraded positive evaluation by both the caregiver and the daughter. As with the prior two extracts, this extract has shown Trudy's difficulty in demonstrating knowledge in a domain of which one is generally expected to have primary access (i.e., Type 1 knowables). Although the hints do work to help Trudy locate the right person, they also seem to mark the growing frustration among the persons in Trudy's close social network that she is taking so long to complete the task and that she might not successfully identify her son.

9.4.2 Displaying Difficulty with Answering

Trudy most often displays difficulty with responding to the first pair part action produced by either the researcher or by someone from her closer social network (e.g., daughter or caregiver/nurse). In this section we explore in detail how these sequences are accomplished by showing (1) how Trudy displays downgraded epistemic access in her response (e.g., by guessing, remaining silent, disengaging from the activity); (2) how co-present interactants pursue a response from Trudy via hints (Nilsson, 2017), encouragers and directives to get Trudy to focus attention on the photo; and (3) how co-present interactants account for or assess Trudy's performance within post-sequences.

9.4.2.1 Guessing: Indexing Downgraded Epistemic Access

Trudy's response sometimes appeared in the form of a Yes/No-interrogative, commonly as '*is it/that X?*' These actions seek confirmation, thus allowing the recipient to take up a K^+ position (Heritage 2013). Two examples of this practice have already been seen in Extract 1, where Trudy asked 'is it you' and 'is that Susi', both utterances receiving disconfirmation. Another example is shown in Extract 4.

Extract 4: R=researcher; Tr=Trudy; D=daughter

```
01   R:    Wer is des.
           Who is that.
     R     points at Tr in the photo

02         (4.4)
     Tr    gazes at the photo then looks over at D

03   Tr:   Bist es du.
           Is it you.

04   D:    ↓Na[i ben's ned.
           ↓No[its not me.

05   Tr:   [Na.
           [No.
     Tr    lateral head movement
     Tr    looks again at the photo
```

The researcher's *wh*-interrogative *who is that* gives Trudy an opportunity to take up increased epistemic rights by supplying the answer to 'who'. Trudy's response of 'is it you' does different kinds of interactional work. First, the interrogative format displays uncertainty (compare with the declarative: 'it's you'), as does the long 4.4-second pause that precedes it. Second, her question opens up another sequence, which not only delays the provision of the answer but also puts the burden of responding/confirming onto the daughter. And third, the two former interactional features index a diminished epistemic stance because Trudy displays uncertainty about the person's identity, and also shows that she must rely on others to confirm or provide the sought-for information. In the next turn, the daughter completes the sequence through disconfirmation ('↓no its not me'), leaving the identity of the person in the photo as yet-to-be determined.

9.4.2.2 Response Pursuit from Recipients

Because Trudy was most often not able to immediately name the person in the photo, the other interlocutors were often found to pursue a response through various interactional practices. These included providing hints, encouraging Trudy to respond and getting Trudy to focus on the photo.

9.4.2.2.1 Hinting

Actions that provide hints generally give an interlocutor a clue or some information that allows the interlocutor to make an appropriate inference. This kind of discursive work is shown in Extract 5, which is a slightly longer version of Extract 4. Trudy is shown a photo of herself, taken many years earlier.

Extract 5: R=researcher; Tr=Trudy; D=daughter

```
01    R:      Wer is des.
              Who is that.
      R       points at Tr in photo

02            (4.4)
      Tr      looks at picture then looks over at D

03    Tr:     Bist es du.
              Is it you.

04    D:      ↓Na[i ben' s ned.
              ↓No[its not me.

05    Tr:     [Na.
              [No.
      Tr                  lateral head movement
      Tr                  looks again at the photo

06            (1.0)

07    D:      Des is mei mutter.
              That is my mother.

08            (0.7)

09    Tr:     Dei mutter.=
              Your mother.=
      Tr      gaze at D
```

From the analysis of Extract 4, it was shown that Trudy displayed uncertainty and, in effect, did not provide an answer to the researcher's initial *wh*-interrogative. After the daughter disconfirmed that she was the person in the photo, followed by an affirming 'no' from Trudy in line 5, a 1-second silence ensued, making a response from Trudy once again relevant. In line 7 the daughter provides a reference to the person's identity ('that is my mother'). Thus, by inference, Trudy is Joanna's mother and it would be assumed that Trudy could make that connection. After a brief pause, Trudy provides a partial repetition of Joanna's prior turn with clause-final intonation while looking at her, a type of *mirroring* (Ferrara, 1994), which could be displaying a form of reflection or 'being thoughtful'.

Hints from Trudy's social network also take the form of providing more detail, or granularity (Schegloff, 2000), or clarifying who the referent may be, as seen in Extract 6, which forms the beginning of Extract 3.

Extract 6 [taken from Extract 3]: Tr=Trudy; D=daughter; CA=caregiver

```
01  D:   Na +wo is dein sohn.
         Well where is your son.
    Tr      +looks towards D

02       (1.8)
    Tr   maintains gaze @ D ->

03  D:   Tsoarg uns.
         Show us.
    Tr   ------------>

04  CA:  Wo is dein #drittes kind Trudy.  [ dein drittes kind.
         Where is your third child Trudy. [ your third child.

05  D:                                    [ Da fesche bua
                                          [ The handsome boy.
    Tr   ------------>
    Tr   #looks back at photo ------------------->

06       (2.0)

07  CA:  Dein brave bub. mm?
         Your good boy. mm?
```

As already discussed in relation to Extract 3, the daughter had initially directed Trudy to identify her son, but as no response was forthcoming, the caregiver and the daughter provided Trudy with further information or hints. Thus the others provided more 'granular descriptions' of the person being referenced, which might make the identification of the person in the picture easier ('your third child; the handsome boy; your good boy').

These practices align with what has previously been identified in CA research as *pursuing a response* (Davidson, 1984; Pomerantz, 1984); that is, following a no-response from the recipient or in the presence of interactional features that presage a dispreferred response such as an inability to answer, practices are set in motion that may facilitate the respondent's capacity to take up epistemic rights and access by providing the preferred response – in this case, the *correct* answer.

9.4.2.2.2 Encouragers

In contexts where Trudy is showing some difficulty with answering, the members of her social network sometimes provide expressions of encouragement, as shown in Extracts 7 and 8.

9 Identifying Family Members in Photographs

Extract 7 [taken from Extract 2]: R=researcher; Tr=Trudy; CA=caregiver

```
25   R:    Probier ma anders- anders foto.
           Let's try a different- different photo.
     Tr    looks directly at photo ─────────>

26         (          4.1          )
     Tr    ─────> looks away towards others in room

27   CA:   ↓Ja::
           ↓Yes::

28   Tr:   [H(h)ah hah hah hah hah hah.

29   R:    [+Wer is des. wer is des.+
           [+Who is that. who is that.+
     R      +points at specific person with tapping motion+

30   CA:   Wer is #das. du kennst zicher. Trudy.
           Who is #that. you know for certain. Trudy.
     Tr          #looks back at photo
```

Extract 8 [taken from Extract 1]: Tr=Trudy; D=daughter; CA=caregiver

```
17   D:    °Wer is des.°
           °Who is that.°

18   CA:   Probier's. (0.5) noch einmal schnell daran denken
           Try it. (0.5) once again quickly think about it
     Tr    looks away from photo then towards others

19         (0.8)

20   D:    Schau das an s' bühdl.
           Look at it the picture.

21         (1.5)
     Tr    looks back at photo

22   CA:   Du kennst zicher zehr gut.
           You know certainly very well.

23         (1.0)
     Tr    moves photo away, in front of her

24   CA:   Deine enkel
           Your grandchildren
```

In Extract 7, following the researcher's *wh*-interrogative of line 29 asking Trudy to identify a person in the photo, in the subsequent turn the caregiver repeats the question and appends an expression that endorses Trudy's epistemic competence ('you know for certain. Trudy'), thus offering encouragement and confidence that Trudy will be able to give the correct answer. During this time Trudy looks back at the photo, showing that she is willing to re-engage with the task. Similarly in Extract 8, after Trudy's repeated delays in responding, the caregiver works to strongly bolster her capacity to identify the person ('you know certainly very well'). On the upside, these expressions of encouragement are a show of confidence ('you know this!') and work to upgrade Trudy's epistemic status. They also work as a response pursuit strategy, maintaining structural alignment on the joint task of getting Trudy to provide the 'right' answer. But on the downside, in cases when Trudy is not able to remember or provides an incorrect answer, they are exposing her lack of epistemic authority, resulting in a situation where Trudy can (repeatedly) lose face.

9.4.2.2.3 Attention-Focus Directives

Response pursuits do not necessarily focus on the person's epistemic status, whether or not they have the ability to access a certain domain of knowledge. At times, response pursuits orient to the person's lack of attention or engagement with the task and call upon the person to become more focused.

Extract 9: [taken from Extract 1]: Tr=Trudy; D=daughter; CA=caregiver

```
08    Tr:    Bist es du.
             Is it you.
      Tr     looks over at others

09    D:     Na schau' s ↓an und dann sagst unsers.
             Well look ↓at it and then tell us.

10    CA:    Noch einmal.
             Once again.
      Tr     looks back at photo

11    D:     Ganz genau anschauen
             Look at it very carefully

12           (1.0)

13    Tr:    Is des Susi.
             Is that Susi.
      Tr     points at photo, repeatedly tapping it with her finger

14    D:     [↓Na::
             [↓No::
```

15	CA:	[Hm hm. des is- [*Hm hm. it is-*
16		(3.4)
17	D:	°Wer is des.° °*Who is that.*°
18	CA:	Probier' s. (0.5) noch einmal schnell daran denken **Try it. (0.5) once again quickly think about it**
	Tr	*looks away from photo then towards others*
19		(0.8)
20	D:	Schau das an s' bühdl. **Look at it the picture.**
21		(1.5)
	Tr	*looks back at photo*
22	CA:	Du kennst zicher zehr gut. *You know certainly very well.*
23		(1.0)
	Tr	*moves photo away, in front of her*
24	CA:	Deine enkel *Your grandchildren*

Following Trudy's guess in line 8 and then shifting her gaze away from the photo, the daughter does not offer confirmation or disconfirmation, but instead directs Trudy to focus on the photograph ('well look ↓at it and then tell us') – the response may imply disconfirmation (i.e., it is not her) and it may also work as a refusal to respond, suggesting that Trudy should answer for herself. Subsequent to this, in line 9, is another directive to engage with the photo, this time from the caregiver ('once again'), immediately followed by another imperative-formatted directive from the daughter, calling on Trudy to focus her attention ('look at it very carefully'). After a confirmation-seeking sequence, comprising a guess from Trudy ('is that Susi') and then a disconfirmation ('↓No::'), her social network again uses focusing-attention directives. First, in line 18, the caregiver begins with a bare imperative ('try it'), followed by a command to focus quickly on the photo. Trudy, however, disengages from the activity by shifting her gaze away from the photo, which leads the daughter, in line 20, to again direct Trudy to look at the photo ('look at it the picture').

To summarize, response pursuits from Trudy's close social network seem to be guided by both epistemic and deontic concerns. Hints work at helping Trudy to 'find' the right answer and demonstrate her ability to remember

Type 1 autobiographical knowledge. Encouragers also focus on epistemics by displaying confidence in her being able to access personal knowledge domains. Attention-focus directives, on the other hand, orient to deontics by urging Trudy to re-engage with and focus on the task at hand. Thus response pursuits both orient to Trudy's difficulty in taking up a K⁺ position concerning Type 1 knowables and in remaining focused on tasks.

9.4.3 Assessments in Sequential Third Position

Following the question- or directive-response sequence, a member of Trudy's social network has the opportunity to produce what may be termed a third position assessment (Schegloff, 2007; see also Table 9.1 for exam questions). These are slots in which family members may account for or assess Trudy's performance. In many of the extracts shown thus far, Trudy's (second position) response was not correct. This resulted in a negative assessment of Trudy's response in third position, such as the daughter's '↓no its not me' seen in Extract 4. This negative evaluation also has important sequential implications. Because Trudy has not yet got it right, the activity of identifying the person on the photo has not come to a close, but rather there is an implication that subsequent talk will orient to getting an eventual identification. Thus, as has been shown, the speakers mobilize various practices in the pursuit of a (correct) response, such as by offering hints, adding more granularity or even getting Trudy to (re-)engage and focus on the photo.

When Trudy provides a correct answer, however, different response types will occur in third position. This is shown in Extract 10.

Extract 10: [from Extract 2]: Tr=Trudy; D=daughter; CA=caregiver

```
30    CA:    Wer is das. du kennst zicher. Trudy.
             Who is that. you know for certain. Trudy.

31           (1.2)

32    Tr:    Joanna. bist des du.
             Joanna. is that you. ((taps finger on photo))
      Tr     taps finger on photo
      Tr     looks towards D, back to photo, then towards D

33    D:     Genau. =des bin i:.
             Exactly. =that's me:.

34    CA:    Super. perfekt. ja:?
             Super. perfect. yes:?
```

Trudy's correct identification of her daughter in line 32 is followed by Joanna's positive assessment ('exactly') and confirmation ('=that's me:'), which gets further upgraded by the caregiver in line 34 with 'super' and 'perfect' (see also Webb, Chapter 15 this volume, and Jones, Chapter 12 this volume, for discussions of similar evaluative third position responses). According to Schegloff (2007), these expressions work as *sequence closing thirds*. As the name suggests, they close off the sequence, thereby licensing the start of a new sequence.

9.4.4 Certainty Displays

Trudy's responses to first position *wh*-interrogatives to identify a person in a photo or first position directives to 'find X' are often hesitant and designed as guesses. She also often disengages with the activity by looking away from the photo. There were instances, however, in which her responses displayed certainty, as in Extract 11.

Extract 11: [a continuation of Extract 5]: Tr=Trudy; D=daughter; CA=caregiver

```
07    D:    Des is mei mutter.
            That is my mother.

08          (0.7)

09    Tr:   Dei mutter.=
            Your mother.=
      Tr    looks at D

10    D:    =Wer is den des.
            =Who is that.

11          (6.8)
      Tr    looks at photo then looks over to D

12    Tr:   i bin des ned.
            It's not me.

13    D:    Na schau das a:n.
            Well look a:t it.

14          (11.0)
      Tr    looks at photo
```

At the beginning of this extract Joanna had provided Trudy with a hint to help her identify the person in the photo ('that is my mother'). It can be recalled that Joanna is actually referring to Trudy (from an earlier period in her life). Although Trudy, in line 9, partially repeats the prior turn through mirroring, thus displaying some form of 'reflection', she does not go on to say that she herself is in the picture. Trudy may thus be conveying slight hesitancy or even incipient disagreement with her daughter. In line 10 Joanna repeats the request to identify using a *wh*-interrogative, leading Trudy to again engage with the photo before looking back up towards Joanna. Trudy then responds with a declarative devoid of modal expressions displaying uncertainty ('it's not me'). In this way, she indicates who the person on the photo is *not*, thus contradicting her daughter. What this disagreement shows is that Trudy has indeed understood the daughter's hint ('my mother' = 'Trudy'), but also that Trudy is not always displaying uncertainty and can take up an upgraded epistemic stance even if her professed knowledge turns out to be incorrect. Nonetheless, her contradiction does expose other cognitive deficits, since it shows that she was not able to 'recognize' a younger version of herself.

Another example in which Trudy denies with certainty that a given person in the picture is not the one that she is looking for is shown in Extract 12.

Extract 12: Tr=Trudy; D=daughter; CA=caregiver; N=Nurse

```
01   N:     Findst du der Joanna ihr' n mo:h.
            Can you find Joanna's hu:sband.

02          (              13.0              )
     Tr     looks at photo, then away
     D                      places a different photo in front of Tr

03   N:     Is a des.
            Is that him.

04   D:     Wer is den des.
            Who is that

05          (      3.2      )
     Tr     pounds on photo with right fist

06   Tr:    [Hhh h(h) ah hah.
07   ?      [Ahhhhh

08   Tr:    Wer is den
            Who is it
     Tr     looks at the others

09   N:     Wer is. sag ↓unsers. schau ihn genau an dann sagst unsers.
            Who is it. tell ↓us. look at him closely then tell us.

10          (5.3)

11   Tr:    D- der Joanna ihr mo:h is des ned. i ke(h)nn d(h)e(h)n
            T- the its not Joanna's hu:sband. I don't kn(h)o(h)w
     Tr     looks at photo, makes a fist and clenches teeth

12          Ü(h)be(h)rhau(h)pt ned.
            H(h)im a(h)t a(h)ll.
     Tr     looks at photo, makes a fist and clenches teeth
```

9 Identifying Family Members in Photographs   217

```
13          (3.0)

14   CA:   Und gestern gut. mama hat       [g' zagt. gestern gut und jetzt.
           And yesterday good. mama had [said. yesterday good and now.

15   D:                                    [ Mm hm.
16          (2.0)

17   D:    Gestern hat' s es kannt.
           Yesterday she could recognize him.
```

In line 1 the nurse directs Trudy to identify Joanna's husband using the 'find X' turn format. The photo shown to Trudy has many people in it and so might prove overly challenging for her. After Trudy has looked at the picture for over 10 seconds, the daughter then places a different picture in front of Trudy containing only one person, Joanna's husband. The nurse then requests confirmation from Trudy ('is that him), followed immediately by a *wh*-interrogative from Joanna ('who is that'). Thus, to respond affirmatively, Trudy needs either to confirm the prior question with 'yes' or state that it is Joanna's husband. Instead, in line 5 Trudy makes a visible emotional display consisting of her pounding her fist on the person in the picture, followed by a brief outburst of laughter and, in line 8 produces a *wh*-interrogative ('who is it'). Trudy's question serves as a *repair initiator* (Schegloff et al. 1977) because she is soliciting help in answering the question, but it also serves as implicit disagreement because it does not offer the preferred variant (confirmation or 'the answer') to the prior questions. In line 9, rather than provide the 'repair', the nurse repeats the question and then produces an attention-focus directive ('look at him closely then tell us'), suggesting that Trudy's inability in answering is due to her lack of attention and not a 'faulty' memory. As a response, however, Trudy makes a certain display of denying that it is Joanna's husband and that she has no knowledge of or any relationship to this person (lines 11–12). While constructing her turn, Trudy also makes various emotional displays of anger or irritation by clenching her teeth and making a fist while looking at the (unknown) person in the photo. In lines 14–17, occurring off-camera, the caregiver and the daughter explain to the researcher that Trudy was able to easily recognize Joanna's husband in the photo on the previous day.

9.4.5 *Displaying Knowledge of Co-present Interlocutors*

The activity of identifying and displaying knowledge of persons appeared to be different when comparing contexts of 'looking at family photos' to 'everyday talk between co-present interlocutors'. Extract 13, which occurred towards the end of the research, shows an example of how Trudy is able to display unsolicited knowledge about personal life events that include her daughter.

Extract 13: R=researcher; Tr=Trudy; D=daughter; CA=caregiver

```
01   D:    [Schau den an.
            [Look at him.

02   Tr:   [Du::.
            [You::.
     Tr    moves hand towards and touches D's leg

03   Tr:   Bist meine erste tochter.
            Are my first daughter.
     Tr    holds lightly onto D's shirt

04   D:    Des stimmt. [ja
            That's right.[yes

05   Tr:                [Ja:.
                         [Ye:s.

06   Tr:   Die hab i g'macht wie i achtzehn jahr oid war.
            You I made when I was eighteen years old.

07   D:    Genau.
            Exactly.

08   Tr:   Ja:.
            Yes:.

09         (1.8)

10   Tr:   [Du bist mei:
            [You are my:

11   D:    [Und wie hoas i?
            [And what's my name?

12   D:    Wie hoas i?
            What's my name?

13         (1.5)

14   Tr:   Joanna.

15   D:    Mm hm.

16         (3.3)

17   D:    Und wie hoast mei bua?
            And what's my boy's name?

18         (2.4)

19   Tr:   Lois.
```

9 Identifying Family Members in Photographs

```
20   D:    Na des is mei ↑mo:h. wie hoast- (0.7) mei ↑bua.
           No that's my ↑hu:sband. what is (0.7) my ↑boy's name.

21         (4.2)

22   Tr:   Hans.
     Tr    looks at D

23   D:    Genau. und hat da Hans a scho a kind.
           Exactly. and does Hans already have a child.
     D     points at Tr

24         (4.5)

25   Tr:   Ja.
           Yes.

26         (2.3)
     Tr    looks at D

27   D:    Genau.
           Exactly.

28   Tr:   Hat er oans oder zwar.
           Does he have one or two.

29   D:    Uh oans hat a.
           Uh he has one.
     D     holds up 1 finger

30   Tr:   Oans hat a.
           One he's got.

31   D:    Und wie hoast ↑der.
           And what's ↑his name.

32         (5.0)
     D     points to person in photo towards end of silence

33   D:    Is des da Hans.
           Is that Hans.

34         (1.6)

35   Tr:   Ja koh eh sein das a der Hans is.
           Yes that's possible that that's Hans
     Tr    looks at photo

36         (4.7)

37   D:    Jaja des is a.
           Yeah yeah that's him.
     Tr    looks at D
```

38	Tr:	((nods))
39	D:	Wann's das sagst, geh
		If you say so, right

In line 1 of this extract, the daughter Joanna is about to initiate another round of person identification by getting Trudy to focus on another photo ('look at him'). At the same time, however, Trudy initiates a different move by verbalizing the second person pronoun 'You::' and non-vocally by touching her daughter's leg. She then continues her turn in line 3 by stating or announcing some biographical information ('are my first <u>daughter</u>'). Thus, in contrast to the other extracts examined so far, Trudy initiates a sequence and shows that she can be a cooperative and engaged participant in the interaction. By doing so, she also takes up primary epistemic rights and access (Heritage, 2013). Following a confirming response from the daughter, Trudy continues to provide even more biographical information ('you I made when I was eighteen years old'). The daughter's response in line 7 confirms what Trudy has said, but it might also be doing additional work. Because Trudy would, by most accounts, have first-hand, primary knowledge of at what age she gave birth to her daughter, Joanna's response of 'exactly', by emphasizing the 'correctness' of what Trudy said, treats this knowledge as contestable; that is, she could have gotten it wrong and this biographical knowledge may not necessarily (or no longer) be in Trudy's epistemic domain. In line 10, Trudy begins a turn in which it appears that she will be launching another statement, thus taking up primary epistemic rights ('you are my:'), but what follows instead are a series of *exam questions* or *known answer questions* (Levinson, 1992; Schegloff, 2007) in which Trudy's knowledge about her personal social network is being tested. For example, the questions directed to Trudy – 'what's my name?', 'and what's my boy's name?', 'and does Hans already have a child' and 'and what's ↑his name' (lines 11, 17, 23, 31) – are obviously all known to Joanna, and her third position responses of 'mm hm' and 'exactly' reveal this. In line 28, after being asked if her grandchild Hans has a child, Trudy displays some uncertainty as to whether he has one or two. After it is confirmed that Hans has only one child, Joanna proceeds to ask Trudy to identify someone in a photograph (lines 31–32) and, following no response, provides a hint ('is that Hans'). Trudy's response is designed with some uncertainty ('yes that's possible that that's Hans'), which is then confirmed by Joanna in line 37. Then, following Trudy's nod of agreement in line 38, Joanna orients to Trudy's uncertainty in being able to recognize or identify Hans ('if you say so, right').

It has often been noted that persons with frontotemporal dementia sometimes have difficulty in initiating sequences resulting in interlocutors doing most of the work to keep the interaction going (Mikesell, 2009). What Trudy displayed at the beginning of Extract 13, however, is the ability to take conversational initiatives and to speak about pertinent aspects of her personal biography – perhaps triggered by the proceeding focused activity of getting her to identify family members in photographs. In doing so, she was also able to take up a position of epistemic authority, to reveal some parts of her epistemic domain. But even though the daughter did at first cooperate with Trudy's initiatives, the conversation eventually reverted to a perhaps more typical conversational agenda in which Trudy is tested on what she knows, with the unfortunate result of often making clear where she is lacking in knowledge.

9.5 Discussion

The use of photographs and what is termed *life story books* have been suggested to be useful devices in stimulating recall and positive emotions, and are thus commonly used as interactive tools for persons with dementia (Elfrink et al., 2018). Family photographs align with the person's Type 1 autobiographical knowledge and thus present themselves as opportunities for persons with dementia to take up epistemic authority and disclose information or events pertaining to their lives.

For this chapter, we chose to examine someone who had difficulty recognizing persons from their close network in photographs for the following reasons. We wanted to study how these 'person recall' activities using photographs were interactively organized, how downgraded epistemic rights and access were displayed, and how interactional difficulties of 'non-recall' were managed. We found systematic practices that oriented to Trudy's difficulty, which other persons with bvFTD also share. Generally, Trudy would respond to questions with *wh*-interrogatives by guessing at the answer, using expressions that conveyed no knowledge of the person's identity or disengaging from the activity by diverting her gaze and attention elsewhere. These kinds of responses to questions or directives helped to construct an epistemic stance that indexed a reduced epistemic domain with respect to her ability in recognizing family members in photos. This led to a variety of response pursuits in which her co-present close social network members would provide hints, encouraging her to keep trying and make positive assessments (when she guessed correctly). Oftentimes, however, Trudy was unable to take up a K^+ position, which had negative implications for face and also her relationships with members of her close social network (see also Webb, Chapter 15 this volume): that is, remembering your family members is a necessary precondition for maintaining these relations, and constantly being 'reminded' that you are no longer competent in this domain (i.e., remembering your children, grandchildren, etc.) may have a negative impact on ways of relating with these people in the future (see also Jones, Chapter 12 this volume). Trudy was, however, able to take up a position of epistemic authority in two important respects. First, she was often able to strongly assert who was *not* in the photo – even though she was not necessarily correct in her assertion – and second, she seemed to find it easier to display knowledge about personal events with co-present persons with whom she had a close relationship.

The activity of looking at family photos did not seem to stimulate much recall for Trudy; that is, she was generally not successful in, for example, naming the people in the photo, stating the relationships between them (and to herself) or even saying something about the context in which the photo was taken. A previous CA study on persons with bvFTD's use of reference terms while looking at photos has shown that these persons may sometimes *over-suppose and under-tell* or, conversely, *under-suppose and over-tell* (Mates, 2010). In the former a person could state the person's name, for example, without clarifying the kinship relations (e.g., my sister, daughter, grandchild, etc.), whereas in the latter a person could provide an excess of referential information in cases where the addressee already knows the information. In this case study, Trudy did not seem to properly align with either of these practices, as she consistently displayed difficulties in accessing this knowledge, although, according to some members of her social network present during the conversation, she has days where she is able to recall the names of her family members much more easily. Thus her epistemic status in relation to this territory of knowledge is not constant, but fluctuates. Further, Trudy's ability to display knowledge of and recognize co-present familiar persons suggests that her capacity to access biographical knowledge may be facilitated by various features pertaining to her everyday present setting or to other people's typical conduct or ways of relating to her (perhaps the manner in which they speak with her or their voice patterns). Difficulties seem to emerge when she is required to display knowledge without the proper contextual scaffolding, as seen when she is asked to look at family photographs. To conclude, on days where persons with bvFTD are finding it especially difficult to take up a K^+ position, there may be a larger 'social payoff' when others in the close social network ease up rather than persist in using (exam-like) strategies to solicit answers.

References

Avineri, N. (2010) 'The interactive organization of "insight": Clinical interviews with frontotemporal dementia patients.' In A. W. Mates, L. Mikesell and M. S. Smith (eds.) *Language, Interaction and Frontotemporal Dementia: Reverse Engineering the Social Mind.* London: Equinox, pp. 115–138.

Clayman, S. E. and Heritage, J. (2014) 'Benefactors and beneficiaries: Benefactive status and stance in the management of offers and requests.' In P. Drew, and

E. Couper-Kuhlen (eds.) *Requesting in Social Interaction*. Amsterdam: John Benjamins Publishing Company, pp. 55–86.

Couper-Kuhlen, E. (2014) 'What does grammar tell us about action?' *Pragmatics*, 24(3): 623–647. doi:10.1075/prag.24.3.08cou.

Davidson, J. (1984) 'Subsequent versions of invitations, offers, requests, and proposals dealing with potential or actual rejection.' In J. M. Atkinson and J. Heritage (eds.) *Structures of Social Action: Studies in Conversation Analysis*. Cambridge: Cambridge University Press, pp. 102–128.

Drew, P. (2018) 'Epistemics in social interaction.' *Discourse Studies*, 20(1): 163–187. doi:10.1177/1461445617734347.

Drew, P. and Couper-Kuhlen, E. (2014) 'Requesting – from speech act to recruitment.' In P. Drew, and E. Couper-Kuhlen (eds.) *Requesting in Social Interaction*. Amsterdam: John Benjamins Publishing Company, pp. 1–34.

Elfrink, T. R., Zuidema, S. U., Kunz, M. and Westerhof, G. J. (2018) 'Life story books for people with dementia: A systematic review.' *International Psychogeriatrics*, 30(12): 1797–1811. doi:10.1017/S1041610218000376.

Ferrara, K. W. (1994) *Therapeutic Ways with Words*. New York: Oxford University Press.

Goffman, E. (1981) *Forms of Talk*. Philadelphia: University of Pennsylvania Press.

Hepburn, A. and Bolden, G. B. (2013) 'The conversation analytic approach to transcription.' In J. Sidnell and T. Stivers (eds.) *The Handbook of Conversation Analysis*. Chichester, UK: John Wiley & Sons, Ltd, pp. 57–76.

Heritage, J. (1984) 'A change-of-state token and aspects of its sequential placement.' In J. M. Atkinson and J. Heritage (eds.) *Structures of Social Action: Studies in Conversation Analysis*. Cambridge: Cambridge University Press, pp. 299–345.

(2013) 'Epistemics in conversation.' In J. Sidnell and T. Stivers (eds.) *The Handbook of Conversation Analysis*. Oxford: Wiley-Blackwell, pp. 370–394.

Jones, D. (2015) 'A family living with Alzheimer's disease: The communicative challenges.' *Dementia*, 14(5): 555–573. doi:10.1177/1471301213502213.

Kendrick, K. H., and Drew, P. (2016). 'Recruitment: Offers, requests, and the organization of assistance in interaction.' *Research on Language and Social Interaction*, 49(1): 1–19. doi:10.1080/08351813.2016.1126436

Kipps, C. M. and Hodges, J. R. (2006) 'Theory of mind in frontotemporal dementia.' *Social Neuroscience*, 1(3–4): 235–244. doi:10.1080/17470910600989847.

Labov, W. and Fanshel, D. (1977) *Therapeutic Discourse: Psychotherapy as Conversation*. New York: Academic Press.

Landmark, A. M. D., Gulbrandsen, P. and Svennevig, J. (2015) 'Whose decision? Negotiating epistemic and deontic rights in medical treatment decisions.' *Journal of Pragmatics*, 78: 54–69. doi:10.1016/j.pragma.2014.11.007.

Levinson, S. C. (1992) 'Activity types and language.' In P. Drew and J. Heritage (eds.) *Talk at Work: Interaction in Institutional Settings*. Cambridge: Cambridge University Press, pp. 66–100.

Mates, A. W. (2010) 'Using social deficits in frontotemporal dementia to develop a neurobiology of person reference.' In A. W. Mates, L. Mikesell and M. S. Smith (eds.) *Language, Interaction and Frontotemporal Dementia: Reverse Engineering the Social Mind*. London: Equinox, pp. 139–166.

Mchoul, A. (1978) 'The organization of turns at formal talk in the classroom.' *Language in Society*, 7(2): 183–213. doi:10.1017/S0047404500005522.

Mehan, H. (1979) *Learning Lessons: Social Organization in the Classroom.* Cambridge, Mass.: Harvard University Press.

Mikesell, L. (2009) 'Conversational practices of a frontotemporal dementia patient and his interlocutors.' *Research on Language & Social Interaction*, 42(2): 135–162. doi:10.1080/08351810902864552.

(2014) 'Conflicting demonstrations of understanding in the interactions of individuals with frontotemporal dementia: Considering cognitive resources and their implications for care and communication.' In R. W. Schrauf and N. Müller (eds.) *Dialogue and Dementia: Cognitive and Communicative Resources for Engagement.* New York: Psychology Press, pp. 147–180.

Mishler, E. (1984) *The Discourse of Medical Interviews.* New Jersey: Ablex.

Mondada, L. (2018). 'Multiple temporalities of language and body in interaction: Challenges for transcribing multimodality.' *Research on Language and Social Interaction*, 51(1): 85–106. doi:10.1080/08351813.2018.1413878

Muntigl, P., Hödl, S. and Ransmayr, G. (2014) 'Epistemics and frontotemporal dementia.' *Ricerche di Pedagogia e Didattica – Journal of Theories and Research in Education*, 9(1): 69–95.

Neary, D., Snowden, J. S., Gustafson, L. et al. (1998) 'Frontotemporal lobar degeneration: A consensus on clinical diagnostic criteria.' *Neurology*, 51(6): 1546–1554.

Nilsson, E. (2017) 'Fishing for answers: Couples living with dementia managing trouble with recollection.' *Educational Gerontology*, 43(2): 73–88. doi:10.1080/03601277.2016.1260911.

O'Keeffe, F. M., Murray, B., Coen, R. F., Dockree, P. M., Bellgrove, M. A., Garavan, H., Lynch, T. and Robertson, I. H. (2007) 'Loss of insight in frontotemporal dementia, corticobasal degeneration and progressive supranuclear palsy.' *Brain*, 130(3): 753–764. doi:10.1093/brain/awl367.

Pomerantz, A. (1980) 'Telling my side: "Limited access" as a "fishing" device.' *Sociological Inquiry*, 50(3–4): 186–198. doi:10.1111/j.1475-682X.1980.tb00020.x.

(1984) 'Pursuing a response.' In J.M. Atkinson, and J. Heritage (eds.) *Structures of Social Action: Studies in Conversation Analysis.* Cambridge: Cambridge University Press, pp. 152–166.

Rossi, G. (2012) 'Bilateral and unilateral requests: The use of imperatives and *mi X?* interrogatives in Italian.' *Discourse Processes*, 49(5): 426–458. doi:10.1080/0163853X.2012.684136.

Sacks, H. and Schegloff, E. A. (1979) 'Two preferences in the organization of reference to persons in conversation and their interaction.' In G. Psathas (ed.) *Everyday Language: Studies in Ethnomethodology.* New York: Irvington Publishers, pp. 15–21.

Schegloff, E. A. (2000) 'On granularity.' *Annual Review of Sociology*, 26(1): 715–720. doi:10.1146/annurev.soc.26.1.715.

(2007) *Sequence Organization in Interaction: A Primer in Conversation Analysis.* Cambridge: Cambridge University Press.

Schegloff, E. A., Jefferson, G. and Sacks, H. (1977) 'The preference for self-correction in the organization of repair in conversation.' *Language*, 53(2): 361–382. doi:10.1353/lan.1977.0041.

Sidnell, J. (2013) 'Basic Conversation Analytic Methods.' In J. Sidnell and T. Stivers, (eds.) *The Handbook of Conversation Analysis*. Chichester, UK: John Wiley & Sons, Ltd, pp. 77–99. doi:10.1002/9781118325001.ch5.

Sorjonen, M.-L., Raevaara, L. A. and Couper-Kuhlen, E. (2017) 'Imperative turns at talk: An introduction.' In M.-L. Sorjonen, L. A. Raevaara and E. Couper-Kuhlen (eds.) *Imperative Turns at Talk: The Design of Directives in Action*. Amsterdam: John Benjamins, pp. 1–24.

Stevanovic, M. and Peräkylä, A. (2014) 'Three orders in the organization of human action: On the interface between knowledge, power, and emotion in interaction and social relations.' *Language in Society*, 43(2): 185–207. doi:10.1017/S0047404514000037.

Stevanovic, M. and Svennevig, J. (2015) 'Introduction: Epistemics and deontics in conversational directives.' *Journal of Pragmatics*, 78: 1–6. doi:10.1016/j.pragma.2015.01.008.

Svennevig, J. and Landmark, A. M. D. (2019) 'Accounting for forgetfulness in dementia interaction.' *Linguistics Vanguard*, 5(s2). doi:10.1515/lingvan-2018-0021.

10 'You Know This Better'

Interactional Challenges for Couples Living with Dementia when the Epistemic Status Regarding Shared Past Events Is Uncertain

Anna Ekström, Elin Nilsson and Ali Reza Majlesi*

10.1 Introduction

In this chapter we analyse an interview with a couple where one of the spouses has a dementia diagnosis. Our detailed sequential analyses are focused on how the couple talks about events when the person with dementia might not always remember the events being talked about. Telling about life with dementia can be a sensitive topic, especially when the topic concerns difficult and problematic experiences due to the disease, or when problems related to the disease become an issue in the telling. In the excerpts analysed for this chapter, the spouse without dementia is the teller of a story in which the spouse with dementia is a main character. As persons with dementia may have trouble remembering the specific details of past events in their own lives, their *epistemic authority* (Heritage & Raymond, 2005) might be questioned (see Landmark et al., 2021; Lindholm & Stevanovic, 2022; also Jones, Chapter 12 this volume; Muntigl & Hödl Chapter 9 this volume). In interactions between couples, therefore, partners of people diagnosed with dementia recurrently have to take into consideration that their spouse may not remember accounts and details of stories they tell, even though the person with dementia may be the main character of the story. In such instances, the person with dementia may not just be a (ratified) official hearer (Dynel, 2011; Goffman, 1981) of a story told by someone else, but can, in Goffman's terms, become an addressed recipient of a story about his or her own life. In those situations, people with dementia may not be positioned as co-tellers of their life stories. Instead, life stories are sometimes designed with the person with

---

* This study has been conducted within the Center for Dementia Research (CEDER), which was funded by the bank of Sweden Tercentenary Foundation between the years 2011–2016 (Grant no. M10–0187:1) and the project Life with Dementia: Communication, Relations and Cognition, which is funded by FORTE: The Swedish Research Council for Health, Working Life and Welfare (Grant no. 2016-07207). A particular thanks go to the people living with dementia and their spouses who participated in the project.

dementia either as an addressed recipient or even as a third-party to whom the plot and the details of the story are news.

How a story is designed is closely related to what the recipients of the story can be expected to know already (Sacks, 1973). Speakers regularly adjust their ways of speaking (including style, vocabulary and content) to who is listening, something often described using the term *recipient design* (Goodwin, 1979; Sacks, 1992). Participants' orientations toward a story and the way stories are designed are intimately linked to the parties' epistemic status regarding their degree of knowledge of the topic (Goodwin, 1979; see Muntigl & Hödl Chapter 9 this volume). In conversation, there is a strong preference for not telling participants stories or information they already know (Goodwin, 1979; Sacks, 1973; Stivers et al., 2011). Most of the time, participants' assumptions about their interlocutors' prior information are correct – participants generally have a good understanding of who knows what, and are therefore able to adjust their telling accordingly (Stivers et al., 2011). As for interaction involving people with dementia, such assumptions are much more difficult to make. What kind of information a person with dementia has access to at a specific moment is often not possible to predict, as this can vary from time to time (Marcusson et al., 2011). A person with dementia might not be able to remember either recent events that happened just moments ago or events that have happened in the more distant past, but could just as well remember details of both the present and the past. Thus the *epistemic status* (Heritage, 2012) of a person with dementia can be both uncertain and fluctuating (see Lindholm & Stevanovic, 2022). What kind of information participants assume that the other has and the distribution of rights and responsibilities among the present parties will be displayed in how their talk is organized and locally managed on a turn-by-turn basis.

In this chapter we use data from research interviews and investigate how a couple, in which one of the spouses is diagnosed with dementia, orient toward and handle interactional challenges in narrations of past shared events that arise when the spouse with dementia has severely limited (or no) access to these events. We show how the spouse who still has access to the events orients to these issues by organizing and reorganizing the participation frameworks in resourceful ways and delicately deals with her spouse's limited or lack of knowledge using a variety of face-saving practices. Drawing on conversation analytic methods (Sacks, 1992) and a detailed and multimodal analysis of interaction (Goodwin, 2018; Mondada, 2016), the chapter aims to provide empirical examples and analytical insights related to the sequentially unfolding of a joint storytelling in circumstances when the epistemic status of one of the co-tellers is unclear. By doing this, the chapter adds to a growing body of literature focusing on issues related to epistemic matters and the management of asymmetric access to knowledge in interaction involving people with dementia (e.g., Hamilton, 2019; Hydén & Samuelsson, 2019; Landmark et al., 2021; Lindholm & Stevanovic, 2022; Muntigl et al., 2014, Nilsson, 2017; Nilsson et al., 2018; Svennevig & Landmark, 2019).

10.2 Participation Frameworks, Participation Status and Interactional Positionings

The concepts of participation framework and interactional positioning are greatly influenced by Goffman, whose work highlights the significance of different interactional arrangements and the different possibilities of participation in such arrangements (Goffman, 1981; see also Rae, 2001). In interactional encounters, participants' engagements cannot adequately be described merely using the roles of "speaker" and "listener". Goffman (1981, p. 137) proposes that "an utterance does not carve up the world beyond the speaker into precisely two parts, recipients and non-recipients, but rather opens up an array of structurally differentiated possibilities, establishing the participation framework in which the speaker will be guiding his delivery". So the participants' engagements in interactions are connected to a range of different statuses. Goffman (1981) describes the term *participation status* as referring to a specific participant's relation to a current utterance: "When a word is spoken, all those who happen to be in a perceptual range of the event will have some sort of participation status relative to it" (p. 3). For speakers, Goffman describes at least three main positionings including animator (utterance producer), author (utterance designer) and principal (responsible for the message). Listeners (or hearers) are divided into ratified (e.g., audience) and unratified (e.g., bystanders or eavesdroppers) positions, as well as addressed and unaddressed (ratified) hearers (Goffman, 1981; see also Goodwin, 1996). The term *participation framework*, then, portrays the collected relations to a specific utterance of all the participants in an activity.

While Goffman's work mainly centres around categories to illustrate participation in interactional encounters, later studies have highlighted the inherently situated and ever-changing nature of participation on a turn-by-turn basis (Goodwin, 1996; Goodwin & Goodwin, 1992, 2004; Rae, 2001). In these studies, and also in this chapter, participation is viewed as interactively accomplished through temporally unfolding courses of action, with constantly changing roles and statuses, rather than a stable structure for the actions undertaken (Rae, 2001). Participation framework and participation status – or rather, *interactional positioning* – are thus considered as significant for analysing the forms of participation and the participants' current engagement in the course of the activity (Goodwin, 1996; Goodwin & Goodwin, 1992). Following this line of work, participation framework and interactional positioning are used in this chapter to describe and analyse the participants' sequentially unfolding engagement of a jointly told story.

10.3 Epistemics and Accountability

In his central work on knowledge in interaction, Heritage (2012) describes three concepts that are especially important for participants and analysts alike: *territories (or domains) of knowledge*, *epistemic status* and *epistemic stance*. Domains of knowledge refer to certain areas of information. According to Pomerantz (1980), there are two types of knowables, constituting different domains: Type 1 knowables and Type 2 knowables. Type 1 knowables concern knowledge from first-hand experience and Type 2 knowables concern indirectly acquired knowledge. A Type 1 knowable includes, for example, a person's feelings and their previous involvements or motives for doing something, and it is commonly associated with specific privileges (Heritage, 2012; Muntigl et al., 2014; Muntigl & Hödl Chapter 9 this volume; Pomerantz, 1980). Participants are considered to have primary rights and access to the information they experienced first-hand and have themselves been exposed to, something that is reflected in how participants design their conversation (Heritage & Raymond, 2005). In general, participants orient to each other as having privileged access to their own opinions and experiences, and also as having specific rights to tell about them (Heritage & Raymond, 2005; Pomerantz, 1980; Sacks, 1973). Type 1 knowables are also associated with certain responsibilities, as a person might be held accountable for not having (or not claiming) access to this kind of information (Pomerantz, 1980; Stivers et al., 2011).

Having or not having access to knowledge about an event helps to shape some specific interactional positionings and builds a particular 'epistemic constellation' (Koole, 2012) where participants show their epistemic statuses regarding that event. Participants' epistemic status refers to a person's position as being more or less knowledgeable in relation to a certain epistemic domain (Heritage, 2012). A similar framework described by Labov and Fanshel (1972) introduces the terms A-events, B-events and A-B events in which A-event knowledge is primarily known to participant A (the speaker), B-event knowledge is primarily known to participant B (the recipient), and A-B events are known to both. Participants recognize each other as more or less knowledgeable in relation to a current domain of knowledge. This status is, however, not a static position but can 'vary from domain to domain, as well as over time, and can be altered from moment to moment as a result of specific interactional contributions' (Heritage, 2012: 4). Closely related to participants' knowledge of specific domains is their epistemic stance, which refers to how the participants position themselves in relation to some specific piece of information. In and through the design of turns, participants can use various linguistic and interactional resources to display their knowledge position: as knowledgeable or not, and also the degree of certainty of their knowledge (Heritage, 2012; Heritage & Raymond, 2005). It should be noted that participants might take a certain epistemic stance vis-à-vis a specific topic to appear more or less knowledgeable than they really are (Goodwin, 1979; Heritage & Raymond, 2005). Claiming forgetfulness can, for example, be used as a way to stimulate talk and support participation (Goodwin, 1987) or to resist responsibility (Muntigl & Choi, 2010).

10.3.1 Epistemics in Analyses of Interaction Involving People with Dementia

In general, people are expected to have access to their own biography and to be able to account for their own past (Muntigl et al., 2014; Pomerantz, 1980). Due to a declining ability to remember, this is not always the case for people with dementia. Issues related to epistemic rights and responsibilities have recently been investigated with a focus on interaction involving people with dementia in several studies (e.g. Black, 2011; Hamilton, 2019; Hydén & Samuelsson, 2019; Landmark et al., 2021; Lindholm & Stevanovic, 2022; Muntigl et al., 2014, Nilsson, 2017; Nilsson & Olaison, 2019; Nilsson et al., 2018; Svennevig & Landmark, 2019; Williams et al., 2019).

Hamilton (2019) outlines a number of identified strategies a person with dementia uses to handle memory problems related to Type 1 knowables. When asked questions related to personal facts that proved difficult to recollect, the person with dementia used both fellow interlocutors and assistance from the material surrounding to be able to provide an answer. In these situations, it was noted that partners of the person with dementia sometimes contradict the answers given by the person with dementia and answer on their behalf (Hamilton, 2019; see also Nilsson et al., 2018). How spouses initiate corrections and repairs related to the epistemic domain of the person with dementia is a specific focus in a study by Landmark et al. (2021). In this study, couples' management of conflicting knowledge-claims and negotiation of epistemic rights was investigated. Three main practices for correcting the person with dementia were identified: for example, the partner without dementia claiming epistemic authority and denying the person with dementia's authority; or inviting the person with dementia to self-correct, thereby attributing some epistemic authority to them. Instances of disagreement where the spouses provided reasons for their alternative claims and displayed a more symmetric epistemic gradient were also found. Nilsson et al. (2018) also showed how spouses with dementia sometimes actively hand over epistemic primacy to their partners by assigning them to be their spokespersons regarding information that they would normally have been expected to know themselves.

Related to the aspects of social sensitivity of handling asymmetries of knowledge (Linell & Luckmann, 1991), Nilsson (2017) argues that the act of prompting, or 'fishing' for Type 1 knowables regarding a specific memory may have a face-threatening and counter-productive effect on the participation of a person with dementia in an ongoing interaction. Managing such a potential face threat due to the difficulty of recollecting, as Svennevig & Landmark (2019) show, may be done through accounts or justifications. Likewise, focusing on a conversation between a person with dementia and her two relatives, Hydén & Samuelsson (2019) have also argued that the participants jointly work to avoid face threats and confrontation when disagreement occurs, not only on factual matters but also on more foundational questions, such as who could possibly be alive at a certain point in time; this is what the authors call 'reality disjunctions'.

In line with the abovementioned studies, Black (2011) examined a conversation between a woman with dementia and her daughter, focusing on how the daughter challenges her mother's statements and takes an epistemic stance as being more knowledgeable in relation to domains of knowledge 'without explicit indication of sensitivity to the fact that the domains of knowledge in question would normally be considered more Sophia's [the mother] than Lucy's [the daughter]' (pp. 84–85). Epistemic authority seems to be underlined through the use of a number of conversational techniques, including specific turn designs (see Muntigl & Hödl Chapter 9 this volume) and the emphasis of subjective experiences, which are sometimes acknowledged by the mother with dementia. Black argues that although the daughter in this way threatens the mother's position as an equal participant in the conversation with the capability of knowing about her own life, the mother manages to participate in the conversation 'without overt loss of face in the form of allowing herself to be corrected or contradicted about her own ability, experience, or knowledge' (Black, 2011: 86).

In another study, Muntigl et al. (2014) analysed clinical interviews with patients with frontotemporal dementia, focusing on how patients position themselves regarding knowledge about their health. When asked about their condition, the patients would either deny being ill without necessarily accounting for their condition, or affirm being ill but display and elaborate on their epistemic stance with varied certainties with regard to direct knowledge and experience of their condition. That is, it is shown that disclaiming knowledge of any problem or claiming it with various degrees of awareness has effects on how people with dementia succeed in displaying themselves as competent social actors (Muntigl et al., 2014).

10.4 Methods and Materials

For this study, we analyse an extended excerpt taken from a collection of interviews with couples, one of whom has been diagnosed with dementia.[1] The

---

[1] Interviews were conducted as part of a research project run at Center for Dementia Research (CEDER) at Linköping University, funded by the bank of Sweden Tercentenary Foundation between the years 2011 and 2016 (Grant no. M10-0187:1).

interviews were conducted at two geriatric clinics by two researchers, and the couples were interviewed together with their spouses. In the interviews, the couples were asked about their current life together, their shared history and their experiences of living with dementia. The specific excerpt analysed comes from an interview with Mike, who was 79 and had been diagnosed with dementia of the Alzheimer's type, and his wife Karen, who was also 79 but did not have a dementia diagnosis. The couple had been married for more than 50 years and they had lived together in the same house during this time. Before data collection, the application for ethical approval to conduct this research was granted by a regional committee for ethical vetting. The data collection was also undertaken in accordance with the ethical guidelines and principles of the Swedish Research Council, which include the couple's written consent to participate in the study.

In the chosen excerpt, Karen is the teller of a story about some past events when Mike did not recognize her as his wife. Apart from memory loss as the basic symptom of Alzheimer's disease, a symptom associated with dementia is agnosia – the difficulty to process sensory information – which might result in an inability to recognize persons or objects. Neurodegenerative illnesses like Alzheimer's disease are also related to Capgras syndrome, in which a person may believe a family member has been replaced by an imposter (Josephs, 2007). Even if, as analysts, we cannot be sure about the reason why Mike did not recognize Karen as his wife, the aforementioned associated symptoms with Alzheimer's disease (and other dementias), such as memory loss, agnosia and Capgras syndrome, correspond to what Karen presents as occasionally happening to Mike. In the story, Mike is one of the main characters. However, as it becomes apparent from the beginning of the story, Mike does not recall these events. By using an extended excerpt from a single interview, it is possible to follow in detail how the couple handle the telling of this story to the interviewers while at the same time attending to the fact that this story is also (at least in parts) new to Mike. The excerpt is analysed by means of multimodal conversation analysis (Goodwin, 2018; Mondada, 2016), and the analyses are informed by concepts related to *epistemics and accountability* (Heritage & Raymond, 2005, 2012; Pomerantz, 1980; Stivers et al., 2011) and *participation frameworks* (Goffman, 1981; Goodwin, 1996; Goodwin & Goodwin, 1992, 2004; Rae, 2001).

10.5 Analyses

The analyses start from the beginning of the story described above. The wife has mentioned that Mike's illness has deteriorated somewhat, and one of the interviewers picks up on this and asks her to elaborate on how Mike's condition got worse. The interview is conducted in Swedish. We show the translation in bold and italics, and the embodied actions are marked with grey background in the

10 Challenges for Couples Living with Dementia 233

transcripts. Symbols like asterisks (*), or circumflexes, also known as carets (^), show the exact moment of bodily actions within the turns of talk (see also the transcription conventions listed at the beginning of this book). The participants in the interview are Karen = K; Mike = M; Interviewers are researchers LC and E (who is also the second author of this chapter).

10.5.1 Introducing the Story

Extract 1

```
01    LC:   *va var de som hände när du (.) säger att de blev lite sämre
            what was it that happened when you (.) say that it got a
            little worse
                *...LC & K -mutual gaze->
02    K:    ((smacks her lips))
03    LC:   va var de som hände
            what was it that happened
04    K:    de hände: (.) väldit (0.2) många gånger (0.7) särskilt på
            it happened (.) very (0.2) many times (0.7) especially in
05          kvällarna att Mike ∧inte trodde att ja va ja. (1.4)
            the evenings that Mike didn't think that I was me.
                                    ∧K...points to herself->
06          utan han trodde att ja (.) han vänta på mej å han
            instead he thought that I (.) he waited for me and he
07          åkte ∧till å me väg å leta efter mej fast att jag va hemma .hh
            even went looking for me even though I was at home .hh
               K->∧,,,
08          (0.7) å han (.) trodde mej inte (0.3) alls utan han sa (0.8)
            (0.7) and he (.) didn't believe me (0.3) at all instead he
            said (0.8)
09          ja fi:ck visa (0.4) vem ja va (å) han titta på körkortet*
            I had to show (0.4) who I was 'n he looked at the driver's
            license
                                                          K->*gaze
            towards M
10    M:    °nä:° va de så?
            °no:° was that so?
11    K:    ja (.) så va de (.) å Laurent *våran son fick komma in å han sa
            yeah (.) it was (.) and Laurent our son had to come over and
            he said
                                    K->*gaze towards LC->>
12          att de ä ju mamma näe (0.4) de ä en annan kvinna som ä här sa
            that it is mommy [ju] no (0.4) it's another woman that is here
13          han.
            he said.
14          (0.5)
15    M:    hm
16          (1.2)
```

In this first sequence, Karen is telling a story about some past events that involved both Mike and herself; they were both present and would both presumably have knowledge of these events from first-hand experience (see Pomerantz, 1980). In this way, this is an A–B event for Karen and Mike, and the knowledge domain should be a Type 1 knowable to both of them. As Karen tells the story, she creates a participation framework with the two interviewers as main recipients of the story. Karen's telling about the past event comes as a response to a question posed directly to her about the deterioration of Mike's condition as the interviewer poses the question using the second person singular pronoun 'you' (line 01) and a direct invitation to her to recount what had happened (line 03). She starts off a story rather straightforwardly, describing the events in which Mike is one of the main characters (from line 04 onwards). In her reference to Mike, she uses both his proper name (line 05) as well as a third person singular pronoun (lines 06, 08 and 09). This is a common way of telling a story for a third, unknowing, party when all involved participants have access to the information being told, and it is also a recurrent pattern in the interview material (Hydén & Nilsson, 2015; Nilsson et al., 2018). In line 10, however, it becomes apparent that Mike does not have access to this story. By posing a confirmation-seeking question, '°no:° was that so?' (line 10), Mike takes an unknowing epistemic stance toward the events being talked about, although the event could be expected to be a Type 1 knowable for him, as he is the one who presumably has performed the described actions. In other words, the event seems like a B-event to Mike, as evidently displayed in his question (line 10) (see Labov 1972: 124).

Mike's positioning of himself as not knowing about, or perhaps even taking a disbelieving stance towards, these events (line 10) does not come with any account of why he does not recognize the story. Instead, he is posing his question without any extra interactional work, marking the event as something out of the ordinary by simply asking '°no:° was that so?' (line 10), and thereby indicating a lack of recollection. Similarly, Karen's response in line 11 is not in any way questioning why Mike does not remember what happened, and she does not hold him accountable for not knowing this. She simply responds to Mike by upholding the claim and elaborates with further details by referring to their son, as he was called over to his parents that evening (and could potentially corroborate the story) (lines 11–13; note the particle 'ju' in line 12, which is used in Swedish to show mutual knowledge or shared information; see Heinemann et al. (2011)). By responding in this way and not treating Mike's lack of recollection as surprising or noteworthy, Karen can be viewed as ratifying Mike's diminished epistemic position. Karen's focus on what happened and not on different experiences of the event seems to tally with other studies (e.g., Hydén & Samuelsson, 2019; Svennevig & Landmark, 2019) that also describe instances of similar discrepancies in terms of shared memory or experience in interaction involving a person with dementia. As Karen continues with the story, the interviewer seems to become her main recipient, as shown by her gaze and orientation toward him (line 11), while she again positions Mike as a present third party by referring to him in the third person (line 13).

10.5.2 Changing Participation Framework

Soon after Mike has positioned himself as unknowing in relation to the events in Karen's story, framing this as a B-event to him, the participation framework for the telling also changes. As Karen continues the story, she now turns toward Mike, looks at him and directly tells him how she felt when he could not recognize her as his wife: 'I was pretty sad then' (Extract 2, line 19). A change of Mike's participation between a ratified hearer, an addressed recipient and a character of the story (a third party present) in the telling (see e.g., Nilsson et al., 2018) can be observed throughout the whole sequence. Such a repeated shift between a second-party and a third-party positioning seems to highlight Mike's interactional position within the epistemic constellation as unknowing. As will be shown, these changes in the participation framework and thus also the epistemic constellations are often accompanied and managed by embodied actions (see also Nilsson et al., 2018).

Extract 2

```
17  K:    å de här va rätt så jobbit faktiskt för ja (.) förstog inte hur
          and this was pretty hard actually cause I (.) didn't understand
18        de
          how it
19        kunde ↑bli så å de va (0.4) *ja va väldi lessen då.
          could ↑be like that so it was (0.4) I was pretty sad then
                              K->*gaze at M, M looks in K's
          direction->
          (0.7)
20  K:    .hh .hh ple
21  M:    va säger Laurent om de där nu då?%
          what does Laurent say about that now then?
                              M->%looks at K->
22  K:    ja*%Laurent: kom ju in: e e sent en kväll de var ju lite upprört
          well Laurent: came [ju] in: e e late one night when [ju] the mood
          was a
          K,M->*%gaze down, K still oriented towards M->
23        (.) stämning hemma.
          little upset at home.
24        (0.5)
25  M:    m:
26        (1.2)
27  K:    å: eh (0.8) en gång kom () (.) *RINGde Sara våran dotter (0.8)
          an_ eh (0.8) one time came () (.) Sara our daughter CALLed (0.8)
                              K->*,,,gaze and orientation towards LC->
28  K:    .hh å en annan kväll när ja* (0.5) då va Mike (0.3)
          .hh and another night when I (0.5) then (.) then Mike was (0.3)
```

```
29      väldit (.)
        very
                        K->*gaze down->
30      då när han-*(.) när han får% (.) när de har varit såna här gå då
        (.) then when he- (.) when he gets (.) when ther've been these
31      ä han
        then he gets
                        K-> *...gaze at LC->
                                M-> %...gaze up to the ceiling->
32  K:  (.) så sträng (1) mot mej. (1.3) *å säger att du ä inte Karen
        (.) so harsh (1) with me (1.3) and says you are not Karen (0.6)
                                                K->*gaze at M->
33      (0.6)*
        K->*gaze down
34          ∧* du kan %inte vara född trettifyra. (0.8) ∧å du: är inte du
        you cannot have been born thirty-four (0.8) n' you're not you
35      ä (.)
        you're (.)
        K-> *...gaze away->
        M->∧fading smile—————————————∧,,,
                M-> %gaze down->
36  K:  nån* annan (0.5) å du vet ja.
        someone else (0.5) and you know [yeah/i]
        K->*gaze at LC & E->
37      (1) * (1)
        K ->*,,,gaze down->
38      å då: m: (0.7) *∧de var en kväll (0.6) då var klockan halv tie
        and then: m: (0.7) it was one might(0.6) it was around half past
        nine
                        K->*∧turns head to M, strokes M's hand->
39      elle nåt sånt då ∧kom*ja på att*ja måste ringa till en (0.3) å
        or so then I remembered I had to call someone (0.3) and say
                        K->∧stops stroking, keeps her hand on M's->
                        K->*gaze at LC, K->*,,,gaze away->
40      säga att ja inte kan komma imorrn .hh (1.0) HHH så ja ringde å
        that I cannot make it tomorrow .hh (1.0)HHH so I called and said
41      sa de här ä karen då tog Mike∧ telefonen * från mig (0.∧3) å
        this's Karen and then Mike took the phone from me (0.3) and (.) it
                        K->∧...opens hand pointing at M,,,∧
                        K-> *...gaze at M->
42      s:å (.) då va de:*
        was then
        K->*gaze at LC——*gaze down->>
43      (.) *mannen där som svara (0.7) å då prata han me Mike å då
        (.) the man who answered(0.7) then he spoke to Mike n' then he
        K->*gaze away->
44      förstog
        understood
45      han att de inte va bra *ska vi komma bort sa han (0.2) så* då
        that it wasn't good shall we come over he asked (0.2) so then
                        K->*,,,gaze back to Inl——————————*...gaze
        at M->
```

```
46    kom dom hem* (0.3) *till oss också°% (0.5) å då va de likadant
      they came over (0.3) to our house too (0.5) n' then it was the same
              K->*...gaze down, head turned in M's direction->
                      M->%gaze at K->
47    att du Into∧ trodde att ja va ja. (0.9) utan du: (0.8) hade
      that you didn't believe that I was I (0.9) instead you (0.8) had
              M->∧gaze up->
48    (1.8) ah du fick för dej att ja Å ∧*ja skulle inte få gå å lägga
      (1.8) ah the idea that I AND I was not allowed to sleep in my own
                      M->∧gaze at K->
                      K->*gaze down, head turned
      forward->
49    i min sång å: (0.6)% (0.2) <for då: sa du att> de kommer inte
      bed and (0.6) (0.2) <'cause then you said that> Karen won't like this
                      M->%gaze away->
50    Karen tycka om när hon kommer hem (1)∧ (1) ∧men på morron ä de
      when she comes home (1) (1) but in the morning it's over [thing's
51    över
      changed]
                              K->∧,,,takes away her hand
                              from M's, clasps hands->>∧
52    så på morron vet *inte Mike% om att de här har hänt.
      so in the morning Mike doesn't know that this has happened.
              K->*gaze at M->>
                      M->%gaze at K->
53    (0.3)% (0.5)
              M->%gaze down->>
54 M: (jaså) (0.4) hm
      (oh really) (0.4) hm
```

When Karen continues, there is a rather long sequence where she describes a specific evening when Mike did not recognize her. In the first part of the telling in Extract 1 (lines 1–16), Mike was positioned in Karen's story as a third party present (Linell, 2009; see also Nilsson et al. (2018) for a discussion of such positioning in interaction involving people with dementia). In the continuation of the telling in Extract 2, at lines 17–19 when Karen talks about her feelings, she actually turns her gaze toward Mike and thereby includes him as an addressed recipient of her talk. This gives an interactional space to allow Mike to enter into the talk again by asking a question (line 21). Karen's change of embodied orientation toward Mike, followed by the question, begins a sequence in which Mike seems to be included as a main addressee (lines 22–23). It is noteworthy that the question that Mike poses in response ('what does Laurent say about that now then?', line 21) heightens his position as someone who is not aware of his own life story and the consequence of his own actions. After Karen's response (lines 22–23), the only reaction from Mike is an acknowledgement token 'm:' (line 25). He does not take any stance on his own involvement in the story. Following the lack of affiliation with the story by Mike, Karen then once more redirects her gaze away from Mike and towards the interviewer (line 27) and continues her story with the interviewer as her main addressee. This change in participation framework is seen not only in Karen's bodily orientation, but also in the way she designs her story by providing an explanation of who Sara, the couple's daughter, is (line 27), information that would be expected to be known by Mike but not the interviewers.

In the continuation of Karen's telling, Mike is again positioned as a present third party by the use of his proper name (lines 28, 41 and 43) as well as the third person singular masculine pronoun (lines 30, 31). In line 47, however, Karen again changes the way she designs her story and addresses Mike by using a second person singular pronoun you (du in Swedish) when describing what happened and tells him what he said, something of which he shows no recollection. In this passage the interviewers are not included as addressed recipients of the story, but participate rather as ratified overhearers, or perhaps unaddressed recipients (Goffman, 1981), as Karen, in lines 46–51, tells a story about Mike that is designed with Mike as the addressed recipient. This way of designing the telling puts Mike in the spotlight as an unknowing party in the story of which he is the main character and of which he should presumably have first-hand knowledge.

In line 52 there is a new change in the participation framework, starting when Karen removes her hand from Mike's hand (see Nilsson et al., 2018: 782–784) followed by a 2.2-second silence. When Karen continues, she is once again referring to Mike, using his proper name (line 52). This can be seen as a change in the primary recipiency of her story. Nevertheless, Mike provides an acknowledgement of Karen's story by saying '(jaså) (0.4) hm' ('oh really'; line 54) and thereby continues to claim a position as recipient of her story. As previously shown in research (e.g., Lindholm, 2016: 835), the Swedish token 'jaså' signals 'accepting the previous turn as news', indicating receiving new and somewhat surprising information (see Heritage, 1984; Wilkinson & Kitzinger, 2006). Mike's 'jaså'-prefaced turn can also be understood in the same way, that is conveying elements of surprise at the previous turn, which highlights that Karen's telling is news to him (see, for example, *third-turn receipts* in Heritage, 1985). This tallies with the analysis that Mike has taken a position of an unknowing party throughout all episodes of talk despite his co-presence in the course of events and first-hand experience of them. With 'jaså', it seems that Mike has taken an unknowing stance toward Type 1 knowables, something that we analyse in more detail in Section 10.5.3.

In sum, the extracts of the interaction have so far shown how the interactional positionings (or participatory status in Goffman's terms) of the person with dementia fluctuate between an addressed recipient of the story and the third person character in the story. The constant change of the participation framework goes hand in hand with the interactional positioning of the person with dementia vis-à-vis the knowable and also the management of him being cast as a character in a story in which he does not remember his involvement. The analysis has also shown how Karen uses embodied resources to manage the social sensitivity of telling this story by directing her gaze and body toward different recipients and also by using 'touch' in handling the third-party positioning of Mike in the interaction (see also Nilsson et al. (2018) for details of the use of embodiment in the management of the speaking on behalf of a person with dementia).

10.5.3 Unknowing Stance towards Type 1 Knowables

As mentioned previously, a person is usually considered knowledgeable and accountable regarding their own experiences as well as their own private health (Heritage, 2012; Muntigl et al., 2014; Stivers et al., 2011). In the previous part of the extract, despite some signs revealing his unknowing position in the telling (e.g., lines 10, 20, 46), Mike has not explicitly stated that he does not know the story or does not have access to the information or the experiences Karen publicly shares with the interviewers. In the following part, Mike is clearly taking a downgraded epistemic position to Type 1 knowables and at the same time positions Karen as having primary access to information regarding his life and health condition.

Extract 3
```
55   K:     *s:å:[men de] ha varit (1.0) °ah° (1.5) väldit of:ta ett tag
            s:o: [but it] has been (1.0) °well° (1.5) very often a while
56          då-
            then
            K->*gaze away-->
57   M:          [(ja)]
                 [yeah]
58   K:     &$$$;men ↑nu har de *inte varit faktiskt på (*%1.2) °ah° säkert
            but now it actually hasn't been for (1.2) well surely (a) two
                        K->*gaze towards M————*,,,towards LC->
                                              M->%gaze towards K->
59          (ett) två tre vecker. (2.4) så de har vari bättre nu.
            three weeks. (2.4) so it's been better now
60          (1.2)
61   K:     .hh
62   M:     har*%de vari normalt den veckan* (be be) [( )]
            has it been normal that week (be be)      [( )]
            K & M->*%mutual gaze————————*K...gaze down->>
63   K:                                            [a: nu har%] de varit
                                                   [yeah now ] it has
                                              M->%gaze down->>
64          normalt du har inte haft dom här problemen på [kvällen.]
            been normal you haven't had those problems in [the evening]
65   M:                                                   [m:]
            ((11 lines omitted))
```

While these episodes of Mike not recognizing his wife used to be rather common (line 55), Karen states that for the last two-three weeks 'it has been better' (lines 58–59), possibly an attempt to tone down the regularity of the problem. This seems to be taken as an opportunity for Mike to take part in the story once more, seeking information and also confirmation about his own behaviour, which has so far been under question throughout the telling. From line 58 onwards, Mike turns to Karen and keeps his gaze towards her while Karen states that Mike's condition in the past two or three weeks has not been as previously described as it has been 'better' (even if perhaps still not good). This description is followed by Mike's upgrading Karen's gloss of being 'better' to being 'normal' when he directly asks whether his own condition has 'been normal' (line 62). By asking this question, Mike takes an epistemic, unknowing stance regarding aspects related to his own biography: he is turning to his wife for information about how he has been and has behaved during the past week (line 62). In response, Karen confirms that 'it has been normal', thereby confirming Mike's upgrading of the description of his own condition from 'better' to 'normal' (lines 63–64). She verifies this description by adding that, lately, Mike has not had the previously described problems. Notably in her response, Karen is not marking Mike's question as extraordinary or noteworthy. Instead, she responds straightforwardly and without any extra interactional work. Moreover, by turning to Mike, she also changes the participation framework once more by directly addressing Mike with a second person pronoun, making him a primary addressed recipient of this turn. Directly addressing Mike and highlighting his lack of awareness of his own health and condition (even though it belongs to his knowledge domain) heightens Mike's positioning as an unknowing party, although Karen does not topicalize Mike's lack of knowledge as a problem and does not make him directly accountable for showing a lack of knowledge of his own past and health (see Hydén & Samuelsson, 2019; Svennevig & Landmark, 2019).

When the story continues in line 77, Karen moves back to using Mike's proper name, once again including the interviewers as the addressed recipients. Karen elaborates on her previous story and describes how Mike sometimes takes the car to go to look for her, even though she is in fact at home trying to convince Mike that she is his wife. Mike again explicitly acknowledges his lack of knowledge (and also evidently some confusion) about the events, and thus once more takes a downgraded epistemic position while positioning Karen as the knowing party in, what would expectedly be, their shared epistemic domain.

Extract 4

77   K: åh (0.3) å Mike blir v- (0.3) väldit t*u*ff mot mej då
          an (0.3) and then Mike gets v- (0.3) very firm with me
          >>*K & M gaze down*->

78		(0.7) ∧de värsta har varit nåra gånger när han (0.3) INTE
		(0.7) and the worst has been a couple of times when he (0.3)
		does NOT
		∧K...moves her torso forward->>
79		%pås- tror att ja ä *hemma (1.%1) å*utan fast ja a där
		sta- believe that I am at home (1.1) 'n but even though I am
		there
		%M...gaze towards K-> *K and M mutual gaze%,,, *K...gaze
		towards LC->
80		å säger ja (0.2) Ä*;R ju här ser du inte de (1.0) så (0.3) har de
		and I say (0.2) but I AM here do you not see that (1.0) so (0.3)
		it has
		K->*gaze down->
81		*hänt att han har tagit bilen å stuckit väg å letar efter mej*
		(0.5)
		happened that he has taken the car and gone looking for me (0.5)
		K->*gaze towards E———————————————————
		———————————————,,,
82		å de ä jobbit tycker ja.
		and that is hard I think.
83		(1%.2)
		M->%gaze down, deep breath in, facing forward->
84	E:	°m:°
85		(2.4)
86	K:	de har v hänt vid ett- nåra tillfällen tre fyra tillfällen.
		and that has happened so- some times three four times
87		(0.9)
88	M:	%ha ja ((harklar))*har ja hittat dej då?
		hav' I ((clears throat)) have I found you then?
		M->%gaze towards K->*...gaze towards M ((mutual gaze))->
89	K:	*@näe[((skrattar))] de har %du inte .hh@
		@no [((laughs))] you haven't .hh@
		K->*gaza down-> M->%gaze down->>
90	M:	[((laughs))]
91	M:	@°(m)°@
92	K:	@du har inte hittat mej *eftersom ja va hemma@ ju
		you haven't found me cause I was home [ju]
		K->*gaze at M->>
93		(0.4)
94	M:	mhm:
95		(0.5)
96	LC:	å å då brukar du komma hem igen Mike? utan å,
		an an then you usually come home again Mike? without,
97		(2∧.5)∧
		∧M...moves his head and torso from side to side∧
98	LC:	((clears throat))
99	M:	%de vet du bättre än ja va
		you know that better than me right
		M->%...gaze towards K ((mutual gaze))->>
100		(0.7)
101	K:	ja du har ju kommit hem
		yeah you have come home

Karen's description of these events is mainly designed with the interviewers as addressed recipients as she is repeatedly using a third person pronoun and a proper name to refer to Mike (lines 77, 78, 81) (however, observe that Karen's gaze is also directed toward Mike in the climax of the story where Karen says that Mike did not 'believe'" that she was at home, line 79). It is also one of the interviewers who provides some minimal feedback to this part of the story (line 84), showing that the interviewer positions herself as a main addressee responsible for responding to Karen's telling. However, in line 88, after being described as a person who was 'firm' with his wife ('and that has happened so- some times three four times', line 86), Mike once again claims a position as recipient to the story by asking Karen for information about how the episodes ended, episodes where Mike himself is the main character. His contribution can be interpreted both as an attempt to bring the story to the end by asking what eventually happened: 'have I found you then?' (line 88), and also as an indication that he has not been following the message of the story and is having trouble understanding the logic of it. Mike would not have asked the question had he kept track of the telling in which Karen describes that she was, in fact, at home when he went looking for her. Whereas the issue so far has been how Mike is positioned or positions himself as an unknowing party in the story about his own past, this sequence does not seem to be just about accessing information. There is also a trouble in understanding what is being talked about.

Mike's question, 'have I found you then?' (line 88), displaying his difficulty in keeping up with the logic of the story, is responded to by Karen with laughter (line 89). Even if Karen provides the information that Mike has requested, she simultaneously does interactional work that may diminish the potential discomfort associated with Mike's problem of recalling the event, as well as his problem following the story. Responding to Mike, she makes him the addressed recipient by using the second person pronoun and accompanies her response (lines 89 and 92) with a smile (shown by the symbol @ in the transcript) and also laughter. Even if the laughter displays that Mike got the story wrong and that it is a laughable matter, the laughter also frames the trouble as something not too serious and may very well be a face-saving strategy adopted in a delicate situation (Saunders, 1998). Mike also joins in the laughter, which perhaps momentarily covers up the trouble at talk (using laughter to manage embarrassing situations has been studied in dementia, e.g., Lindholm (2008); see also laughter in talk with people with aphasia in Wilkinson, 2007).

As in previous excerpts, Mike does not frame his questions as extraordinary or unexpected. He poses his questions straightforwardly without any account for why he asks Karen for information about whether he found her or not. While not knowing about one's own past is recurrently something that needs to be accounted for (Muntigl et al., 2014; Pomerantz, 1980), this seems not to be the case here. Neither Mike nor Karen marks Mike's downgraded epistemic stance to this Type 1 knowable as extraordinary or something for which Mike should be held accountable.

In what follows, one of the interviewers poses a direct question to Mike about the events Karen has talked about (line 96). This is followed by a 2.5-second silence where Mike gazes towards the interviewer, moving his head from side to side, and Karen gazes towards Mike (line 88). As seen in lines 97–99, Mike does not answer the question as to whether he usually comes home. Instead, he turns to Karen, stating that this is something she knows better: 'you know that better than me right' (line 99). When taking the turn in line 101, Karen first addresses Mike, confirming to him that he does indeed usually come home. She uses the particle 'ju', which shows that she expects Mike to know this, even if he seems to be incognizant of it. By handing over the question to Karen, stating that this is in fact something she knows better, Mike relinquishes epistemic authority to his own biography and positions Karen as the more knowledgeable about what he did at the time in question.

10.6 Discussion

In the analysed extended extract, Karen is the teller of a story featuring Mike as the main character. Karen is the one doing almost all the talking and she also takes primary responsibility for orchestrating the activity. The frame for this activity is a research interview where Karen and Mike are asked about their life together and how Mike's disease became noticeable in their daily activities. As it turns out, Mike does not remember the events being talked about and Karen therefore has to adapt her telling to this fact. The design of this type of talk is complex as the interactants must keep track of both the content of the story and, at the same time, get it across to others, as well as manage the potential sensitivity of telling a story that should already be known to their spouse. Throughout the telling of the analysed story, Karen alternates between designing her story with the interviewers as her main recipients and also structuring her telling so that Mike, to whom the information is (presumably) also news, becomes an addressed recipient. The way Karen tells her story makes relevant at least two altering participation frameworks (Goffman, 1981) for the activity. In the first framework, Karen is telling her story with the interviewers as her addressed recipients, and Mike as mainly a (ratified) official hearer. In this framework, she is referring to Mike using a third person singular pronoun or his proper name, and she also includes explanatory information directed to the interviewers, for example explanations of who the couple's children are. In the other framework, Mike is positioned as an addressed recipient of Karen's story and the interviewers are instead positioned as ratified official hearers. In this framework, Karen addresses Mike directly with the use of the second person singular pronoun, making him a primary addressed recipient. However, in both these frameworks all participants are in a sense recipients of Karen's story even when they are not discursively positioned as a main addressed recipient (see Goodwin & Goodwin, 1992, 2004). When Karen is addressing Mike using the second person singular pronoun, the story told is also made available to the interviewers as part of Karen's response to their questions. Similarly, when Karen is telling her story with the interviewers as main recipients, the information is also available to Mike, who occasionally claims a position as recipient also in these instances by, for example, producing tokens of acknowledgement, posing follow-up questions or asking for clarifications. Therefore, the participation frameworks are, in this sense, both a dynamic and multilayered moment-to-moment accomplishment of the participants (see Goodwin, 1996; Goodwin & Goodwin, 1992, 2004; Rae, 2001), shaped and reshaped according to the management of the topic and its potential sensitivity for the participants, particularly for the person with dementia as a co-present character of the story.

Changing the participation framework and directly addressing the person with dementia when talking about his challenges are interactionally (and socially) consequential. Although Mike seems unaware of his actions and the event portrayed in the telling throughout the analysed sequence, it seems that his unknowing position is upgraded when he is positioned as an addressed recipient in second party positioning. As shown and argued in the analysis (see lines 11, 39–43, 55–56, 80–83), when Karen addresses Mike directly while talking about his actions about which he does not display knowledge, his position as unknowing is foregrounded and the epistemic asymmetry between the spouses becomes more prominent (see, Landmark et al., 2021; Nilsson et al., 2018). This highlighting of Mike's unknowing position makes the social situation even more sensitive and elicits extra interactional work. As shown in the analysis, Karen uses several resources such as touch (lines 33–43), smile and laughter (e.g. lines 80–83), together with the direction of her gaze and head movements to include Mike in the talk, and to mitigate and manage a possibly embarrassing situation, something that can be considered a face-saving act (see Nilsson et al. (2018) for an analysis of similar patterns).

From the interview with Karen and Mike, it may be suggested that both Karen and Mike orient toward a *joint access* to (some of) Mike's Type 1 knowables. In the extract, Karen is providing information on behalf of Mike, both in relation to the biographic information and in relation to his health condition, but her actions are not unwarranted. There are instances where Mike asks Karen for information that belongs to his epistemic domain (Type 1 knowables to him) (lines 10, 20, 54, 79), and he even explicitly states that Karen is the one who is more knowledgeable in relation to some of this information (line 90). For Karen and Mike, Mike's biographic knowing is distributed between the two of them, and when Mike does not remember a specific event, he can turn to Karen for assistance (see Hamilton, 2019). In previous studies of spouses taking a superior epistemic stance in relation to the epistemic domain belonging to a person with dementia, potential problems and risks of such conduct have been foregrounded (e.g., Black, 2011; Hamilton, 2019; Landmark et al., 2021). This study, following Nilsson et al. (2018), highlights the nuances of practices involved in managing epistemic access to Type 1 knowables for people with dementia and the potential benefits of collaborative activities through which a spouse takes over some of the epistemic responsibilities of the person with dementia.

In sum, Mike's appreciation of Karen's access to the event without challenging her version of the story, together with Karen's non-confrontational approach that does not question Mike's unknowing stance nor explicitly asks him about his recollections (see. Williams et al., 2019), makes the interactional activity proceed smoothly. The interview questions are co-operatively answered, although dominantly by Karen. Despite the delicacy of revealing Mike's behaviour and his diminished epistemic status, with Karen's skilful recipient design (Sacks, 1992) of her telling and her seamless shifting between participation frameworks throughout the interview, the sensitiveness of the topic is mitigated. Even when Mike is sometimes directly addressed as a recipient of his own life story and his position as an unknowing party is hence drastically heightened, Karen manages to attenuate the impact of telling as a face-threating act through the use of embodied resources and engaging with Mike in the conversation while telling the story to the interviewers. Her body posture, gaze direction, putting her hand on Mike's hand and orienting towards him, time and again, are used as mitigating devices. Moreover, Mike is never interactionally positioned as accountable for his unawareness of his actions and Karen takes the responsibility for talking on behalf of both of them without challenging Mike's unknowingness or difficulty remembering his role in the story. Finally, even if positioned as an unknowing party about his own biographical story, Mike is also provided with interactional space to remain active as a participant in the interaction and his needs and requests for information about his own life are simultaneously responded to.

10.7 Conclusions and Potential Implications for Practice

The analyses in this chapter highlight how issues related to knowledge and dementia can benefit from using an interactional and distributed perspective. While access and rights to knowledge are usually divided between participants depending on the knowledge domain and the participants' relation to the topic, where a participant has a dementia disease, a more flexible approach toward such divisions could be advantageous. As it might be difficult to project what kind of information a person with dementia has access to at a specific moment, the result of this study suggests the benefit of applying an adaptable approach regarding the framework for a specific interactional activity and the participants' interactional positionings in that event. Living with dementia recurrently means that the details of one's own life sometimes become uncertain or totally disappear (for longer or shorter periods of time). Our study demonstrates that conversational practices where an interactional partner refrains from holding a person with dementia accountable for their loss of memory, and instead enables the person with dementia to pose questions regarding their own life, may be understood as an increased appreciation of their contingencies in interaction. Moreover, engaging with people with dementia through various communicative practices would reduce the impact of the sensitivity of talking about their condition in their co-presence, which in turn could also potentially lead to the alleviation of some distress associated with such experiences. Making room for questions and dialogue, and providing the requested information in a way that minimizes the possible face-threatening aspects of such exchanges, are important aspects to prioritize in conversations with persons with dementia.

References

Black, R. (2011) 'Dementia and epistemic authority: A conversation analytic case study.' *Studies in Applied Linguistics and TESOL*, 11(2): 65–93.

Dynel, M. (2011) 'Revisiting Goffman's postulates on participant statuses in verbal interaction.' *Language and Linguistics Compass*, 5(7): 454–465.

Goffman, E. (1981). *Forms of Talk*. Philadelphia: University of Pennsylvania Press.

Goodwin, C. (1979) 'The interactive construction of a sentence in natural conversation.' In G. Psathas (ed.) *Everyday Language: Studies in Ethnomethodology*. New York: Irvington Publishers, pp. 97–121.

(1996) 'Transparent vision.' In E. Ochs, E. A. Schegloff and S. A. Thompson (eds.) *Interaction and Grammar*. Cambridge: Cambridge University Press, pp. 370–404.

(2018) *Co-operative Action*. Cambridge: Cambridge University Press.

Goodwin, C. and Goodwin, M. (1992) 'Context, activity and participation.' In P. Auer and A. di Luzio (eds.) *The Contextualization of Language*. Amsterdam: John Benjamins, pp. 77–99.

(2004) 'Participation.' In A. Duranti (ed.) *A Companion to Linguistic Anthropology*. Maldan, MA: Blackwell, pp. 222–244.

Hamilton, H. (2019) *Language, Dementia and Meaning Making. Navigating Challenges of Cognition and Face in Everyday Life*. London: Palgrave Macmillan.

Heinemann, T., Lindström, A. and Steensig, J. (2011) Addressing epistemic incongruence in question–answer sequences through the use of epistemic adverbs.' In T. Stivers, L. Mondada and J. Steensig (eds.) *The Morality of Knowledge in Conversation (Studies in Interactional Sociolinguistics)*. Cambridge: Cambridge University Press, pp. 107–130. doi:10.1017/CBO9780511921674.006.

Heritage, J. (1984) 'A change-of-state token and aspects of its sequential placement.' In J. Maxwell Atkinson and J. Heritage (eds.) *Structures of Social Action: Studies in Conversation Analysis*. Cambridge: Cambridge University Press, pp. 299–345.

(1985) 'Analyzing news interviews: aspects of the production of talk for an "overhearing" audience.' In T. A. van Dijk (ed.) *Handbook of Discourse Analysis*. London: Academic Press, vol. 3, pp. 95–117.

(2012) 'Epistemics in action: Action formation and territories of knowledge.' *Research on Language & Social Interaction*, 45(1): 1–29.

Heritage, J. and Raymond, G. (2005) 'The terms of agreement: Indexing epistemic authority and subordination in talk-in-interaction.' *Social Psychology Quarterly*, 68(1): 15–38.

Hydén, L-C. and Nilsson, E. (2015) 'Couples with dementia: Positioning the "we".' *Dementia*, 14(6): 716–733.

Hydén, L. C. and Samuelsson, C. (2019) '"So they are not alive?": Dementia, reality disjunctions and conversational strategies.' *Dementia*, 18(7–8): 2662–2678.

Josephs, K. A. (2007) 'Capgras syndrome and its relationship to neurodegenerative disease.' *Archives in Neurology*, 64(12): 1762–1766.

Koole, T. (2012) 'The epistemics of student problems: Explaining mathematics in a multi-lingual class.' *Journal of Pragmatics*, 44: 1902–1916.

Labov, W. and Fanshel, D. (1977) *Therapeutic Discourse: Psychotherapy as Conversation*. New York: Academic Press.

Landmark, A. M. D., Nilsson, E., Ekström, A. and Svennevig, J. (2021) 'Couples living with dementia managing conflicting knowledge claims.' *Discourse Studies*, 23(2): 191–212.

Lindholm, C. (2008) 'Laughter, communication problems and dementia.' *Communication & Medicine*, 5(1): 3–14.

(2016) 'Boundaries of participation in care home settings: Use of the Swedish token *jaså* by a person with dementia.' *Clinical Linguistics and Phonetics*, 30(10): 832–848.

Lindholm, C. and Stevanovic M. (2022) 'Challenges of trust in atypical interaction.' *Pragmatics and Society* 13(1): 109–127.

Linell, P. (2009) *Rethinking Language, Mind, and World Dialogically: Interactional and Contextual Theories of Human Sense-making*. Charlotte, NC: Information Age Publishers.

Linell, P. and Luckmann, T. (1991) '*Asymmetries in dialogue: Some conceptual preliminaries*.' In I. Marková and K. Foppa (eds.) *Asymmetries in Dialogue*. Hemel Hempstead, UK: Harvester Wheatsheaf, pp. 1–20.

Marcusson, J., Blennow K., Skoog I. and Wallin A. (2011) *Alzheimers sjukdom och andra kognitiva sjukdomar* [Alzheimer's disease and other cognitive diseases]. Stockholm: Liber AB.

Mondada, L. (2016) 'Challenges of multimodality: Language and the body in social interaction.' *Journal of Sociolinguistics*, 20(3): 336–366.

Muntigl, P. and Choi, K. T. (2010) 'Not remembering as a practical epistemic resource in couples therapy.' *Discourse Studies*, 12(3): 331–356.

Muntigl, P., Hödl, S. and Ransmayr, G. (2014) 'Epistemics and frontotemporal dementia.' *Journal of Theories and Research in Education*, 9(1): 69–95.

Nilsson, E. (2017) 'Fishing for answers: Couples living with dementia managing trouble with recollection.' *Educational Gerontology*, 43(2): 73–88.

Nilsson, E. and Olaison, A. (2019) 'What is yet to come? Couples living with dementia orienting themselves towards an uncertain future.' *Qualitative Social Work*, 18(3): 475–492.

Nilsson, E., Ekström, A. and Majlesi, A-R. (2018) 'Speaking for and about a spouse with dementia: A matter of inclusion or exclusion?' *Discourse Studies*, 20(6).

Pomerantz, A. M. (1980) 'Telling my side: "Limited access" as a "fishing" device.' *Sociological Inquiry*, 50: 186–198.

Rae, J. (2001) 'Organizing participation in interaction: Doing participation framework.' *Research on Language and Social Interaction*, 34(2): 253–278.

Sacks, H. (1973) 'On some puns with some intimations.' In R. W. Shuy (ed.) *Sociolinguistics: Current Trends and Prospects*. Washington DC: Georgetown University Press, pp. 135–144.

(1992) *Lectures on Conversation*. Vols. I & II, G. Jefferson (ed.). Oxford: Blackwell Publishing.

Stivers, T., Mondada, L. and Steensig, J. (2011) 'Knowledge, morality and affiliation in social interaction.' In T. Stivers, L. Mondada and J. Steensig (eds.) *The Morality of Knowledge in Conversation*. Cambridge: Cambridge University Press, pp. 3–24.

Svennevig, J. and Landmark, A. M. D. (2019) 'Accounting for forgetfulness in dementia interaction.' *Linguistics Vanguard*, 5(s2): 1–12.

Wilkinson, R. (2007) 'Managing linguistic incompetence as a delicate issue in aphasic talk-in-interaction: On the use of laughter in prolonged repair sequences.' *Journal of Pragmatics*, 39(3): 542–569.

Wilkinson, S. and Kitzinger, C. (2006) 'Surprise as an interactional achievement: Reaction tokens in conversation.' *Social Psychology Quarterly*, 69(2): 150–182.

Williams, V., Webb, J., Dowling, S. and Gall, M. (2019) 'Direct and indirect ways of managing epistemic asymmetries when eliciting memories.' *Discourse Studies*, 21(2): 199–215.

11 Maintaining Personhood and Authority in Everyday Talk of a Family Living with Dementia

Lyndsay M. Lindley

11.1 Introduction

Owing to increased awareness and opportunities for diagnosis of dementia (Gauthier et al., 2021), there has been a move toward recognising the importance of maintaining abilities, independence and quality of life for people with dementia (Department of Health, 2009; Mok & Müller, 2014; Sabat & Lee, 2011). This chapter, part of a wider study of family interaction (Lindley, 2016), focuses on the interactional competence of a person with dementia and some ways in which her independence is facilitated, and her personhood[1] validated, by her interlocutors. Drawing on a corpus of 15 hours of conversation, the study investigates the interactional practices of a woman diagnosed with dementia (seven years prior to participation in this project) in conversation with a variety of interlocutors including family caregivers, teenage grandchildren and community service providers. Recording took place over a period of three months, in a range of naturally occurring settings. The interaction is explored primarily through applied conversation analysis (Antaki, 2011) and supported by caregiver interviews and extensive ethnographic observations.

The overwhelming character of the conversations in these data is that of a person with dementia who is capable and assertive. Adopting a competence-based model (Coupland et al., 1991) of life with dementia, the study reveals how the social environment empowers the person with dementia to demonstrate her competence and expertise and that the practices of the conversational partners enable and support this. Where previous studies have focused on how conversational partners collaborate in co-constructing competence (Hamilton, 1994; Jones, 2015; Müller & Mok, 2014; Orange, 2001), this study additionally demonstrates evidence that a person with dementia has the ability to negotiate epistemic authority and often reorient herself following episodes of memory lapse, confusion and disorder. The negotiation of epistemics is central

---

[1] The term 'personhood' here follows the definition set out by Kitwood (1997: 8): 'It is a standing or status that is bestowed upon one human being, by others, in the context of relationship and social being. It implies recognition, respect and trust.'

to how people conduct their social interaction (Heritage, 2013). However, the scope of epistemics does not (necessarily) involve the cognitive state of knowing or not knowing, but rather refers to an individual's authority to access 'bodies or types of knowledge' (Drew, 1991: 45). That is, epistemic status relates to what each individual in conversation is entitled to know, share or assess in relation to other participants in the interaction (Heritage, 2013).

From my personal experience of interacting with people with dementia, I have developed a belief in the importance of valuing the person and their wisdom, and supporting their independence and competence. Nevertheless, when preparing to collect conversational data for this study, I had certain preconceptions as to the linguistic features and deficits I would encounter; for example, word-finding difficulties, circumlocution and repetition (Orange, 2001), as well as the potential for diminished self-worth and social withdrawal (McCarthy, 2011; Sabat, 2001). While some of these features are present, the nature of the conversations recorded was that of a capable woman who is treated with great respect by all those who interact with her.

The person at the centre of this study is Dana, an 88-year-old woman living with dementia. The aim of the research was to explore the data to discover features of Dana's conversations which characterise her as an authoritative interlocutor. Sequences of everyday conversations were explored, revealing certain environments in which authority and assertiveness are made relevant, including reminiscence and advice-giving. I consider how the person with dementia employs certain interactional practices to present herself as authoritative, and even when confusion and delusion do arise, how she skilfully extricates herself from this and returns to reality in the here and now. The family setting provides opportunities for shared reminiscence (Fivush, 2008). Where forgetting becomes relevant in interaction (Goodwin, 1987; Muntigl & Choi, 2010), conversational partners cooperate to prompt and evoke collaborative remembering (Hydén, 2011; Hydén & Örulv, 2009; Norrick, 2019, 2020).

11.2 Methods

11.2.1 Participants in Interaction

The central two participants were a woman (referred to as 'Dana'), who was 88 years of age and living alone in her own home, and her primary caregiver (her son, referred to as 'John'). The names of all participants have been anonymised. Following the initial meeting with the dyad, in which I received written consent to conduct my study, further conversational participants from the family and community agreed to take part (see Table 11.1). This provided the opportunity to gather a unique data set with the person with dementia in

Table 11.1 *Participants' demographic information*

Participant pseudonym	Age	Relationship to Dana	Role	Settings
Dana	88		Person with dementia	All
John	61	Son	Primary Caregiver	At home, mealtimes, car journeys, watching TV
Maureen	59	Daughter-in-law	Caregiver	At home, mealtimes
Emma	33	Granddaughter		Emma's house
Mick	51		Visiting chiropodist	Dana's house
Hal	–		Hairdresser	Hairdressing salon
George	50	Son	Caregiver	Family meals at George's house
Trudy	–	Daughter-in-law	Caregiver	Family meals at George's house
Chloe	15	Granddaughter		Family meals at George's house
Barney	13	Grandson		Family meals at George's house

conversation with a wide range of conversational partners in a variety of settings. This data set was the basis for a larger project (Lindley, 2016, 2020) on which this chapter builds. Ethical approval for this study was received from the University of York, St John: Reference: UC/3/9/12/LL.

11.2.2 Data

The data collected in this study are everyday conversations between a woman living with dementia, her family and members of the community. Conversations were recorded on an audio recording device. It was relatively simple to operate and was demonstrated to the participants, then left with them to record at their convenience. The device was small and portable, giving ample flexibility to the participants to carry it with them on trips or moving from room to room. I visited Dana at home periodically to exchange the memory card in the device, and each time I ensured that I had listened to the previous week's recordings in order to familiarise myself with the content and to be aware of any problems with recording or issues with consent or confidentiality.

Since the aim of the data collection was to obtain, as near possible, natural conversations, it was explained to the participants that they could record any part of their daily life and interactions. I stressed that constant dialogue was not necessary and there was no need to do any special activities or discuss specific topics. The family recorded as they wished over a period of three months, resulting in a total of 15 hours of audio data. The recordings were transcribed following the conventions of conversation analysis (Jefferson, 2004). The full corpus of recordings included mealtimes, watching television, car journeys, a visit from the chiropodist and a recording of one of Dana's weekly appointments at her hairdresser's salon. Noticing sequences involving reminiscence and advice-giving, especially in multigenerational conversations, I analysed these with respect to epistemics. Sequences were carefully inspected, exploring how the person with dementia was able to display primary epistemic rights and access.

11.3 Findings

Examination of the data revealed that Dana was able to assert epistemic authority (Stivers et al., 2011) in different activities such as advice-giving and narrating autobiographical events. I explore how, by using contextual cues of sequential implicativeness (Schegloff & Sacks, 1973), Dana successfully collaborates in reminiscence sequences initiated by her co-participants. On occasions when Dana displays confusion or lapses in memory, I show how she manages the interaction to reclaim authority.

Many of the recorded conversations involved Dana reminiscing about her working life and, in particular, as a young person growing up in Belfast. Dana vividly describes the streets and places of interest in the city as well as the characters she remembers from her youth. Dana is, of course, the expert in facts relating to her own life history; being allowed the opportunity to demonstrate this can contribute hugely to her feeling of self-worth (Fivush et al., 1999). Also, Dana is the only person in these recorded conversations with access to memories of her youth, so she can confidently hold the floor on these topics and is rarely contradicted. As well as reminiscence and life story sequences, Dana engages in advice-giving as an interactional vehicle to demonstrate her expertise.

11.3.1 Advice-Giving as a Means to Demonstrate Competence

Giving advice to a co-participant in conversation is a way to position the advice-giver as holding greater authority on a subject than the advice recipient (Vehviläinen, 2001). Extract 1 is taken from a dinnertime conversation between Dana and her son's (George's) family. Trudy is Dana's daughter-in-law and Chloe and Barney are teenage grandchildren. Following a similar mealtime conversation a few days earlier, seemingly a point of confusion for Dana is the work/school habit of Chloe, who is 15. Dana frequently asks about Chloe's occupation and is reminded that she is still at school but has a part-time job as a waitress.

11 Maintaining Personhood and Authority

Extract 1

```
1                ((George talks on the phone in the background))
2    Dana        .Hh I didn' t- I thought she worked there period.
3    Trudy       Hh NO: n no she just on a Sunda:y cz she still at schoo:l
4                (0.4)
5    Dana        Oh,
6                (0.3)
7    Dana        U- bwell (0.3) u yu learning anything
8                (1.1)
9    Chloe       ↑Yes:↑
10   Dana        Ye:s:
11               (0.3)
12   Trudy       How to wash up (0.3) hu[hahe  ]
13   Chloe                              [Ss hss]
14   Dana        Oh wll[she knows that already]
15   Trudy             [I think it's all good c]ustomer
16   Trudy       ser[vice isn't it]
17   Dana           [It- it-      ] yea it are you learning how to say
18               hello: and bye[bye]
19   Trudy                     [Eh ] [heheh ]
20   Barney                          [Tchuuc][ghuu   ]
21   Dana                                    [Or is it]
22   Chloe       >I learnt that when< I
23   Chloe       [Was a little girl £ actually: huhu £]
24   Trudy       [Ah hahah                            ] ha ha ha
25   Dana        Ah yeah but then and then you have
26   Dana        [To be able] to say to a customer
27   Chloe       [Ah ha ha  ]
28   Barney      [(                              °)]
29   Dana        [Is it- can I get you something el:se]
30   Chloe       £Yea:h£
31               ((1.0) Trudy and Barney talking quietly))
32   Dana        You know if theh if they're playing about with their menu:
33   Chloe       Y-[yea:h                  ]
34   Dana          [N they don' t kn]ow what they' re talking about .hhh they
35               say
36               (0.4)
37   Dana        But you say w- (.) would you like[me to] get something=
38   Chloe                                        [Yea:]
39   Dana        =Else for you
40   Trudy       Yea: s:[s' all] good lear[ning int it]
41   Dana               [Yeah  ]          [Uh- u- o-  ]
42   Dana        Or if you r if you: read the menu an you YOU: understand the
43               menu .hh you can say that' s very: .h (.) that- if youw if
44               you were thinking about something that' s very nice
45   Dana        [We do that] nice .hh you don' t have to go into a rig' morole
46   Trudy       [Mmm       ]
47   Chloe       [Yea ]
48   Dana        [You j]ust say:
49               (((0.8) George on phone))
50   Dana        Er- oh- ahw- we' d we do tha:t n its very nic:e=
51   Trudy       =↑Ye[a↑::h]
```

```
51  Chloe    [Yeah     ]
52  Dana     >[Its veh-]< its very populah
53  Chloe    Mmm
54  Trudy    Gramndma gu's >good at this< she's that was your job wasn't
55           it from: how ol w' from your age Chloe
56  Dana     ↓From being a wee gir:l↓
57           (0.2)
58  Dana     Defi[nitely]
59  Trudy        [Ye[a::h]]
60  Chloe            [(Yea)]
61           (0.2)
62  Dana     .Hhh
63  Trudy    V' always been a[waitress haven't yer]
64  Dana                     [Yea:h al            ] ways but or-
65  Dana     you've a:lways got to be r:eady(.)[for] people
66  Chloe                           .            Mm [mmm]
67           (0.5)
68  George   RI:GHT COME ON THEN MOTHER AV GOT TO GO:
```

The overall sequence in Extract 1 is delivered as advice to Chloe but is simultaneously a reminiscence for Dana about her own time working as a waitress. Dana's reminiscence sequence bears similarities to storytelling since the reminiscence is 'locally occasioned' (Jefferson, 1978: 220) and topically coherent as it follows news of Chloe's waitressing job. Hydén et al., (2013) observed that storytelling in family conversations can be fulfilling for a person with dementia, supporting the identity of the teller. After a shaky start, Dana displays her epistemic authority as she draws on her many decades working as a waitress to offer advice to Chloe. There are four co-participants in this conversation: Chloe is the chief recipient and Trudy and Barney intermittently participate in this interaction or continue their own two-party conversation simultaneously. Such intermittent schism in multi-party talk is systematically achieved without impeding the ongoing conversation (Sacks et al., 1974), and although Dana seems to be directing the advice to Chloe, Trudy also maintains a supporting role in this conversation.

A common language characteristic of people with dementia (Hamilton, 1994, 2019; Orange, 2001) is circumlocution, a means of delivering meaning indirectly in order to overcome problems with lexical access. Dana's use of circumlocution can be seen to cause difficulties in conversation on occasion. Further analysis of Extract 1, in which Dana is having a mealtime conversation with her daughter-in-law and two teenage grandchildren, demonstrates potential problems associated with circumlocution. In the opening to this extract when Dana was reminded that Chloe is still at school and has a weekend job as a waitress, Trudy seems to attempt to deflect the topic when she utters a 'laughable' followed by laugh particles in line 12 and Chloe joins her mother by producing laugh particles in overlap. Glenn (1989: 136) describes 'laughables' as 'those items in reference to which people laugh'. Dana, however, does not laugh but utters further serious talk. At lines 17–18, Dana goes on to expand on her earlier question saying 'are you learning how to say hello and bye bye', which I have classified as circumlocution. This problematic turn is treated as a laughable by each of Dana's co-participants: see their laughter in lines 19 and 20.

Laughter itself does not directly relate to coded linguistic meaning, but the sequential environment in which it occurs reveals the affiliative or non-affiliative characteristics of the sequence (Glenn, 2003; Jefferson, 1979). Glenn (1995, 2003) distinguished between the practices of *laughing at* and *laughing with* co-participants. An interlocutor producing a first laugh at their co-participant's troubles or producing an antagonistic laughable towards an interlocutor would be said to be laughing *at*. The 'butt' of the laughter (Glenn, 2003: 64) can then join the laughter and attempt affiliation or decline and continue with serious talk.

Dana's interlocutors laugh together (lines 19–27) but Dana continues with serious on-topic talk. The laughter produced by Dana's co-participants has the characteristics of 'laughing at' since the first laugh, in response to Dana's circumlocution, was produced by Trudy and overlapped by laugh particles from Barney (line 20). An extension of the laughable was then produced by Chloe in lines 22–23, delivered with smile-voice and turn-final laughter. This sequence seems to be face-threatening (Goffman, 1967 [1955]) to Dana and undermines her epistemic authority. Dana's continuing with on-topic serious talk without any hint of laughter or smiling voice suggests that she has not aligned with the laughable nature of the topic and has treated the laughter as *at* her expense.

At line 25 Dana addresses Chloe directly 'ah yeah but then and then you have to be able to say to a customer'; the use of *you* in this utterance appears to be both directed at Chloe, as recipient, and be a general use of *you* (Sacks 1992) as in *waitresses in general*. Indeed, Dana is not advising that Chloe says 'can I get you something else', but that she should *be able* to make such an offer. By being able to do this, she could fulfil the complex dual role of a waitress in serving her customers and increasing sales on behalf of her employer. Dana now has Chloe's attention, as can be seen from the minimal response in line 30. The delivery of Chloe's utterance has the quality of a smile-voice, denoted by the £ symbol, which appears to be following laughter from Chloe and Barney earlier in the sequence, which may well have been as a result of Dana's circumlocution.

Following a one-second pause (line 31), Dana initiates a more detailed advice sequence. This is prefaced, in lines 32–34, by setting up a scenario in which the customers are 'playing about' and 'don't know what they're talking about'. Dana aligns with Chloe by saying 'you know', which sets apart the waitresses (Dana and Chloe) from the customers, who are in need of guidance.

Chloe acknowledges this scenario with a minimal token in line 33, which projects that Dana can continue with the advice sequence (Goodwin, 1986; Schegloff, 1981). This time Dana delivers the advice by directing Chloe with 'you say' and then performing a courteous offer to the customer (lines 36–38): 'would you like me to get something else for you'. The performance quality of this utterance can be heard in a switch in register, towards Standard English rather than the Northern Irish accent that Dana regularly uses in family conversation. In addition, Dana has now performed the same offer as in line 29 but with the more formal lexical structure 'would you like me to get' rather than 'can I get'. This performative delivery sets the scene in Dana's demonstration (Clark & Gerrig, 1990; Hydén & Örulv, 2009) as she enacts (Kindell et al., 2013) her part as a professional waitress.

Trudy now re-enters the conversation (line 39). Trudy uses the same formulation as before (lines 15–16) 'it's all good [...] isn't it', but this time she refers to 'good learning', which was adumbrated at the start of the sequence with talk about school and Dana's question 'are you learning anything'. Although this chapter is not primarily concerned with repetition (a common characteristic of conversations with persons with dementia), it is interesting to note that repeated formulations and ideas are being produced by Trudy, a participant with no known cognitive impairment. Repetition is common in interaction among participants with shared histories (Norrick, 1997) and can be found regularly across the entire data set, in particular in talk about food, service and working life. Non-impaired interlocutors contribute to, and are coerced into producing, repetition in conversation as familiar topics arise.

In lines 41–52, Dana continues with her advice. She demonstrates (Clark & Gerrig, 1990) to Chloe how to deal with customers: 'that's very nice, we do that nice, we do that and it's very nice' and finally 'it's very popular'. These turns are again delivered with a Standard English accent. After having repeated the adjective 'nice' three times, it seems as though nothing new is forthcoming in this sequence, but then the final demonstration given by Dana, in line 52, is delivered with an almost triumphant Received Pronunciation 'po̱pulah', which is then acknowledged by both Chloe and Trudy. Chloe receipts these recommendations with a minimal token 'mmm', but Trudy validates the advice and Dana's authority to deliver it (lines 54–55). Dana has achieved this sequence in conversation by displaying access to her autobiographical memories. It is delivered in an appropriate manner as advice to a novice waitress, and Dana has received recognition for her authority and expertise in this role.

Furthermore, Dana is ultimately validated as an expert when Trudy says 'you've always been a waitress haven't you' (line 63). Although this turn is addressed to Dana, it is also designed for the other co-present participants to hear, which further upholds Dana's authority and self-worth in this matter.

What is particularly noticeable about the construction of Trudy's turn is the present perfect continuous tense – have [always] been – which imbues Dana's occupation with a sense of continuing professionalism. It is all too easy when speaking to an older person to design one's turn with a sense of what *had been*. As De Beauvoir (1972: 294) observed in her study of old age, there is a feeling of being 'flung from the active into the inactive category'. Trudy has validated, not only the sense of what Dana once was, but also her authority to advise Chloe in the *here and now*.

As Dana delivered her advice, Chloe showed her participation in the conversation with a minimal token 'mmmmm' (line 66), expressing her alignment with Dana's continuation. The sequence ends abruptly as George completes his telephone call and has to leave urgently, taking Dana with him. Although Chloe's lexical contribution to this sequence is minimal, her participation in the interaction has offered Dana an opportunity to advise, remember and be validated as a 'usable participant' (Goffman, 1967) – and, indeed, an expert on her working life.

11.3.2 Shared Reminiscence: Claiming Knowledge

This section explores a sequence in which Dana responds to memories, reminiscences and assertions produced by interlocutors. Whereas Dana's self-initiated reminiscence sequences are often fluent and assertive, reminiscence initiated by others is not treated by Dana with the same authority. She can, however, design her turns as sequentially relevant to come off as *doing remembering*.

Extract 2

```
1    Trudy    Seems like five minutes ago when you came to
2             visit her in Castleford d' you rememb[er tha]t
3    Dana                                         [Go:d ]
4             (0.7)
5    Dana     ˚Gohd bless us?˚
6    Trudy    You came to see me in the hospit[al   ]
7    Dana                                     ↑[Yea]:h↑
8             (0.5)
9    Trudy    >>↑↑Hmemem↑↑<<
10   George   Hggh[gghh  ] ((possible cough))
11   Dana         [>Hu hi] hu<
12   Dana     <˚Ghod    [love her]˚>
13   Trudy    She had a [shock of] black hair d' you 'member=
14   Dana     =£Yeah[oh ho ho huh £                            ]
15   George         [ (>Y' right<) she had black hair]
16   George   [When she w born di' nt she [ Chloe]]
17   Dana     [Hi hi hi                   [Hi hi]hi  ]
18   Trudy                                [[Ye::]a::h]
19   Dana     .Hhh £yeah£
```

```
20              (0.6)
21    Dana      God love her e' she was £gorgeous£ ah heh
22    Trudy     I kno:w: >at least Teddy< got to see her
23              Di[dn' t he] =he was still alive then wasn't he
24    Dana      [Yeah    ]
25    Dana      Yeah=
26    Trudy     =You and Teddy came throu:gh in y
27              li[ttle white] Hond[ a ]
28    Dana        [˚Yeaȟ    ]     [He] he he he
```

During the reminiscence sequence in Extract 2, Dana's is twice asked 'do you remember?' Caregivers and families are often advised not to use this phrase (Alzheimer's Society, 2024) as it is thought to challenge a person with dementia, cause distress and have a negative effect on their self-esteem by exposing memory impairment. In Extract 2, as in other instances of this question found in the data, this is asked without any such difficulties arising. Dana can successfully use the interactional context to sustain her conversation; she is able to align with the projected preference of the question (Pomerantz, 1984) by affirming, or at the very least not disconfirming, that she remembers. Dana is thus ratified as a participant in the shared reminiscence.

In Extract 1 reminiscence sequences were explored that involved Dana's autobiographical memories about her long career as a waitress. Sequences from Extract 1 were packaged as advice to Chloe, the young waitress, but all involved Dana's primary access (Drew, 1991; Heritage, 2012a; Labov & Fanshel, 1977; Pomerantz, 1980, 1984) to knowledge about her own experiences, told by her to others who have only secondary access to the stories. Extract 2 differs from the earlier example in that this is a reminiscence of shared experiences between George, Trudy and Dana; they each have equal epistemic authority (Heritage, 2012a, 2012b; Heritage & Raymond, 2005; Stivers et al., 2011) relating to a shared experience. Furthermore, this reminiscence sequence is initiated by a person other than Dana; she has not 'found' this memory for herself.

Just prior to the start of Extract 2, Dana asked the age of her granddaughter, Chloe. Trudy answered the question, telling Dana she is fifteen and followed up with an assessment of the intervening years having passed so quickly: 'seems like five minutes ago'. This is the start of a reminiscence sequence initiated by Trudy, and she goes on to provide some details of the event: Dana 'came to visit her in Castleford' in line 2, 'came to see me in hospital' line 6 and 'she [Chloe] had a shock of black hair' in line 13. Dana aligns with Trudy's telling with fitted contributions including 'god bless us' in line 5, 'yeah' in lines 7 and 14, and laughter throughout. At line 12, Dana utters the phrase 'God love her'. By using the female pronoun, it seems that Dana is on track in terms of the referent of the conversation, that is Chloe. However, it may not be clear to Dana at this stage that they are speaking about the Chloe of fifteen years ago. There is no explicit mention of the baby or birth until lines 15 and 16 when George brings together the implicit facts given in the sequence so far and states 'she had black hair when she was born didn't she, Chloe'. Dana laughs (line 17) in overlap with George's utterance. Following Trudy's response 'yeah' in line 18, Dana also responds to George's assertion by uttering the word 'yeah', which is delivered with a smile voice. This quality in Dana's voice may be attributed to having just completed a stream of laughter, but it also appears to lend an element of grandmotherly nostalgia to the utterance.

George and Trudy have, collaboratively, provided Dana with an assessable referent. They have described the baby 'she had a shock of black hair' and some of the events occurring at the time of her birth – 'you came to visit her in Castleford' and 'you came to see me in hospital' – but they have not, themselves, made an assessment of the baby's characteristics. For example, they did not say she had *lovely* black hair. Chloe's parents have 'seeded the ground' (Goodwin, 2003: 157) for Dana to make the first assessment, which she does in line 21: 'God love her she was gorgeous'. As Pomerantz (1984) noted, making assessments is related to rights of experiential access to an event or referent. In addition, Heritage and Raymond (2005) state that by uttering the first assessment, an interlocutor is claiming epistemic rights over the assessable. In this case, it has been put to Dana that she was present at the hospital and that she saw the baby. Dana has the right to assess, and by doing so, demonstrates that she has personal access to details of the event.

We cannot know whether Dana actually remembers this event for herself. Given that she is a fluent speaker and her talk is rich with description of events in her self-initiated reminiscence sequences, there seems to be a marked lack of detail in her contribution in this example. Positive assessments of babies, and grandchildren in particular, are culturally relevant and expectable owing to Dana's status as a grandmother (Raymond & Heritage, 2006). Comparable with Jones' (2015: 564) concept of 'answering without knowing', it is possible that Dana cannot access this memory herself but is relying on the interactional context to design her assessment. Dana's interlocutors have, incrementally, created an interactional environment in which Dana can share in a joint reminiscence sequence. Despite the taboo surrounding the phrase *do you remember*, when it is produced, in lines 2 and 13, it provides the sequentially relevant slot for Dana to affirm that she does remember. This question has not exposed Dana's memory impairment or caused upset or interactional difficulties. On the contrary, by exploiting the subtle processes of 'sequential implicativeness' (Schegloff & Sacks, 1973: 296), Dana has demonstrated that she is a competent and authoritative participant in this reminiscence.

11.3.3 Resolving Interactional Problems Involving Confusion

In this section I inspect how Dana's failing understanding leads to interactional breakdowns and the ways she and her co-participants manage to recover her authority. Firs, some background to Extract 3 is required. The Fortes referred to in the conversations are the family who became famous for a large, multinational chain of hotels and restaurants. The name 'Forte' is, therefore, retained so as to preserve the sense of what is being discussed and because the name is publicly known. For the same reason, some names of establishments in Belfast are retained, but all other names of people and private addresses are pseudonyms.

Extract 3

```
1    Dana    That was Belfast .hhh[ (nea:r the)           ]
2    John                         [ So that wasn' t the] f- Fortes then
3                (0.6)
4    Dana    Fortes:sh yes it was the Fortes yeah
5    John    >Cz yu< said mister and missus Finley
6    Dana    Oh- yeah, mister and missus Fin:ley (0.2) yeah=
7    John    =Yeah
8            (0.2)
9    Dana    Ayeah
10           (1.3)
11   Dana    An:d urm
12   John    W' l' oo were mister and missis Finley then
13   Dana    .Hhhh their parents
14           (1.5)
15   John    Parents of:
16           (0.2)
17   Dana    Ba:rney
18           (1.8)
19   Dana    Uug ↑>mhmhmm<↑
20           (0.7)
21   Dana    .Pt you' re m(h)ixing me up £now£
22           (1.3)
23   Dana    .Hhh[hhh          ]
24   John        >[You' re on a]bout< mister Sykes now ar' yuh
25   Dana    <~Mister sykes:~>
26           (1.3)
27   John    At the society club o:r no- >we' re talking about
28           Belfast[ aren' t we]<
29   Dana           <°[Bel      ] fast°>
30           (1.4)
31   Dana    .Hh °°who ws- u- who was there°°
32           (0.3)
33   John    Cz I always thought you said it w- the Café Grande was
34           owned by: u- (0.5) Fortes
35   Dana    Fortes
36   John    Yeah y' knowu- (.) ended up m:assive in this
37           cun-b-m-b- Fortes restaurants
```

```
38              (0.2)
39      John    On the mo:torways n stuff
40              (1.8)
41      John    No:
42              (0.5)
43      Dana    I don't know: no:
44              (1.5)
45      Dana    But I wor̲ked in the Café Gra̲:nde
```

The uncertainty in this sequence arises from John questioning some details relating to Dana's reminiscence (not shown) about working in the Café Grande in Belfast. Dana mentions her employers, the Finleys and the Fortes, and John is trying to understand the relationship between the two.

Lines 2–15 involve a sequence in which John is probing for information about the relationship of the two families, the Finleys and the Fortes. Dana does not seem to understand what he is asking or, perhaps, considers that the question has been satisfactorily answered. After a pause in line 10, Dana produces a turn 'and uhm' which suggests she is projecting a resumption of her earlier topic. Local (2004) showed that turn-initial 'and uhm' is a device to signal that the upcoming turn would not be sequentially relevant to the immediate prior, but a move to resume an earlier topic. Dana, however, does not complete the turn and John continues with his questioning about the Fortes and the Finleys, which leads to Dana becoming confused, as evidenced in line 21. Dana is consistent in the fact that the Finleys are parents of the Fortes, but what John wishes to clarify is how they came to have different names. Elsewhere in the data John and Dana discuss this problem: for example, John says: 'Mr and Mrs Finley must have been Frank Forte's inlaws'. While Dana repeatedly offers the same information, answering John's questions with sequentially relevant and consistent facts, she does not seem to understand the complexities of the overall project that John is proposing, which is that the Finley's son would, according to British custom, take the same surname as his parents.

John's probing for information seems to result in Dana's uncertainty. In line 15 John invites a collaborative completion (Lerner, 2004) from Dana to try to elicit the information. Dana answers 'Barney' with intonation that has an abrupt quality, the start of the single word being of increased amplitude. This is followed by perturbations from Dana and in line 21 she actually states 'you're mixing me up now', delivered with laugh particles and smile voice. The indication of laughter signals a light-hearted recognition of her incompetence (Haakana, 2010; Jefferson, 1984; Wilkinson, 2007) and John continues with a serious account of whom she may be referring to in line 24.

Further questioning from John on the matter does not elicit an answer. In lines 25, 29 and 35, Dana simply repeats parts of John's prior turns. In line 36 John initiates a side-sequence (Jefferson, 1972) to elaborate on the Forte question. He uses the phrase 'you know', which is a marker of knowledge management in conversation (Schiffrin, 1987). *You know* refers to knowledge which is either generally known or which is expectedly shared between the co-participants. John incrementally delivers the information about the Forte family, who are known in the hotels and motorways services businesses. After a pause of 1.8 seconds in line 40, he modifies his assumption that Dana should know about this and utters 'no', which seems to signify an abandonment of the side sequence. At line 43 Dana utters 'I don't know no', confirming that she does not know about the Fortes' chain of restaurants.

This is the point at which Dana achieves the transition from uncertainty back to authority. By clearly stating that she *does not know*, the sequence is closed and nothing further is added by John as a 1.5 second pause ensues. The subsequent turn is constructed with a turn-initial *but*, indicating a referential contrast (Schiffrin, 1987) between the referent that Dana does not know about (the Fortes dilemma) and that which she does know (the Café Grande). Dana's turn in line 45 'I worked at the Café Grande' is delivered with declarative syntax, claiming ownership of knowledge. Her lexical choice *but* simultaneously manages various features of the ongoing talk: (1) it connects her statement to the prior talk, showing that it is sequentially relevant, (2) it projects the contrast of the actions *not knowing* to *knowing*, (3) it signals the speaker's pursuit of an earlier topic (Schiffrin, 1987) – a return to the topic last referenced in line 1. The latter feature is crucial for Dana, it seems, since she returns to talk about autobiographical events over which she has primary authority and can confidently hold the floor.

11.4 Discussion

This chapter has explored situations in which a person with dementia can present herself as authoritative. The social setting empowers Dana to demonstrate her competence and expertise, facilitated through interaction with her extended family and members of the community. Dana's reminiscences are not merely formulaic, perseverant monologues, but are sequentially relevant topic transitions and sustained through her epistemic primacy relating to the memories.

Dana uses advice-giving as a way to demonstrate her epistemic authority in certain situations. By advising her granddaughter, Chloe who is working as a part-time waitress, Dana presents herself as an expert waitress. She even uses this authority to recover from a lapse in interactional competence when her verbal fluency momentarily fails and seems to prompt laughter from her interlocutors. Dana does not affiliate with the laughable nature of the sequence but generates an interactional environment in which further advice was sequentially relevant. During the advice-giving, Chloe utters little more than minimal tokens. However, Chloe's sustained attention and her very presence at the family dinner table have provided the relevant opportunity for Dana to advise and be validated as expert.

Dana's diminished understanding was exposed when she could not answer John's complex questions about the names and relationships of the families she had worked for in Belfast. Eventually, after a great deal of uncertainty, Dana expressed her authority and restored her epistemic status (Heritage, 2012a, 2012b; Stivers et al., 2011) by stating that she did *not know* about that subject but, by contrast, returned to a topic over which she could claim primacy.

I examined a sequence from a family mealtime conversation in which participants talked about a shared reminiscence of the birth of Dana's granddaughter fifteen years earlier. During this sequence, Trudy repeatedly used the phrase *do you remember* as a tag question to incrementally declared details of the event. Contrary to general advice that this question should be avoided, this practice actually supported the sequential flow and overall project of the interaction, allowing Dana to align with the action of the current talk: family reminiscing. The words 'do you remember', it seems, do not necessarily cause interactional breakdown. It is the action underlying the utterance which could have this effect. As evidenced in Extract 3, in which John probes Dana for information about the Finleys and the Fortes, we can see that actions such as probing, testing and asking a person with dementia to prove that they remember may result in a breakdown of interaction and lead to feelings of diminished self-worth. On the other hand, the question 'do you remember', used in a supportive interaction, helped Dana to contribute to the family talk about shared experiences. Though it seems likely that Dana did not, at first (if at all), remember the details of the shared memory of Chloe's birth, she was able to sustain the conversation. Her co-participants incrementally and collaboratively supplied details about the event and Dana demonstrated, by assessing the 'gorgeous baby', that she could competently *do* remembering.

References

Alzheimer's Society (2024) 'What not to say to somebody with dementia.' https://www.alzheimers.org.uk/blog/language-dementia-what-not-to-say.

Antaki, C. (2011) 'Six kinds of applied conversation analysis.' In C. Antaki (ed.) *Applied Conversation Analysis: Intervention and Change in Institutional Talk*. Basingstoke: Palgrave Macmillan.

Clark, H. H. and Gerrig, R. J. (1990) 'Quotations as demonstrations' *Language*, 66(4): 764–805.

Coupland, N., Coupland, J. and Giles, H. (1991) *Language, Society and the Elderly: Discourse, Identity and Ageing*. Oxford: Blackwell.

De Beauvoir, S. (1972 [1970]) *Old Age*. London: Penguin.

Department of Health (2009) *Living Well with Dementia: A National Dementia Strategy*. https://assets.publishing.service.gov.uk/media/5a7a15a7ed915d6eaf153a36/dh_094051.pdf.

Drew, P. (1991) 'Asymmetries of knowledge in conversational interactions.' In I. Markova and K. Foppa (eds.) *Asymmetries in Dialogue*. Hemel Hempstead: Harvester Wheatsheaf, pp. 21–48.

Fivush, R. (2008) 'Remembering and reminiscing: How individual lives are constructed in family narratives.' *Memory Studies*, 1(1): 49–58.

Fivush, R., Haden, C. and Reese, E. (1999) 'Remembering, recounting and reminiscing: The development of autobiographical memory in context.' In D. C. Rubin (ed.) *Remembering Our Past: Studies in Autobiographical Memory*. Cambridge: Cambridge University Press, pp. 341–359.

Gauthier, S., Rosa-Neto, P., Morais, J. A. and Webster, C. (2021) *World Alzheimer Report 2021: Journey through the Diagnosis of Dementia*. Alzheimer's Disease International. www.alzint.org/resource/world-alzheimer-report-2021/

Glenn, P. J. (1989) 'Initiating shared laughter in multi-party conversations.' *Western Journal of Speech Communication*, 53(2): 127–149.

(1995) 'Laughing at and laughing with: Negotiations of participant alignments through conversational laughter.' In P. ten Have and G. Psathas (eds.) *Situated Order: Studies in the Social Organization of Talk and Embodied Activities*. Lanham, MD: University Press of America, pp. 43–56.

Glenn, P. (2003) *Laughter in Interaction*. Cambridge: Cambridge University Press.

Goffman, E. (1967 [1955]) 'On face-work.' In E. Goffman, *Interaction Ritual: Essays on Face-to-Face Behavior*. New York: Pantheon Books, pp. 33–40.

Goodwin, C. (1986) 'Between and within: Alternative sequential treatments of continuers and assessments.' *Human Studies*, 9(2–3): 205–217.

(1987) 'Forgetfulness as an interactive resource.' *Social Psychology Quarterly*, 50(2): 115–131.

(2003) 'Recognizing assessable names.' In P. Glenn, C. LeBaron and J. Mandelbaum (eds.) *Excavating the Taken-for-Granted: Essays in Social Interaction*. A Festschrift in honour of Robert Hopper. Mahwah, NJ: Lawrence Erlbaum, pp. 151–161.

Haakana, M. (2010) 'Laughter and smiling: Notes on co-occurrences.' *Journal of Pragmatics*, 42(6): 1499–1512.

Hamilton, H. E. (1994) *Conversations with an Alzheimer's Patient: An Interactional Sociolinguisitc Study*. Cambridge: Cambridge University Press.

(2019) 'Now what was that called?' In *Language, Dementia and Meaning Making*. Cham: Palgrave Macmillan, pp. 21–56.

Heritage, J. C. (2012a) 'Epistemics in action: Action formation and territories of knowledge.' *Research on Language and Social Interaction*, 45(1): 1–29.

(2012b) 'Epistemic engine: Sequence organization and territories of knowledge.' *Research on Language and Social Interaction*, 45(1): 30–52.

Heritage, J. (2013) 'Epistemics in conversation' In J. Sidnell and T. Stivers (eds.) *The Handbook of Conversation Analysis*. Chichester: Wiley-Blackwell, pp. 370–394.

Heritage, J. and Raymond, G. (2005) 'The terms of agreement: Indexing epistemic authority and subordination in talk-in-interaction.' *Social Psychology Quarterly*, 68(1): 15–38.

Hydén, L. C. (2011) 'Narrative collaboration and scaffolding in dementia.' *Journal of Aging Studies*, 25(4): 339–367.

Hydén, L. C. and Örulv, L. (2009) 'Narrative and identity in Alzheimer's disease: A case study.' *Journal of Aging Studies*, 23(4): 205–214.

Hydén, L. C., Plejert, C., Samuelsson, C. and Örulv, L. (2013) 'Feedback and common ground in conversational storytelling involving people with Alzheimer's disease.' *Journal of Interactional Research in Communication Disorders*, 4(2): 211–247.

Jefferson, G. (1972) 'Side sequences.' In D. N. Sudnow (ed.) *Studies in Social Interaction*. New York: Free Press, pp. 294–338.

(1978) 'Sequential aspects of storytelling in conversation.' In J. N. Schenkein (ed.) *Studies in the Organization of Conversational Interaction*. New York: Academic Press, pp. 219–248.

(1979) 'A technique for inviting laughter and its subsequent acceptance/declination.' In G. Psathas (ed.) *Everyday Language: Studies in Ethnomethodology*. New York: Irvington, pp. 79–96.

(1984) 'Laughter organization in talk about troubles.' In J. M. Atkinson and J. Heritage (eds.) *Structures of Social Action: Studies in Conversation Analysis*. Cambridge: Cambridge University Press, pp. 346–369.

(2004) 'Glossary of transcript symbols with an introduction.' In G. H. Lerner (ed.) *Conversation Analysis: Studies from the First Generation*. Amsterdam: John Benjamins, pp. 13–31.

Jones, D. (2015) 'A family living with Alzheimer's disease: The communicative challenges.' *Dementia, The International Journal of Social Research and Practice*, 14(5): 555–573.

Kindell, J., Sage, K., Keady, J. and Wilkinson, R. (2013) 'Adapting to conversation with semantic dementia: using enactment as a compensatory strategy in everyday social interaction.' *International Journal of Language & Communication Disorders*, 48(5): 497–507.

Kitwood, T. (1997) *Dementia Reconsidered: The Person Comes First*. Maidenhead: Open University Press.

Labov, W. and Fanshel, D. (1977) *Therapeutic Discourse: Psychotherapy as Conversation*. London: Academic Press.

Lerner, G. H. (2004) 'Collaborative turn sequences.' In G. H. Lerner (ed.) *Conversation Analysis: Studies from the First Generation*. Amsterdam: John Benjamins, pp. 225–256.

Lindley, L. (2016) 'Competence in Everyday Interaction: A Conversation Analytic Approach to Repetition, Confusion and Getting Things Done when Living with Dementia.' PhD thesis, University of Leeds, Leeds, UK, White Rose eTheses Online: http://etheses.whiterose.ac.uk/14314/.

(2020) 'Foregrounding competence in interaction with a person with dementia: Co-participant responses to disordered talk.' In T. Stickle (ed.) *Learning from the Talk of Persons with Dementia*. Cham: Palgrave Macmillan, pp. 111–134.

Local, J. K. (2004) 'Getting back to prior talk: And-uh(m) as a back connecting device in British and American English.' In E. Couper-Kuhlen (ed.) *Sound Patterns in Interaction: Cross-Linguistic Studies of Phonetics and Prosody for Conversation*. Amsterdam: John Benjamins, pp. 377–400.

McCarthy, B. (2011) *Hearing the Person with Dementia: Person-Centred Approaches to Communication for Families and Caregivers*. London: Jessica Kingsley Publishers.

Mok, Z. and Müller, N. (2014) 'Staging casual conversations for people with dementia.' *Dementia*, 13(6): 834–853.

Müller, N. and Mok, Z. (2014) '"Getting to know you": Situated and distributed cognitive effort in conversations with dementia.' In R. W. Schrauf and N. Müller (eds.) *Dialogue and Dementia: Cognitive And Communicative Resources for Engagement*. Hove: Psychology Press, pp. 61–86.

Muntigl, P. and Choi, K. T. (2010) 'Not remembering as a practical epistemic resource in couples therapy.' *Discourse Studies*, 12(3): 331–356.

Norrick, N. R. (1997) 'Twice-told tales: Collaborative narration of familiar stories.' *Language in Society*, 26: 199–220. http://dx.doi.org/10.1017/S004740450002090X.

— (2019) 'Collaborative remembering in conversational narration.' *Topics in Cognitive Science*, 11(4): 733–751.

— (2020) 'The epistemics of narrative performance in conversation.' *Narrative Inquiry*, 30(2): 211–235.

Orange, J. B.(2001) 'Family caregivers, communication and Alzheimer's disease.' In M. Lee Hummert and J. F. Nussbaum (eds.) *Aging, Communication and Health: Linking Research and Practice for Successful Aging*. London: Lawrence Erlbaum Associates, pp. 225–248.

Pomerantz, A. (1980) 'Telling my side: "Limited access" as a "fishing" device.' *Sociological Inquiry*, 50(3–4): 186–198.

— (1984) 'Agreeing and disagreeing with assessments: Some features of preferred/dispreferred turn shapes.' In J. Maxwell Atkinson and J. Heritage (eds.) *Structures of Social Action: Studies in Conversation Analysis*. Cambridge: Cambridge University Press, pp. 57–101.

Raymond, G. and Heritage, J. C. (2006) 'The epistemics of social relations: Owning grandchildren.' *Language in Society*, 35(5): 677–705.

Sabat, S. R. (2001) *The Experience of Alzheimer's Disease: Life through a Tangled Veil*. Oxford: Blackwell.

Sabat, S. R. and Lee, J. M. (2011) 'Relatedness among people diagnosed with dementia: Social cognition and the possibility of friendship.' *Dementia*, 11(3): 315–327.

Sacks, H. (1992) *Lectures on Conversation*, volumes I and II. Oxford: Blackwell.

Sacks, H., Schegloff, E. A. and Jefferson, G. (1974) 'A simplest systematics for the organization of turn-taking for conversation.' *Language*, 50(4): 696–735.

Schegloff, E. A. (1981) 'Discourse as an interactional achievement: Some uses of "uh huh" and other things that come between sentences.' In D. Tannen (ed.) *Analyzing Discourse: Text and Talk* (Georgetown University Round Table on Languages and Linguistics 1981), Washington DC: Georgetown University Press, pp. 71–93.

Schegloff, E. A. and Sacks, H. (1973) 'Opening up closings.' *Semiotica*, 8(4), pp. 289–327.

Schiffrin, Deborah (1987) *Discourse Markers*. Cambridge: Cambridge University Press.

Stivers, T., Mondada, L. and Steensig, J. (2011) 'Knowledge, morality and affiliation in social interaction.' In T. Stivers, L. Mondada and J. Steensig (eds.) *The Morality of Knowledge in Conversation*. Cambridge: Cambridge University Press, pp. 3–24.

Vehviläinen, S. (2001) 'Evaluative advice in educational counselling: The use of disagreement in the "stepwise" entry to advice.' *Research on Language and Social Interaction*, 34(3): 371–398.

Wilkinson, R. (2007) 'Managing linguistic incompetence as a delicate issue in aphasic talk-in-interaction: On the use of laughter in prolonged repair sequences.' *Journal of Pragmatics*, 37(3): 542–569.

Part 5

Communicative Challenges in Everyday Social Life

12 Language and Cognition in Conversations with a Person with Alzheimer's Disease

Danielle Jones

12.1 Introduction

Alzheimer's disease, the most common form of dementia, is a degenerative and progressive disability in which the anatomy and physiology of the brain becomes increasingly damaged over time. The person's ability to remember, understand, communicate and reason will gradually decline, and the symptoms will become progressively more marked (Alzheimer's Society, 2020a). Memory impairment is one of the earliest and most significant symptoms of Alzheimer's disease: 'Memory loss is a distressing part of dementia, both for the person with dementia and for those around them ... it will gradually become apparent that the memory problems are becoming more severe and persistent' (Alzheimer's Society, 2020b). During the earlier stages of the disease, people may start to become increasingly confused, disorientated with time and place, forgetful about recent conversations or events, repetitive, and lose interest in others (ADI, 2020), often with consequent feelings of upset, anger and frustration. In the later stages of Alzheimer's, the ability to identify who they are, what they are doing and who the people around them are decreases[1] (Kennard, 2009). This decline impacts the type and quality of communication people can sustain.

The relationship between communication and cognition has been extensively explored within a variety of disciplines including psychology, linguistics, sociology, neurosciences and cognitive sciences (see Potter & te Molder, 2005). Early ethnomethodological positions espoused a detachment between *action* and *intent*, concluding that language does not provide an entry into cognition, nor does it offer insight into actual cognitive states (Wittgenstein, 1958; Schegloff, 1991; Edwards & Potter, 1992; Lynch & Bogen, 2005). Working broadly within this approach, conversation analytic (CA) researchers 'are not primarily concerned with what happens in the minds of

---

[1] While these are common symptoms of Alzheimer's, it is important to remember that people experience dementia in different ways, and symptoms appear and decline at different rates, depending on factors such as their physiology, their emotional resilience, and their access to quality support and treatment.

conversationalists but rather with the evidenced behavior' (Sacks, 1992; Bogels & Levinson, 2017: 71). For example, in CA, attributions (or self-attributions) of cognitive states (e.g., 'I can't remember') are not treated as reflecting actual cognitive events but rather as accomplishing a range of social activities. However, there has been an increasing interchange between CA research and psycholinguistics, supported by neuroimaging, which changes our understanding of the relationship between language and cognition. Using neuroimaging, such as electroencephalogram (EEG) and functional magnetic resonance imaging (fMRI), researchers can measure the underlying cognitive processes enabling people to understand and produce language (Bogels & Levinson, 2017; Gisladottir et al., 2018). It is acknowledged that there may be a closer connection between interaction and cognition, recognizing interaction as a 'source' of cognition, through the identification of cognitive 'moments' in interaction (Drew, 2005a; Heritage, 2005). Viewing language and interaction as a window to cognition is especially relevant for exploring the effects of cognitive decline as a result of Alzheimer's disease, through the changing patterns of language in interaction. This chapter explores this intersection between cognition and interaction by longitudinally analyzing the cognitive abilities (and the change in those abilities) of a person with dementia, examining how memory loss is reflected in verbal conduct during everyday family communication.

12.2 Data and Methods

The data are audio recordings of 70 naturally occurring telephone conversations (identified using the prefix ALZ 1-70) between a woman with Alzheimer's (pseudonymized as 'May') and her family members (daughter 'Natalie' and son-in-law 'Bill'). They were collected between February 2006 and June 2008 as part of a wider investigation into family interactions and the impact Alzheimer's disease has on family communication and relationships (Jones, 2012, 2015). Of these 70 recordings, 20 calls from the beginning of the recording period will be used as the 'early calls' (ALZ1–ALZ20). These were recorded over a period of one month spanning February and March 2006. Within this chapter, these initial calls will be compared with 10 calls recorded at the end of the recording period between March and June 2008 (ALZ60–ALZ70). The conversations analyzed in this chapter therefore span two years and four months. A recording device was attached to the family's telephone, and they manually operated the device to record May's calls. In 2006, when recording began, May was 72 years old and had received a formal diagnosis of Alzheimer's in 2001. May was resident at 'Lilly Hill', a residential home from mid-2005 to May 2008 (for 66 out of the 70 calls – including all the 'early calls', ALZ1–ALZ20 and calls ALZ60–ALZ66 from the later comparative subset). Towards the end of the recordings, May moved to 'Searle Court', a specialist care home for people living with dementia where the final four calls were recorded (ALZ67–ALZ70 from the comparative subset).

To make and receive calls at Lilly Hill, May used the residential home's payphone. This frequently caused problems for May as she struggled to insert coins upon hearing the call had connected. The calls between May and her family became the main medium of communication through which their relationships were played out. May repeatedly called Natalie and Bill several times each day, predominantly to make a request to return home, which was subsequently and repeatedly denied, creating anxiety and distress for everyone. May's symptoms progressed fairly markedly during this time period. The most noticeable change was the degeneration of her short-term memory.

CA was used as a method for analyzing the data (see Drew, 2005b; Sidnell, 2010). The recordings were transcribed using conventions widely adopted in CA (Jefferson, 1983, 2004). All the names of people and places are pseudonymized. As previously highlighted, this chapter explores a deeper connection between language and cognition than hitherto acknowledged in CA studies, shifting away from analyzing the interactional organization of cognition as it is displayed in talk to exploring actual cognitive states as revealed and made relevant in interaction. It explores May's actual cognitive abilities and the change in her cognitive faculties over time by examining how memory loss (amongst other symptoms) is reflected in verbal conduct. This approach changes the status of both data and analysis, in that here I am not looking at practices or patterns of interaction per se. Instead, I'm using excerpts to illustrate possible cognitive decline, privileging content over structure for what it can tell us about states of brain functionality. Ultimately, Alzheimer's disease is a cognitive impairment and results in the loss of cognitive functioning, and so we would expect to find indicators of that in talk. It is therefore through the analysis of conversation that we can say something about cognition. This exploration of language and its relationship to cognition, through the investigation of May's changing interactional patterns, will be the focus of this chapter.

12.3 Analysis

Observing the changing symptoms of May's disease (as manifest in talk) from the beginning of the recording in February 2006 to the end in June 2008 shows signs that May experienced considerable and degenerative short-term memory loss. The main purpose of May's repeated calls was to make a request to return home, as she was unable to remember where she was living or to recognize the current establishment in which she found herself as home. In 41 of May's calls the request featured as the main business. This alone is evidence of her memory deficits, as she habitually called several times each night over a two-and-a-half-year period to make this same request.[2] May's memory lapse between calls is evident throughout the progression of the disease. However, at the earlier stage (in the *earlier calls* – recorded between February and March 2006) there is some evidence of memory retention between calls and definite retention within each call itself. At the later stage (in the *later calls* – recorded between March and June 2008) there is very little evidence of memory retention between calls and much evidence of memory loss within each call. The decline of May's memory is particularly apparent at the later stages when she was unable to retain information within seconds of being told it. This provides evidence of the diminishing functionality of May's short-term memory.

Alongside increasing confusion and memory problems, May demonstrated other common symptoms such as becoming disoriented with regards to her own location, losing interest in others, developing a readiness to blame others and a marked inability to adapt to change. She seldom enquired about her family's well-being and displayed little interest when told information about their lives. She blamed her daughter for placing her in residential care by saying things like 'I can't understand what you're doing to me at the moment. You're bunging me in here', and she refused to accept that she was living in residential care when informed by her family, responding with 'I certainly don't want to stay here', 'I think the answer is I would like to come home. Definitely' and 'In fact I'll start walking down'. These features made for difficult interactions and placed a strain on social relationships.

In analyzing and discussing my findings in the following section, I explore four elements of the interaction relevant to memory retention/loss:

(1) May's early calls – May displays some memory retention between calls.
(2) May's early calls – May demonstrates memory retention within calls.
(3) May's later calls – May exhibits little or no memory retention between calls.
(4) May's later calls – May demonstrates no memory retention within each call.

First, I consider how May's ability to retain information between her earlier calls varies.

---

[2] It is important to note that people with Alzheimer's often struggle with the concept of 'home', which may evoke memories or emotions of a time or place where the person felt comfortable or safe, or of a home that no longer exists, making it difficult for people to identify or accept their current surroundings as home (Alzheimer's Society, 2020b).

12.3.1 May's Early Calls: Memory Retention between Calls

In 2006, during the earlier calls between May and her family, May demonstrated the ability to retain information between conversations, independently of being informed by her interlocutors. As identified, throughout all the calls in the corpus, May repeatedly contacted her family to make a request to return home. Six of the first seven recordings featured such a request, and in each case the request was designed with no orientation to their status as a repeated request and with embedded presuppositions that she would return home so the issue was *when* (e.g., 'When am I coming home' and 'When on earth can I get home'). When informed that she was living in the care home, May frequently, with surprise, admitted having forgotten (e.g., 'Oh bloody hell. I'd forgotten'). This lack of displayed awareness of her ongoing situation provides evidence of her memory loss, even at the earlier stages of the disease. There are a few other examples of May's memory lapses between calls in 2006. However, these are not as frequent as the memory loss May exhibited in 2008. In the earlier calls, there is evidence to suggest that May was sometimes able to retain information over time, thus providing some evidence of her intact cognitive functioning.

In Extract 1, May demonstrates some memory retention. During a previous conversation, which occurred about five minutes before this, Bill (son-in-law) informed May (person with dementia) that Natalie (May's daughter) was at a council meeting. In this call (Extract 1), following an enquiry about her residential arrangements, May continues to display an awareness that Natalie is out at the meeting without having been informed about it during this call.

Extract 1 (ALZ04: Feb 2006)
```
01 MAY  I do apologis[e. I gather] Natalie's at a
02 BIL              [I kno::w.   ]
03 MAY  council meeting.
04       (0.6)
05 BIL  Yes. She is. Ye::s.
```

May is able to display that she is aware of Natalie's attendance at the meeting, 'I gather Natalie's at a council meeting' (lines 1–3). 'I gather' suggests that she has been informed about Natalie's attendance at the meeting during some prior interaction (which interaction we cannot tell), but it is not inferred from the current conversation. This is a clear example of May's ability to produce information from memory, therefore leading to a more 'positive' interaction, with Bill being able to confirm that May has got something right.

The following two extracts feature talk about Natalie's leg. In February 2006 Natalie broke her leg in an accident, a fact that May often forgot. However, in these early extracts May was still able to be solicitous from memory, showing care to her daughter. This capacity to be other-attentive is a feature of human sociality that appears to deteriorate with the progression of the disease. If one has no recollection of an event (such as one's daughter breaking her leg) one will not be able to topicalize it in conversation nor display any signs of caring (see Drew & Chilton, 2000). The degeneration of the functionality of May's memory, and thus deterioration in her ability to display caring, is evident in the later calls. However, here she displays memory retention between calls and is solicitous about her daughter's well-being.

Extract 2: (ALZ11: March 2006)
```
01   MAY    How are you love an' how' s yo- everything going
02          going the:re. How' s your le:g.
03   NAT    .hh It' s alright. hh It' s not so much longer
04          until I can get the plaster off it so
05          that' ull be good.=
06   MAY    =Oh good love.
07   NAT    .hh That' ull be a great relie:f [ I think]
08   MAY                                     [  I'm  ] su:re
09          it will darling.
10   NAT    Hhh
11   MAY    £Honestly you hh poor th(h)ing.
```

Extract 3 (ALZ07: Feb 2006)
```
01   BIL    How ar' you.
02          (0.6)
03   MAY    .hh huh °d' yu really want to kn(h)ow.° huh
04   BIL    N(h)o. N(h)o I kn(h)ow. .hhh huh .h Natalie' s
05          out at the moment.
06   MAY    Right.
07          (0.3)
08   MAY    So how i:s she:,
09   BIL    She- she' s oka:y. Yeah she' s not too bad.
10          Still hobbling arou:nd.=
11   MAY    =Ye:s qui:te.
```

In Extract 2, May demonstrates recollection of Natalie's broken leg by explicitly enquiring about it during the 'how are you' sequence of the call opening (Schegloff, 1986; Kitzinger & Jones, 2007). May starts with a general enquiry about Natalie's well-being, 'How are you love' (line 1), before continuing with 'an' how's yo-' (line 1). Although one could suggest that May was heading for the explicit enquiry about the broken leg, before completing her turn May abandons it in favour of another more general enquiry, 'how's everything going there' (lines 1–2). She then continues with the explicit enquiry about the broken leg, 'How's your leg' (line 2). May is claiming to have remembered Natalie's misfortunes and is demonstrating her ability to be solicitous, to show her care and concern for her daughter. This extract not only demonstrates May's capacity to remember information about her family's lives but that she also actively takes an interest in them as she continues to display sympathy for Natalie's situation, 'Honestly you poor thing' (line 11). Evidence of empathic displays and 'social talk' were increasingly absent in May's later calls, which presented problems for the relationships between her and her family members.

Extract 3 is similar in that May displays recollection of the broken leg and enquires about her daughter's well-being, which orients to an understanding about some particular problem. However, this problem is not explicitly stated. Initially May does not produce a 'no-news' reply to Bill's 'how are you' enquiry and instead asks 'Do you really want to know?' (line 3). This displays that there is in fact 'news' to tell and implies that this news is not good (Jefferson, 1980). May manages this with laughter, which works to delete the hearable social troubles. Bill's next turn is responsive to this in that he reciprocates the laughter, aligning with an awareness of the delicate nature of the prior utterance and displaying sympathy and understanding towards May's bad news, 'No. No I know' (line 4). He then continues to say, 'Natalie's out at the moment' (lines 4–5), accounting for why it was he who called her back and displaying a stance that Natalie would be the best person to talk to about her troubles. May's next turn 'Right' (line 6) receipts and accepts this account. May subsequently departs from the routinized sequence of call-openings (see Schegloff, 1986) in favour of recipient-designing her next turn to display a special concern for Natalie, 'So how *is* she' (line 8). May is again being solicitous by enquiring about the well-being of her daughter, and she displays an understanding that when speaking to/about someone with a special claim to concern (as Natalie has a broken leg), 'howaryou' questions should *not* be done in the routinized way: instead, they should be done with particular emphasis, as May does here. In producing this turn May is implicitly displaying her ability to remember her daughter's special concern. She understands that it warrants a special acknowledgement and engages competently in caring and social graces. Bill eventually addresses the special concern in his next turn by stating that Natalie is 'Still hobbling around' (line 10), which indexes the problem with Natalie's leg. May next receipts the news that Natalie is hobbling around, 'Yes' (line 11), and further claims that it was that specific aspect of Natalie's well-being that she was enquiring about with 'quite' (line 11). During this sequence May displays quite considerable and sophisticated social and interactional competence and intact memory functioning, which contributes to the maintenance of meaningful relationships.

I have shown three instances during May's earlier calls where she exhibited intact memory functioning between calls. In *all* her later communications, May was unable to retain information between conversations like this. Another feature of May's earlier calls was that she displayed a capacity to retain information within calls. She was often able to summarize and recount information during conversations. This was something (which we will see later) May was unable to do as the disease progressed.

12.3.2 May's Early Calls: Memory Retention within Calls

As well as being able to retain information between calls, at the earlier stages May displayed the ability to retain information within calls. This meant that her short-term memory was still functioning reasonably well. On the face of it, being able to summarize a conversation during closing, or topicalize something which was said earlier in the talk, would seem unremarkable in 'ordinary' conversation. However, when compared with May's memory loss exhibited in the later calls, these features constitute a retained competence. Extract 4 shows how May is able to retain information throughout the duration of a conversation.

Extract 4 (ALZ03: Feb 2006)

```
01    MAY    Well yes n' no:.=>I think I-< aren' t I coming
02           home tomorro:w.
03           (0.4)
04    BIL    .hh erm (0.3) NO:: Natalie' s broken her
05           leg[you' re the::re,]
06    MAY       [  Oh:   yes    ] of course she ha::s.
07           (0.8)
08    BIL    Ye::s.=
09    MAY    =Oh I' m staying on here,=
10    BIL    =Ye:s.
11           (.)
12    MAY    I pl-presume the staff here kno:w.
13           (0.8)
14    BIL    Yes.
15    MAY    They do.=
16    BIL    =Ye::s. Oh yes they do. Ye:s.
17    MAY    So I' m no:t coming home yet.
18    BIL    No:.
19           (0.9)
20    MAY    ↑Oh.
21    BIL    No:.
22           (0.6)
23    MAY    Oka::y.
24           (1.4)
25    MAY    I' m sorry I' m such a nuisance if Natalie=I mean
26           I'm< (0.9) I wud- (0.3) t- tr- you' d 've thought
27           I could have been a bit of help to Natalie:.
28    BIL    .HHH[HHHH    HHHH    ]
29    MAY        [No:. Alright Bill.] But I- I'm- (0.3)
30           would be very happy to get home as soo:n as
31           possible plea:se.
32    BIL    Ri::ght. Oka:y. .hh I' ll- I' ll tell Natalie
33           you' ve rung.
34           (0.8)
35    MAY    Thank you Bill.
36           (0.3)
```

```
37   BIL   >Is that alri:ght.< You alright otherwi:se.
38         (0.5)
39   MAY   ↑Well h[ hhh ] ye:s. But I: must admit I thought
40   BIL          [No::.]
41   MAY   I was coming tomorrow. And it's hhh (0.3).h well
42         been a very very VEry major shock to me::.
43   BIL   °Oh right.°
```

The information that May recalls during this conversation is the fact that she is not returning home the next day from the residential facility where she now resides. May's initial presupposition to be returning home, 'aren't I coming home tomorrow' (lines 1–2), is a sign of May's early memory loss, as she is unable to remember that she has been living in residential care for about eight months. However, after Bill bluntly informs her that she will not be returning home, 'No' (line 4), and produces an inability account, 'Natalie's broken her leg' (lines 4–5), referring to Natalie's incapacity as the reason why May is unable to return home, May retains this information during the remainder of the call. She demonstrates this memory by asking questions about the information, 'I presume the staff here know' (line 12), and offering an 'upshot' of the information she has received, 'So I'm not coming home yet' (line 17). This is confirmed, to which May displays surprise, 'Oh' (line 20). Although May is orienting to this information as surprising 'news' and this is evidence of her memory loss, May nevertheless continues to display memory retention later in the call. There were 44 seconds between May's request to return home being declined (line 4) and her topicalizing this non-granting when asked later if she is 'alright otherwise' (line 37). May's response, 'Yes but I must admit I thought I was coming tomorrow' (lines 39–41), displays recollection of her being informed (during this call) that she is not returning home. As stated before, in 'ordinary' conversation this would be unremarkable. For May, this level of recollection is an achievement; at the later stages May tended to forget information like this within seconds of being told it.

I have analyzed features of May's memory functionality both between and within her earlier calls. During this earlier period, I have shown that May was sometimes able to remember important information about her family, which improved the quality of personal interaction they could achieve and enabled her to engage in the socially gracious act of being solicitous, thus contributing to the maintenance of social relationships. I will now shift the focus to the later calls, where May's cognitive degeneration became increasingly apparent as the disease progressed. May was not only unable to recall information between calls, but her short-term memory had also declined to a state where she was unable to remember information within a conversation, seconds after she had been told it.

12.3.3 May's Later Calls: Memory Loss between Calls

May's short-term memory impairments became increasingly apparent as her disease progressed and she was unable to retrieve experiences or retain information between calls. The decline in her memory capacity is especially evident in Extracts 5–8. They occurred within the final 10 calls in the corpus in 2008 and are taken minutes after one another, all occurring within approximately half an hour. The time lapse between Extracts 8 and 9 of 10 minutes is the longest temporal distance between the calls. May's inability to remember the day's events is particularly remarkable and impacts the interaction she is able to engage in with her family. Extract 5 is the first of four calls in which May is unable to remember the day's events (see Jones, 2012 for further analysis).

Extract 5 (ALZ61: 21.03.08)
```
01   NAT   Goo:d. Have you had a nice da:y,
02         (0.2)
03   MAY   I think so dear.= Well (.) the usual sort
04         of da:y. Nothing special.
05   NAT   Well I thought Laura and Jack came toda:y,
06         (1.0)
07   MAY   Sorry?
08   NAT   I thought you'd been out with Laura and
09         Jack toda:y,
10         (1.2)
11   MAY   Oh blimey. What day is it today.
12   NAT   .hhh Well today is Good Friday but I
13         think you di:d.
14   MAY   Sorry?
15         .h Today is Good Friday.
16         (2.4)
17   MAY   Ri:ght. Well if I- if you say I have
18         I have darling and thoroughly enjoyed it.
```

In this extract May claims to having had 'the usual sort of day' (lines 3–4), which Natalie knows is not accurate and can therefore surmise that May has forgotten about the day's events. Natalie's report that May's other daughter and son-in-law (Laura and Jack) had visited makes May's claim to have done 'nothing special' inappropriate, as spending a day with one's daughter 'should be' special. Jones (2012) identified this as 'answering without knowing' – where deficits of May's inability to remember are exposed in the interaction while she simultaneously demonstrates competency in understanding the requirements to produce a relevant next response. The marked delays in producing an appropriate response (lines 6, 10 and 16) and the lack of displayed remembering about her family's visit are indicative of May's memory deficits. Often in her attempt to disguise her forgetfulness, and 'buy herself time' to try and remember, May employs operations of repair, such as 'sorry' (lines 7 and 14), or seeks further information with which to establish the knowledge of the events that she has forgotten, 'What day is it today' (line 11). Perhaps if it was a significant occasion, such as a birthday or Christmas Day, May could deduce that it is likely that her family would have visited, therefore she could claim to remember the occasion. However, after discovering that it is 'Good Friday', May displays that she is still unable to remember the events of the day by conceding that Natalie must be right and she must have had a visit from her daughter, 'If *you say* I have I have' (lines 17–18). May is orienting to the asymmetry of Natalie's knowledge about her life, over which she should have epistemic primacy, but is here orienting to not remembering and thus relying on Natalie's epistemic primacy (Heritage, 2012).

This extract alone demonstrates May's memory deficits as she is citing the source of her new awareness of the events of the day as coming from information Natalie has given her and not from her own memory. Despite her inability to remember, May orients to remembering by assenting to have 'thoroughly enjoyed' her day with her family, which is built to avoid claiming that she recalls it. She is not independently assessing the quality of the day but is instead attributing a positive character to it, contingent on what she has now been informed about it. Analyzed independently, this call already highlights May's memory impairments. When examined as part of a group of calls, the severity of her memory decline becomes more evident, as the next three conversations show.

Extract 6 (ALZ62: 21.03.08, three minutes after the call shown in Extract 5)

```
01    NAT    Why:, What's the trouble,
02    MAY    I've just had enough.
03           (2.0)
04    NAT    Well (0.2) you've had a lo:vely da:y
05           toda:y,
06    MAY    Have I:,
07           (0.6)
08    NAT    Well do you not think so,
09    MAY    Natalie I just can't remember. ([    )]
10    NAT                                   [We:ll]
11    NAT    tha- that's the trouble. You had lovely
12           da:y' cause you went out with Laura and
13           Jack to Bishop Fountain,
14           (0.8)
15    MAY    Oh blimey. Of course I did.
```

Just before the start of this extract May had asked Natalie to come and get her 'out of this establishment', which Natalie refused to do. Natalie proceeds to enquire about the basis of the request, 'What's the trouble' (line 1), in answer to which May claims to have 'had enough' (line 2). May often professed to be 'at the end of my tether' and 'completely at my wits end' with living in care, which habitually provided the source of her repeated requests to return home. Natalie subsequently tells May that she had 'had a lovely day today' (line 4), which functions to undermine May's request on the grounds that she has 'had enough'. May's next turn, 'Have I' (line 6), highlights her declining cognitive functioning, as she declares she is unaware of the 'lovely day' she has had, which prompts a telling from Natalie. Again, May is orienting to the asymmetry of knowledge held by both her and Natalie about the events of her life and relies on Natalie's epistemic primacy. This is additionally remarkable as this call was recorded about three minutes after Extract 5 in which May has already been informed about her other daughter's visit that day. Natalie next targets the 'quality' of the day, as opposed to furthering the issue of actual existence of the event, which May has undermined in soliciting the information from Natalie. By stating 'do you not think so' (line 8), Natalie is treating May's prior utterance as a challenge to the 'loveliness' of the day rather than a claim to not remembering the events altogether. May then explicitly claims not only having forgotten the 'quality' of her day but also the events that have taken place, 'Natalie I just can't remember' (line 9). Natalie informs May that her poor memory is 'the trouble' (line 11) and reason why she is continually fed up, as she is unable to remember the 'lovely days' she has with her family. Natalie proceeds to remind May again that she has been out with her daughter and son-in-law. May's subsequent display of surprise (see Wilkinson & Kitzinger, 2006), 'Oh Blimey' (line 15), conveys the unexpectedness of this information. The 'oh' preface marks this 'change-of-state'. With 'oh', May is claiming to have transformed from an uninformed to an informed position (Heritage, 1984). In the next component of her turn, 'Of course I did' (line 15), May is *claiming* now to remember the events of the day.

This conversation clearly shows May's inability to remember information about her daily events, which she had been told about three minutes previously. The following call (Extract 7) comes 10 minutes later.

Extract 7 (ALZ63: 21.03.08 10 minutes following the call in Extract 6)

```
01   MAY   Oh Natalie I hh just seem to be wasting
02         my hhh (.) flipping time here.
03   NAT   Why:,
04         (0.2)
05   NAT   What's: >the trouble, .hh You've had a
06         lovely day today. Do you not remember
07         what you've done today.
08         (0.2)
09   MAY   No: frankly.
10         (0.5)
```

```
11   NAT    .hh We:ll you went out for lunch with
12          Jack and Laura and Lee and Andy.
13   MAY    Oh of course I di:d.
```

This call has very similar features to the previous call. May is complaining about 'wasting (her) flipping time' (lines 1–2), to which Natalie tells May again that she 'had a lovely day today' (lines 5–6). This again challenges May's assessment of 'wasting her time'. Natalie then orients to having to remind May about her day by asking May directly if she remembers the day, with a negatively valanced question 'do you not remember what you've done today' (lines 6–7) (Heritage, 2002). This embodies an embedded presupposition that May will be unable to remember the events of the day. May's response is fitted to the preference structure of the question when she admits to not remembering, 'No frankly' (line 9). Despite two calls occurring within the previous 15 minutes where May is told about her family's visit, she is unable to retain this information between the calls and must admit that she has forgotten what she has done that day. After being informed again, May claims to now remember 'Oh of course I did' (line 13), and later again proceeds to orient to social niceties by claiming to have had 'a super day' with her family, thus retracting her claim to be 'wasting her time'. The final example (Extract 8) occurs 4 minutes later.

Extract 8 (ALZ64: 21.03.08 4 minutes after the call in Extract 7)

```
01   NAT    .hh And we've: spoken two or three
02          times this evening already.
03   MAY    Oh heavens I'm sorry Natalie.
04   NAT    That's alright.
05          (0.4)
06   MAY    I'll leave you in peace darling.
07   NAT    We:ll (.) I'm just try- I reminded
08          you last time that you'd been out to
09          lunch with Laura and Jack toda:y.
10          (0.3)
11   MAY    Oh blimey.
12          (0.5)
13   NAT    Hhhhh
14          (1.4)
15   MAY    °Oh yes hh I do remember that now.
16   NAT    Do you,= Do you remember where you
17          went.
18          (0.5)
19   MAY    No:.
20          (0.8)
21   NAT    I think you went to Bishop Fountain
22          today.
23          (0.6)
24   MAY    Oh thank you. Yes of course we did.
```

Prior to the extract May asked, 'What am I doing here', and in response Natalie informed her that she had lived in care for 'a while now'. Natalie continues to undermine May's implicit complaint about her residence by telling May that they have 'spoken two or three times this evening already', to which May responds with surpirse, 'Oh heavens'. Not only is she unable to remember her day, but she is unable even to remember speaking to her daughter 'two or three times' earlier in the evening (about the same issues). May displays more forgetfulneess and surprise after being informed that she had already being reminded during the last call that she had been 'out to lunch with Laura and Jack today' (lines 8–9). Again, 'oh blimey' (line 11) conveys surprise and the unexpectedness of this information, and marks May's 'change-of-state' from an uninformed to an informed position. After some delay May claims to 'remember that now' (line 15). She is orienting to remembering the time spent with family. She is also using the resource of claiming to remember (but not proving/displaying memory) as a strategy to disguise her memory loss, so she can engage proficiently in conversation. May's claim to remember is questioned by Natalie, as she asks May if she remembers where she went. This displays Natalie's scepticism about May's ability to remember and further exposes May's strategies for coping with communication. May again has to inform Natalie that she is unable to remember by producing a stated token of forgetfulness, 'No' (line 19), as she is unable to prove her memory by offering details of her day. This is the fourth call in a row where May's diminishing cognitive functionality becomes apparent. Despite being told three times within the previous 20 minutes that she had spent the day with her family, she was still unable to remember. This provides evidence of the effects of May's Alzheimer's on her ability to retain information and thus engage in interactions about daily events.

These four calls provide evidence of May's memory deterioration as the disease progressed. In the earlier calls I have shown that May was sometimes able to remember information between calls, such as her daughter's broken leg or her attendance at a council meeting. These calls demonstrate that in the later stages of May's disease, she was increasingly unable to retain information. This became distressing for everyone involved, as May forgot about the time she spent with her family, which impacted the quality of interaction she could sustain with others. This provides evidence of the progressive symptoms of the disease as manifest in talk and how it can impact people's everyday lives.

I will now highlight the remarkable decline of May's short-term memory; in the later calls she was unable to retain information told to her even during a particular call (within a matter of seconds). I will use one conversation from the later recordings to exemplify the severity of May's memory dysfunction.

12.3.4 May's Later Calls: Memory Loss within Calls

Memory loss is likely to become more severe as Alzheimer's progresses. At the later stages, people may no longer be able to find their way around familiar surroundings. If the person does not recognize their present environment as 'home', then it is not home for them.[3] This is compounded by the fact that the concept of 'home' might evoke memories of a time or place where the person felt comfortable or safe, or of a home that no longer exists, making it difficult for people to identify their current surroundings as home (Alzheimer's Society, 2020b). In the following extracts, May is told, to her surprise, four times in four minutes that she has a room in the residential facility that she has lived in for some months, and that it is room 15. Each time she is told, May claims not to remember this information and displays that she is surprised by it (Wilkinson & Kitzinger, 2006). These extracts come from one call and are necessarily long as the first and all subsequent discussions of her residence need to be considered.

Extract 9 (ALZ68: Part 1 June 2008)
```
01   MAY   How- Where abouts do I live in this (.) place.
02   NAT   Well you've got a room the:re.
03         (0.2)
04   NAT   With all your things in it.
05         (.)
06   MAY   Oh have I,
07         (0.2)
08   MAY   Oh I must try and find them[sometime.]
09   NAT                              [.hhh     ] Well you
10         li- your room's what number is it. Room fifteen.
11         (.)
12   NAT   .h And if you didn't keep taking the notice off the
13         doo:r and the photographs from the thing outsi:de
14         you'd probably recognize it.
15         (0.8)
16   MAY   hhh Wul (.) can I just go home for tonight then.
17   NAT   No you can't 'cause your house is let to somebody.
18   MAY   WHAT LE:T.
19         (0.3)
20   NAT   Wul yes Mother. You know tha:t.
21   MAY   I'd clea:n forgotten about it. When are they going.
22   NAT   .hh Well I don't know. Not at the moment.
23         (0.3)
24   MAY   Bloody Hell.
25         (1.1)
26   MAY   Oh Natalie:.
27   NAT   .hh But you've been looked afte:r. You've been in
```

---

[3] As evidenced in May's case by her recurrent requests to return 'home'.

```
28              care for nearly three years no:w.
29     MAY      .hhhh
30     NAT      So it's nearly three years since you stayed at
31              ho:me.
32              (1.1)
33     MAY      I would still like to go home. I've had enough of
34              this (.) pacing round and (0.4)
35     NAT      Well you don't have to pace round. You've got a
36              lo:vely room with your things in it.
37     MAY      Whe- in wh- where abouts.
38     NAT      WELL in that BUILDing. I:n room fifteen in that
39              building. Go up in t[he  lift  and  ] it's the one
40     MAY                          [This building,]
41     NAT      straight opposite the door.
42     MAY      The one that I'm here,
43     NAT      ↑Ye:s.
44              (0.2)
45     MAY      Bloody Hell.
```

Extract 9 shows the first time in this call that May, to her surprise, is reminded about her residence in the care home (lines 35–36). Although she has clearly forgotten that she lives there during the beginning of the call, as she has to ask 'where abouts' she lives 'in this place' (line 1), this information was given to her outside this call and demonstrates her memory loss between calls. The short-term memory loss within this call is highlighted when Natalie reminds May that she has a 'lovely room' there (lines 35–36), which is met again with surprise, 'Bloody Hell (line 45). This is the second time in this call Natalie tells May about her room, but the first that demonstrates May's memory loss within this call.

At the beginning of the extract May is told, for the first time in this call, that she has 'got a room there' with all her things in it and that it is 'room fifteen' (lines 2–4 and 10). May claims not to be aware that she has her own room, 'Oh have I' (line 6), which marks May as newly informed. Natalie accounts for May's confusion over the location of her room by detailing the steps the family have taken to ensure that she recognizes it by placing photographs and notices by her door. Natalie informs May that if she had not removed these aids, she would not get so confused and therefore would not need to rely on Natalie to provide such information. May modifies but nevertheless pursues her request to return home just 'for tonight then' (line 16), which Natalie rejects on the grounds that her house is let. May has discussed the letting of her house numerous times within the corpus and indeed was given this information moments earlier in the call immediately preceding this conversation, yet she is still shocked to hear the news that her house is not available for her to move in to. Again, this signals May's deficits, as she is unable to recognize/accept her current residence as home, she is unable to remember not only that she is in care, but also where in the building she lives, and she cannot recall that her house is let. The display of shock in May's response about the status of her house is made accountable by Natalie when she informs May that 'she knows that' already (line 20). In doing this, Natalie is telling May that this is 'nothing new'. May proceeds to account for her display of surprise by indexing her memory problem and claiming to have 'clean forgotten' (line 21), hence making the surprise a fitted response and orienting to the informing as 'news' to her. This asymmetry of knowledge causes interactional difficulties as Natalie is continually having to inform May of information about her own life which she has been told before but forgets within seconds.

Following some talk about the length of time she has been in care, May reiterates that she would 'still like to go home' (line 33) as she has 'had enough of this pacing round' (lines 33–34). In providing an account for why May doesn't need to pace around, Natalie reminds May, for the first time within this call, that she has 'a lovely room' (lines 35–36) in the care home. It has been only 40 seconds since May was initially told (in this call) that she has a room and that it is number 15, and she now demonstrates that she cannot recall it. May makes another enquiry about the location of her room, 'where abouts' (line 37). After being given directions, May yet again displays that she is unaware of the room and its location by asking if it is in the building she is in, 'This building. The one that I'm here' (lines 40–42). After Natalie confirms that May's room is in that building, the response token 'Bloody Hell' (line 45) displays both surprise and an unfavourable stance towards the surprising news of her room.

In the intervening talk between Extracts 9 and 10 (not shown here) May's distress at not only being unable to recognize her current location as home but also her inability to retain information about her residence became evident as she began to cry. The level of upset became clear as she suggested that she will 'just get rid' of herself as she 'can't go on any longer'. Shortly after this was the third occasion on which May was unable to recall her room. Extract 10 comes 72 seconds after the last time she was informed of its existence (in Extract 9). After Natalie reminds May about her room, 'as I say you've got a lovely room there' (lines 77–78), May reiterates her complaint about the 'enormous' scale of her location. May is implying that the room she is in (which is a large communal sitting room) is her room. This again highlights May's memory deficits, as Natalie had already suggested May's room is elsewhere in the building.

Extract 10 (ALZ68: Part 2)

```
77    NAT    And you ha- as I say you've got a lovely room
78           the:re.
79           (0.3)
80    MAY    Well I don't like it on this (.) sca:le. I mean
81           this enor[ mous ]
```

```
82    NAT         [.hh W]ell you don't have to stay on
83                that scale. Your room is your room and it's
84                not a huge room. It's just a nice room
85                with y[our things in it.]
86    MAY             [Is it in a particu]lar building.
87    NAT         .hh It's in the building you're in. It's just
88                upstairs from where you are.
89                (0.5)
90    MAY         Okay love.
((Lines omitted as May unsuccessfully seeks help from a nurse))
105   NAT         .hhhh But you've- in room fifteen.=So you just
106               need to go up in the lift and it's the room
107               opposite the[li:ft.]
108   MAY                     [Oka:y] Natalie. And I've to ke-
109               stay there over night.
110               (0.5)
111   NAT         Ye:s.
112   MAY         Only over night.
113   NAT         .hh Well that's where you're sleeping ye:s.
114               (0.4)
115   MAY         Thank you.
116               (0.4)
117   MAY         Eleven.
118   NAT         NO. Fifteen.=
119   MAY         =I beg your pardon. Fifteen.
120               (0.6)
121   MAY         Okay Natalie I'l[l-
122   NAT                         [Room Fifteen. hh Oka:y,
123               (0.6)
124   MAY         I will go and find it. And stay there.
125   NAT         Al:ri:ght.
126               (.)
127   NAT         Okay,
```

Natalie tells May again that it is a smaller 'room with your things in it' (lines 84–85). Natalie contrasts the enormity of the room May is complaining about (line 80) with the relatively smaller private room she has mentioned before. Displaying a complete lack of memory about its location, May again asks 'Is it in a particular building' (line 86). This, for the third time in a matter of minutes, demonstrates May's significant memory impairment. After some intervening talk about the whereabouts of a nurse who could help May find her room, Natalie orients to May forgetting once more and informs May that it is room 15 and offers her directions (lines 105–107). Seconds later, May checks that she has her room number correct, 'Eleven?' (line 117). Although she is demonstrating that she remembers she has a room, she gets the number wrong, and Natalie corrects her, providing her with her room number yet again, 'No. Fifteen' (line 118).

In Extract 11, towards the end of the call, May once more displays her lack of awareness about her room.

Extract 11 (ALZ68: Part 3)

```
143  MAY   And ha- And I'm sure hh .hh[your house'll
144  NAT                              [Well I'll see you
145  MAY   be cosier  ] than anything that I can imagine.
146  NAT   soon anyway]
147  NAT   You what,
148        (.)
149  MAY   I said your house would be cosier than anything
150        I can imagine I'm going to go through.
151        (0.4)
152  NAT   .hh Well your room's lovely the:re.
153        (1.5)
154  NAT   I[ don-] if you could just remember it you'd- well=
155  MAY    [(    )]
156  NAT   =go and find it. You'll find how nice it is.
157        (0.2)
158  MAY   Where am I going again.
159  NAT   Your room in that (0.2) pla:ce where you're
160        staying.
161        (1.0)
162  MAY   ↑My room↑.
163  NAT   You've got a room the:re with all your thi:ngs
164        in it.
165        (0.5)
166  MAY   Wh- Where I am now,
167  NAT   Yes of course where you are now. That's where
168        you li[ve. ]
169  MAY         [Well] (.) Do they- do I d- do this often.
170  NAT   You live there. Ye:s.
171        (0.4)
172  MAY   Blimey. Okay. Thank you dear.
173        (0.8)
174  MAY   I will go and find it. Wh Wh er Wha- is it a
175        number or anything.
176  NAT   It's room fifteen.
177        (0.2)
178  NAT   A[nd we kee]p putting your name on the door and=
179  MAY    [Thank you]
180  NAT   =things in the thing outside but you keep taking
181        them do:wn. Which is why you probably can't find
182        your room.
183        (0.3)
184  MAY   Room fifteen.
185  NAT   Ye:s.
186  MAY   Okay love.
187  NAT   It's upstairs and straight opposite the lift. Oka:y,
```

The fourth time in this call when May is unable to recall her living arrangements comes at line 152 when Natalie rebuts Mays complaint that Natalie's house will be cosier than anything she could imagine by stating that May's 'room's lovely'. This then, once more, launches the discussion about the location of May's room.

May displays confusion when she asks, 'Where am I going again' (line 158), 'My room?' (line 162) and 'do I do this often' (line 169). Natalie again must tell May that 'You've got a room there with all your things in it' (lines 163–164), following which May asks 'Where I am now' (line 166). She also further asks, 'is it a number or anything' (line 174). Finally at the end of the call, after Natalie has told her five times that her room is number 15, May correctly remembers the room number, 'Room fifteen' (line 184).

This call provides evidence of May's declining memory functioning and performance. The level of her cognitive impairment has degenerated to a stage where she is unable to retain information within seconds of being told it. This was obviously upsetting and frustrating for everyone involved in the interaction, most notably for May, whose memory deficits were exposed within these interactions. It was evidently difficult for her family members to reproduce the same information several times in one call and it be received by May as shocking news each time it was delivered. There was no 'social' talk and the conversation was consumed by distress and upset.

I have shown that, in the earlier stages of recording, May was able to retain information both between and within calls. In the two-year period of recording there is significant evidence to show May's cognitive deterioration. During this time May's memory had become increasingly and considerably impaired. There were obvious signs of the progression of her disease and its effects on her memory (and interaction) during the later calls, where she was unable to recall information both between and within conversations. May forgot important information about where she was living and events that she had been part of within seconds of being told about them. This was distressing for both her and her family members and impacted the quality of communication that she could engage in.

12.4 Conclusion

This chapter has explored the progressive features of Alzheimer's disease, as displayed in changing patterns of interaction over time. The longitudinal nature of the data collected affords a unique insight into what makes communication *different* for those with an advancing cognitive impairment such as dementia. It has acknowledged a closer relationship between language and cognition, one that goes beyond more orthodox conversation analytic approaches, by examining how memory and memory loss are displayed in verbal conduct. It has shown that, through the analysis of conversation, we can say something about cognition. This approach has enabled us to observe May's significant and decreasing memory loss in patterns of interaction. May's degenerative memory impairments become increasingly apparent as the disease progresses.

Much of the prior literature on dementia and interaction has taken a predominantly deficit-focused approach, identifying the *problems* dementia poses for that person's language skills. Although May undoubtedly experienced deficits due to her declining cognition, which impacted her abilities within interaction, May also displayed competence and achievements in her interaction in other ways. She displayed competence with turn-taking and action formation (for example apologies and gratitude with 'thank you'), and indeed often developed quite sophisticated strategies to accomplish other tasks such as displaying shock. Indeed, May was still able to achieve these more routine elements of communication into the very late stages of the disease. Furthermore, she compensated for her memory deficits by *answering without knowing* – producing relevant next actions (despite these often subsequently being exposed as being 'incorrect') in the correct sequential environments. In line with Mikesell's analysis (Chapter 5 this volume), these features of interaction blur the boundaries between *deficit* and *skill*. It is unavoidable to notice the cognitive deficits exposed in these interactions, but at the same time there are interactional skills being mobilized by both participants. While conversation analysis research has played an important role in changing perceptions about the *abilities* of people with dementia (and the collaborative nature of interaction), perhaps these binary concepts (competence *versus* incompetence) are not useful in defining our analysis of complex cognitive issues and interactional events, and possibly do not reflect the complexities of these social encounters.

It is also important to state that I am not suggesting there are discrete *stages* of Alzheimer's disease. Although May's abilities/inabilities were fairly constant and declined steadily (i.e., these patterns identified here were recurrent – May did not have periods of greater/lesser insight), this does not represent all those with a diagnosis of Alzheimer's. I want to reiterate that symptoms such as memory loss are not stable or homogenous – people will experience them differently and at different rates/times. However, gaining this longitudinal insight into a family dealing with Alzheimer's can help provide a deeper understanding of how memory, communication and indeed relationships may be affected.

This chapter points to the usefulness of interaction as a window to understanding cognition and Alzheimer's disease, and offers us a credible tool to highlight the potential degenerative consequences of the disease and how to understand such communication as co-participants in interaction. Only by understanding the difficulties faced in interaction can we help people to develop strategies to communicate differently in order to enhance the quality of that communication (Jones, 2012). Moreover, this approach has enabled me to explore another perspective on memory loss and cognitive decline associated with the progression of Alzheimer's disease.

References

Alzheimer's Disease International (ADI) (2020) 'Symptoms of dementia.' Available at: www.alz.co.uk/info/early-symptoms.

Alzheimer's Society (2020a) 'The Progression, signs and stages of Dementia.' Available at: www.alzheimers.org.uk/about-dementia/symptoms-and-diagnosis/how-dementia-progresses/progression-alzheimers-disease-dementia.

(2020b) 'Memory loss and dementia.' Available at: www.alzheimers.org.uk/about-dementia/symptoms-and-diagnosis/symptoms/memory-loss-dementia.

Bögels, S. and Levinson, S. C. (2017) 'The brain behind the response: Insights into turn-taking in conversation from neuroimaging.' *Research on Language and Social Interaction*, 50: 71–89.

Drew, P. (2005a) 'Is *confusion* a state of mind?' In H. te Molder and J. Potter (eds.) *Conversation and Cognition*. Cambridge: Cambridge University Press, pp. 161–183.

(2005b) 'Conversation Analysis.' In K. L. Fitch and R. E. Sanders (eds.) *Handbook of Language and Social Interaction*. London: Lawrence Erlbaum Associates Publishers, pp. 71–102.

Drew, P. and Chilton, K. (2000) 'Calling just to keep in touch: regular and habitualised telephone calls as an environment for small talk.' In J. Coupland (ed.) *Small Talk*. Harlow: Pearsons Education Ltd, pp. 137–162.

Edwards, D. and Potter, J. (1992) *Discursive Psychology*. London: Sage Publications.

Gisladottir, R. S., Bögels, S. and Levinson, S. C. (2018) 'Oscillatory brain responses reflect anticipation during comprehension of speech acts in spoken dialogue.' *Frontiers in Human Neuroscience*, 12: Article 34.

Heritage, J. (1984) 'A change-of-state token and aspects of its sequential placement.' In J. M. Atkinson and J. Heritage (eds.) *Structures of Social Action: Studies in Conversation Analysis*. Cambridge: Cambridge University Press, pp. 299–345.

(2002) 'The limits of questioning: negative interrogatives and hostile question content.' *Journal of Pragmatics*, 34: 1427–1446.

(2005) 'Cognition in discourse.' In H. te Molder and J. Potter (eds.) *Conversation and Cognition*. Cambridge: Cambridge University Press, pp. 184–202.

(2012) 'The epistemic engine: Sequence organization and territories of knowledge.' *Research on Language and Social Interaction*, 45(1): 30–52.

Jefferson, G. (1980) 'On "trouble-premonitory" response to inquiry.' *Sociological Inquiry*, 50(3/4): 153–185.

(1983) 'Issues in the transcription of naturally-occurring talk: Caricature versus capturing pronunciational particulars.' *Tilburg Papers in Language and Literature*, 34: 1–12.

(2004) 'Glossary of transcript symbols with an introduction.' In G. H. Lerner (ed.) *Conversation Analysis: Studies from the First Generation*. Philadelphia: John Benjamins, pp. 13–23.

Jones, D. (2012) *Conversations with a person with Alzheimer's disease: A conversation analytic study*. Unpublished Ph.D. dissertation. University of York, UK.

(2015) 'A family living with Alzheimer's disease: the communicative challenges.' *Dementia*, 14(5): 555–573.

Kennard, C. (2009) 'Alzheimer's disease: everything you need to know.' Available at: www.healthcentral.com/alzheimers/c/57548/78464/caregiver-tips.

Kitzinger, C. and Jones, D. (2007) 'When May calls home: The opening moments of family telephone conversations with an Alzheimer's patient.' *Feminism & Psychology*, 17(2): 184–202.

Lynch, M. and Bogen, D. (2005) 'My memory has been shredded: A non-cognitivist investigation of "mental" phenomena.' In H. te Molder and J. Potter (eds.) *Conversation and Cognition*. Cambridge: Cambridge University Press, pp. 226–240.

Potter, J. and te Molder, H. (2005) 'Talking cognition: Mapping and making the terrain.' In H. te Molder and J. Potter (eds.) *Conversation and Cognition*. Cambridge: Cambridge University Press, pp. 1–54.

Sacks, H. (1992). 'Lecture 1. Rules of conversational sequence.' In H. Sacks and G. Jefferson (eds.) *Lectures on Conversation* (Vol. I). Oxford: Blackwell, pp. 3–11.

Schegloff, E. A. (1986) 'The routine as achievement.' *Human Studies*, 9: 111–151. (1991) 'Conversational analysis and socially shared cognition.' In L. B. Resnick, J. M. Levine and S. D. Teasley (eds.) *Perspectives on Socially Shared Cognition*. Washington, DC: APA.

Sidnell, J. (2010) *Conversation Analysis: An Introduction*. Chichester: Wiley-Blackwell.

Wilkinson, S. and Kitzinger, C. (2006) 'Surprise as an interactional achievement: Reaction tokens in conversation.' *Social Psychology Quarterly*, 69(2): 150–182.

Wittgenstein, L. (1958) *Philosophical Investigations*. Oxford: Blackwell.

13 Using Digital Communication Support in Interaction Involving People with Dementia
Interactional Strategies to Facilitate Participation and Engagement

Christina Samuelsson and Anna Ekström

13.1 Introduction

In dementia, many abilities gradually deteriorate, typically causing a decline in communicative skills in the later stages. As dementia is not usually associated with specific speech impairments, communication support is not a primary need as a speech-generating device. Rather, those communicative functions in need of support are related to aspects such as the ability to keep track of conversational topics and initiate new topics, and as a support for memory (Alm et al., 2004; Astell et al., 2010). This is usually done with the aid of communication support materials such as newspapers, books and specifically chosen objects, and by materials to encourage reminiscing such as memory books or photos. As pointed out by Bourgeois and Hickey (2009), the goal of intervention in communication support in dementia is primarily to maintain functional communication and improve quality of life by strengthening social relations. Digital technology is an expanding area within the field of communication support for people with dementia (Astell et al., 2004, 2018; Ekström et al., 2017). Today, several digital inventions are available that are specifically designed to support communication for people with dementia.

In a number of studies it has been argued that using digital communication support in interaction with people with dementia may be beneficial (e.g., Astell & Parsons, 2010; Ekström et al., 2017; Smith & Astell, 2018). In a review by Hitch and colleagues (2017), it was concluded that although the evidence that tablets can be used as a compensatory method is inconclusive, there are promising results demonstrating that digital aids may support meaningful engagements in activities. Compared to traditional communication support, communication support based on a multimedia system has been shown to stimulate joint attention by the interlocutors and may possibly also be more enjoyable for both people with dementia and caregivers (Alm et al., 2004; Astell et al., 2010). There are also results indicating that the use of touchscreen computers in communicative activities may strengthen social relationships between carers and people with dementia (Astell et al., 2010).

In what ways communication support – digital or not – affects interaction and how the participants experience the conversation is, of course, largely determined by how the interlocutors act and engage with each other. Similar to traditional augmentative and alternative communication (AAC), a device of itself does not solve a communication problem or compensate for participants' difficulties (Higginbotham et al., 2007). It is *how* the participants make use of the communication support and how they integrate the aid into their interaction that define in what ways a communication support might be beneficial for the participants' communication.

In this chapter we will examine video recordings of conversations involving people with dementia where digital communication support is used, and discuss how such conversations can be organized to promote participation and involvement by a person with dementia. The digital applications described in this chapter include photos, video clips and music. The focus is on two central features of how interaction around a digital communication support evolves – carers' use of questions and the management of the communication support device. In all our recordings of people with dementia interacting with carers when using digital communication support, carers ask the persons with dementia a lot of questions – typically about the content of the communication support. As questions make an answer the expected next action (Sacks, 1992; Schegloff, 2007), the form and content of questions greatly influence the sequential structure and the topics of a conversation. Another prominent feature for interactions revolving around a digital communication support is how the device itself and the included materials are navigated and handled. Due to the design of the application used, it is necessary to, in one way or another, manage the content of the application and decide when and how to change this, for example which photo to view. How this is done and organized is also highly significant for the sequential structure of the interactions and how the conversation proceeds. For this study, these two aspects are explored with the use of empirical examples illustrating a variety of different practices – both beneficial and less beneficial for supporting conversation. The examples are analysed with a focus on the ways the dyads organize their interaction and the consequences of these ways for the continuation of the conversation. By doing this, the chapter aims to further the understanding of strategies used by carers to promote participation and involvement in communication for persons living with dementia.

13.2   Communication and Dementia

Communication is arguably one of the most substantially impacted areas for people with a dementia disease (Alm et al., 2004; Azuma & Bayles, 1997) and is also one of the areas in which people with dementia and their significant others have indicated that the biggest challenges lie (Johansson, 2015; Murphy et al., 2010; Saunders et al., 2011). To quote Guendouzi and Davis (2014: 2): 'As it is through language that memory and family ties are expressed, it is, perhaps, in language use by persons with dementia that unimpaired persons find the most grievous and even startling changes'. In dementia, communicative problems gradually increase. Initially, persons with dementia might find it difficult to keep track in conversation and to remember what has just been said, something that leads to unfinished utterances and repetition (Bayles, 2004). As a dementia disease progresses, abilities to initiate and maintain interactions with other people tend to gradually decline (e.g. Baker et al., 2015; Evans et al., 2007; Örulv & Nikku, 2007). It is also common to have difficulty in retrieving words and phrases, which may lead to substitution of words or the use of semantically weak terms or semantically empty placeholders such as 'you know' or 'whatever you call it', making communication seem vague (Davis & Guendouzi, 2014). In the advanced stages of dementia, the potential to initiate and take part in conversations is often almost non-existent and only isolated vocabulary and formulaic expressions are used (Bayles & Tomoeda, 2014; Hydén, 2018; Wray, 2010). It is, however, important to remember that the pathology of diseases leading to dementia does not cause consistent levels of communicative (or cognitive) impairment for all individuals, and the level of difficulty can also vary from day to day (Prince & Jackson, 2009; Wray, 2010).

Communicative problems make people with dementia particularly vulnerable to social exclusion (Wray, 2010). Interactional partners are crucial for upholding conversational activities involving people with dementia, and the communicative responsibilities are often asymmetrically distributed (Alm et al., 2004; Astell et al., 2010; Baker et al., 2015; Bourgeois & Hickey, 2009; Jansson, 2016). Loneliness and social isolation are significant problems for people living with dementia (e.g. Saunders et al., 2011). Moreover, difficulties in communication can also affect the quality of care that a person with dementia receives. In a report from 2007, the Alzheimer's Society states that 'care staff perceive communication problems as one of the biggest challenges in providing good dementia care' (p. 4).

13.3 Communication Interventions for People with Dementia

There is yet no pharmacological cure for dementia; accordingly, strategies to compensate for functional impairment and to reduce problems experienced are crucial to minimizing the negative impact of the disease for people with dementia and their significant others. When it comes to communicative problems, visual support has been shown to positively affect the potential for people with dementia to participate in communicative activities (Bourgeois & Hickey, 2009). Support in the form of, for example, pictures, communication books and photo albums have proven useful in compensating for communicative difficulties in dementia, and their positive effects on understanding as well as on expressive abilities have been seen. This, in turn, has reduced behavioural problems and made participation in everyday activities more meaningful (Beukelman et al., 2007; Bourgeois & Hickey, 2009; Yasuda et al., 2009). Communicative support might enhance access to cognitive abilities or work as a semantic prime to improve the ability to find words for people with Alzheimer's Disease (AD) (Fried-Oken et al., 2012). More generally, it has been shown that external memory aids, for example notebooks, communication boards and photos, have the potential to improve communication for people with dementia at all stages of the disease (Fried-Oken et al., 2012; Murphy & Boa, 2012). One type of intervention that has been argued to be particularly useful for people with dementia and their caregivers is reminiscence activities (Brooker & Duce, 2000; Finnema et al., 2000). In these kinds of activities, photo albums and scrapbooks containing personalized information may act as both memory aids and communication support. In a review article of 11 studies on speech and language pathologists' interventions for people with dementia, it was concluded that there is preliminary support for communication intervention for people with moderate to severe dementia (Swan et al., 2018). Gains were not maintained following naming therapy, but two studies utilizing AAC and caregiver training reported some maintenance effects on reduction in frequency of repetitive verbalizations (Swan et al., 2018).

The body of research on the use of technology in dementia care in general, and touchscreen technology in particular, is growing, and in a recent scoping review of the use of touchscreen tablet technology by people with dementia (Hitch et al., 2017) a range of exploratory research related to the use of tablets by people with dementia was identified. While conclusions regarding the potential for touchscreen tablets to compensate for communicative and cognitive difficulties were diverse, Hitch and colleagues (2017) conclude that there are encouraging results, showing that touchscreen technology could support meaningful engagement in social activities. Some findings have also indicated that tablets may improve relationships and interaction between carers and people with dementia (Upton et al., 2013). In a pioneering study by Astell and colleagues (2004) examining a previous version of one of the communication tools studied in this chapter, CIRCA, it was shown that this tool prompted and supported conversations between a person with dementia and care providers (including family members) (Alm et al., 2004; see also Astell et al., 2010). Gowans and colleagues (2004) report that interactional activities where CIRCA was used included more stories from people with dementia that were new to their interlocutors. The conversations were also more symmetrical in terms of communicative contributions as well as the responsibility taken for initiating and upholding conversational topics. In comparison with traditional reminiscing activities, using a multimedia system is argued to include more initiatives and choices made by people with dementia. It has also been demonstrated that multimedia systems promote joint attention by the interlocutors and that it may be more enjoyable for both people with dementia as well as caregivers (Alm et al., 2004; Astell et al., 2004; Astell et al., 2010). Multimedia systems are said to provide 'a richness of interaction that is particularly appropriate for those elderly people with diminishing sensory and intellectual capabilities' and 'provide a livelier and more engaging activity for people who struggle with spontaneous interactions' (Alm et al., 2004: 122).

In a study of an application similar to CIRCA but based on personal photos, Ekström and colleagues (2017) demonstrated that although tablet computers may encourage communication for people with dementia and their conversational partners, the results also highlighted some potential pitfalls that may be associated with the use of personalized material instead of general material (see also Astell et al., 2010). The conversations often had the characteristics of a test, where the conversational partner asked the person with dementia to name the people in the photos, something that has previously been put forward as a potentially face-threatening activity if the person with dementia is not able to correctly identify, for example, close relatives (see Small & Perry, 2005).

13.4 The Applications CIRCA and CIRCUS

In this study, two web-based applications called CIRCA and CIRCUS were examined in interactions between people with dementia and caregivers. The latter were either professional caregivers or family members. While both applications are designed to stimulate communication by providing photos, videos and music that could function as an inspiration for finding topics to talk about as well as to help participants with dementia to keep to the topic, the two applications differ in regard to what kind of material they provide. Whereas CIRCA is populated with generic material that potentially could be of interest to 'anyone' (e.g. pictures of animals and flowers, video clips of famous actors and popular songs), CIRCUS has an uploading function and users populate the application with their own materials (e.g. personal photos, favourite video clips and much-loved songs).

13.4.1 CIRCA

CIRCA (Astell et al., 2004; Astell et al., 2010) is a web-based application developed from a previous version for stand-alone devices. CIRCA is

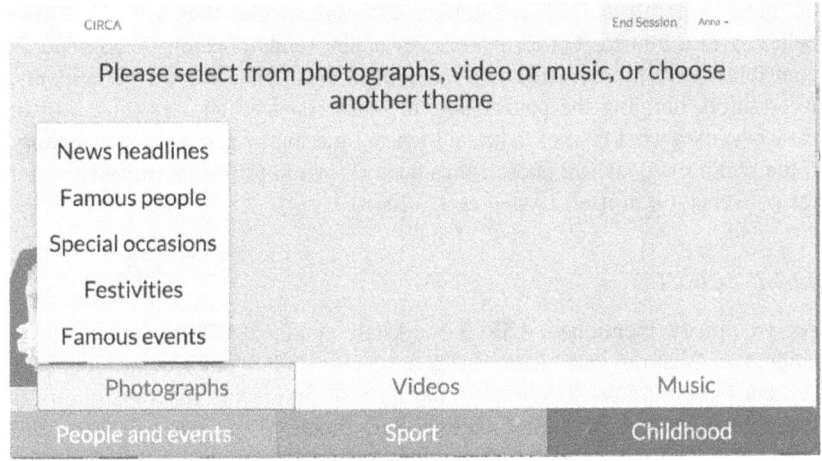

Figure 13.1 Screenshot from CIRCA showing the different categories.

connected to a large database of pictures, videos and music files belonging to six different main categories: childhood, sports, entertainment, recreation, people and events, and everyday life. For each main category, the photo material is sorted into five subcategories (each item can belong to more than one category and subcategory) (see Figure 13.1). When starting the application, three randomly selected main categories appear on the screen and the users are asked to select one. Having selected a category, the users are presented with the choice of viewing photos, watching video clips or listening to music. If the users choose to view photos, they are then presented with five subcategories for the chosen main category (e.g., for the photographs category, the subcategories 'news headlines', 'famous people', 'special occasions, 'festivities' and 'famous events' can be selected). A Swedish version of CIRCA was used in this study (Figure 13.1).

The category system and the randomized selection of topics in CIRCA were chosen for several reasons. First of all, randomizing, and thereby to some extent constraining the participants' choice of category, is believed to make the topics more varied. Conversational partners of people with dementia have a tendency to come back to the same topics and ask the same questions when talking to a person with dementia. By constraining the topics to choose from, the risk of conversational partners limiting the possibilities of topical variation for persons with dementia is believed to be reduced. Moreover, persons with dementia have a tendency to tell the same stories over and over again (Hydén, 2018; Searson et al., 2008), something that is recurrently portrayed as a problem by conversational partners (Cook et al., 2009). By providing a set of three randomly chosen categories, this conversational behaviour is also believed to diminish. On an overall level, the randomization is assumed to contribute to a more varied conversational experience for all participants. In addition, obliging the participants to make repeated choices (first a main category, then what kind of material to view, and finally perhaps a subcategory if the photo materials are chosen) has been shown to provide a fruitful ground for conversation in itself (Astell et al., 2018).

13.4.2 CIRCUS

As previously mentioned, CIRCUS (Astell et al., 2018) has personalized content of pictures and videos from a specific individual's or group's past and current everyday life. CIRCUS has a simple uploading function and users can upload any kind of digital material they choose. They can scan their (old) paper photos, use pictures from the tablet's photo album, find materials on the Internet, photograph favourite recipes, and so on. In CIRCUS, the material is organized in a tree structure of categories where each level consists of three categories (Figure 13.2). For each category, the user can add as many items as they wish. On the top level, an individual user might, for instance, choose the categories 'family', 'holidays' and 'old times'. On the next level, the category 'family' might consist of the three categories 'my children', 'my husband' and 'my parents', and so on. How the material is organized and what kind of

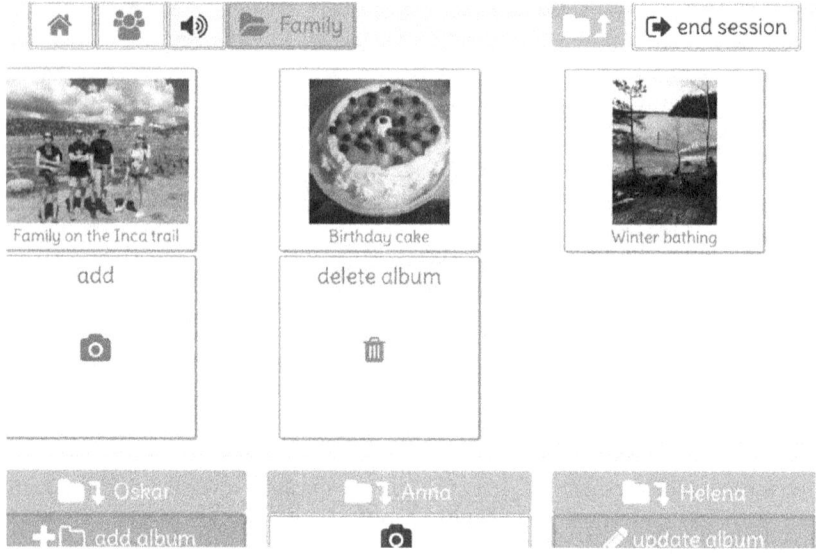

Figure 13.2 Screenshot from CIRCUS showing different personal categories.

categories to include is entirely up to the users. The flexibility of the application makes it possible to use it not only for individual purposes but also to customize it for a group of users.

13.5 Method, Materials and Analytical Approach

This chapter builds on data collected through a number of projects investigating the use of digital communication support in interaction with people with dementia.[1] Within these projects, a large collection of video recordings has been created involving both dyadic and group interactions where digital communication support is used. Our analysis focuses on two general practices – the use of questions and the management of communication support – and explores the variability with which these activities are accomplished. The persons with dementia appearing in the examples (Ada, Liv, Isa, Gun, Jon and Lee) all lived in residential care homes for people with dementia and were well acquainted with the participating members of staff. No formal testing was conducted to assess speech, language and communication or cognitive abilities. Swedish was the first language of all participants. For an overview of the data, see Table 13.1.

The recordings took place in the wards/rooms of each participant at times chosen by the participating carers. The carers received basic instructions on how to use the tablet and the applications, but no specific instructions were given regarding how to use the applications in conversation. For Ada and Isa, a shared CIRCUS application was created comprising 3 albums with 48 pictures of the care home, common activities among the residents and various members of the staff. In addition, Ada and Isa also had one specific personal album each, containing pictures from their private photo albums. For Liv, a personal version of CIRCUS was created using photos from her private photo albums.

The analyses are based on the sequential organization of the interaction presented in the examples where an interactional contribution is viewed as both context dependent and context renewing (Heritage, 1984). In other words, social interaction is considered to be organized as sequences of actions building on each other, where an action is a response to what went on previously in the interaction while, at the same time, it brings about new (re)actions that are organized as responses to how this first action was understood. It is in the response to an action that the recipients of this action display their understanding of what is going on. The sequential organization of interaction provides the participants with a next-turn proof procedure (Sacks et al., 1974) to evaluate whether or not their understanding of what is going on is shared. Monitoring the unfolding of an activity's sequential organization is primarily a source for

---

[1] All projects were associated with Center for Dementia Research, CEDER, Linköping University

Table 13.1 *Number and length of recordings with CIRCA and CIRCUS for the dyads*

	With CIRCA			With CIRCUS	
	Length of recording (min:sec)	Participants		Length of recording (min:sec)	Participants
1	11:34	Ada & Carer	1	13:06	Ada & Carer
2	12:09	Ada & Carer	2	14:15	Ada & Carer
3	13:15	Ada & Carer	3	14:14	Ada & Carer
4	11:27	Ada & Carer	4	12:47	Ada & Carer
5	12:09	Ada & Carer	5	11:14	Ada & Carer
6	15:41	Liv & Carer	6	16:43	Isa & Carer
7	12:22	Isa & Carer	7	14:05	Isa & Carer
8	13:33	Isa & Carer	8	17:43	Isa & Carer
9	12:54	Isa & Carer	9	17:02	Isa & Carer
10	06:07	Isa & Carer			
11	22:48	Isa & Carer			
12	21:16	Isa & Carer			
3	19:05	Jon & carer			
14	19:19	Gill & Carer			
15	09:38	Gill & Carer			
16	17:02	Lee & Relative			
17	17:14	Lee & Relative			
	244:33			**131:09**	

participants themselves to work out an understanding of the actions being undertaken. Being a public affair, however, the sequential organization of displayed understandings is also available for professional analysis, providing scientists with 'a proof criterion (and a search procedure) for the analysis of what a turn's talk is occupied with' (Sacks et al., 1974: 45).

13.5.1 Ethics

Written consent to participate in the project was obtained from all participants. Since persons with dementia experience cognitive and memory problems, the research aims and terms of participation were restated to them prior to each recording. The project was approved by the regional board of ethics in Linköping (Dnr 2016/247-32).

13.6 Results

Our focus here is how questions are used and handled, and how the management of materials in the applications are organized in regard to deciding what to view and when to change material. In relation to this, we will argue for the benefits of carers to (a) put priority on conversation over factual correctness, and (b) be sensitive to the conversational trajectory of the person with dementia.

Throughout all our recordings, posing questions regarding the displayed material constitutes a substantial part of interactions between carers and people with dementia. When a new photo is displayed on the screen, an initial turn from the carers is usually a question to the person with dementia as to whether they hold knowledge about something in the picture being viewed. A much-discussed area in interaction with people with dementia is whether or not to ask factual questions. The use of questions more generally has been put forward as a way to improve communication and to facilitate the participation of people with dementia in social interaction (Perkins et al., 1998; Small et al., 2003). However, there are arguably differences in the affect of questions on interaction depending on what kind of questions are used. Small et al. (2003) found, for example, that the use of yes/no questions as opposed to open-ended questions seems to reduce communicative problems, but that open-ended questions could be used successfully if the question did not require involvement of impaired memory systems (Small et al., 2003: 364). Elsewhere, we have argued that asking a person with dementia what a picture shows, or whether or not the person remembers the event depicted, might risk highlighting problems associated with the disease (Ekström et al., 2017). This is, however, related to the domain of topic within which the question is being asked. While not recognizing or remembering a celebrity or a public building does not necessarily involve any face threat, as this could be ascribed to a more general forgetfulness, not remembering close relatives or significant places could be potentially sensitive (see Astell et al., 2010).

In our material there are examples of successful as well as less successful ways of posing questions regarding specific pictures or personal experiences related to pictures. How initial questions are followed up is also crucial for the possibilities for the persons with dementia to be an active participant in the interaction. In Extract 1, which demonstrates a successful example of posing a specific question regarding a personal experience, Lee is talking to his daughter about a picture of Skansen, a well-known open-air museum in Stockholm. The picture appeared randomly in CIRCA, where the pictures are generic and not personalized.

Extract 1
L=Lee (person with dementia), R=relative
```
01   R:   skansen (0.4) va du uppe på skansen?
          skansen (0.4) did you go to skansen
02   L:   aha
          yea
03   R:   aha okej (0.5) [.hh]
          yea okay (0.5) [.hh]
04   L:                  [pappa] jobba ju farfar jobba ju där vet du
                         [daddy] worked there granddad worked there you
          know
05   R:   ja:: han gjorde de, Donald
          yea:: he did, Donald
06   L:   a:
07   R:   ja: (1.5) ((sighs)) va mysit
          yea (1.5) ((sighs)) that's so nice
```

At the beginning of the extract the daughter asks her father whether he has been to Skansen (line 1), and Lee confirms that he has (line 2). The daughter acknowledges his answer and there is a pause of about half a second. Lee then provides some additional information about his father, who used to work at Skansen. The daughter receives this with a response that marks the information as something she had forgotten but has now been reminded about. After some more silence where Lee and his daughter look at each other and smile, the daughter provides a positive assessment, potentially of the story and the moment they share.

In Extract 1, asking the person with dementia a specific, factual question related to the material elicits a story about a common relative, which then results in a seemingly positive shared experience of remembering this person. As Lee does not only remember whether or not he has been to Skansen but is also able to provide a story of his own related to this topic, the initial question results in a sequence where the person with dementia shares information from his past.

Questions, of course, do not always prompt personal stories. In Extract 2 a carer is talking to Gill about some pictures of houses from her childhood.

Extract 2
C=Carer, G=Gill (person with dementia)
```
01   C:   va ä de här nånstans=
          where is this
02   G:   =de där e va nåra torp som vi hade (0.5) på somrarna
          that's e were cottages we had (0.5) in the summers
03   C:   okej
          okay
04   G:   jaa=
          yea
05   C:   =va låg dom nånstans da
          where were they then
06   G:   de låg i (1.0) ja va hette de nu (1.6) ja ha glömt bort de också=
          they were in (1.0) yea what was it called now (1.6) I've
          forgotten that too
```

```
07    C:     =men va de i närheten av småköpin=
             but was it close to smalltown
08    G:     =ja::e (.) de va så mycke fiskmåsar
             yea:: (.) there were a lot of seagulls
```

This sequence starts with the carer asking where some small cottages in the picture are located. As seen in line 2, Gill does not really respond to this question but instead responds with a description of the cottages and her relation to them – 'some cottages we had in the summers'. While this might not be an answer to the specific question, it is nevertheless a response that moves the conversation forward, other than just saying, for example, 'I don't know'. However, the carer only gives a minimal response in line 3, and then continues with the project of finding out where the cottages were located by posing another question regarding this issue in line 5. In line 6, it becomes evident that Gill has problems providing the location of the cottages. She begins a response but stops to search for the name of the place before concluding that she does not remember the name of the place where the cottages were located. The carer then provides a general suggestion of where the cottages might have been located in the form of a question that might have provided a clue for Gill (line 7). Gill confirms the suggested location, although with some hesitation, and then closes the topic by describing some other characteristic of the place (line 8). After this turn, they change pictures.

In contrast to Extract 1, Gill does not really seem to have any recollection of the location asked about, and when given the opportunity, she closes the topic by saying something that she does know and moves on to something else. While the interactional consequences of asking factual questions in these two examples are closely related to whether or not the person with dementia remembers the events talked about, they can still serve as a point of departure for discussing more general issues. A first point is, of course, to always be prepared for a person with dementia not to have any recollection of previous events or significant others, but also to be aware that the person might just as well not only remember the events but also be able to elaborate on such topics. This poses a delicate dilemma for conversational partners of people with dementia. On the one hand, if a conversational partner asks factual questions regarding personal matters, there is a risk that the person with dementia does not remember them, which would potentially put the person with dementia in a position of lower epistemic status, both interactionally and emotionally. On the other hand, if conversational partners never pose any questions regarding personal memories and experiences, there is a risk that potential for important stories and shared moments of personal significance are lost, and conversations with persons with dementia will never reach beyond the general and unspecific. To better understand these alternatives, we further elaborate on some of the details of our two examples as a way to highlight aspects of the sequences that might prove helpful in handling such delicate interactions.

In Extract 1 we can see that after Lee's initial question confirming that he has been to Skansen, his daughter leaves some interactional space for Lee to pick up on this topic and thereby lead the conversation in a direction of his choice. At the point of the silence, Lee and his daughter have established a conversational topic, Skansen, which to some extent has been suggested by the application, and they have also established that Lee has been to Skansen (and that he remembers that he has been there). From this point, the conversation could go anywhere, and it is not an easy task for the daughter to know what area of this topic to explore if she were to pose another question. She does not seem to know very much about Lee's visits to Skansen, and she does not know if he remembers anything else about these events. By refraining from asking another question immediately and leaving some interactional space for Lee to take over the conversational floor, this sequence evolves into a seemingly nice moment for both Lee and his daughter, and gives Lee the opportunity to share his memories of the current topic. In Extract 2, the sequence develops differently. As the carer does not get any information about where the cottages were located, but rather a description of Gill's relationship to the cottages, one way to continue might have been to let the issue of the location go and continue by exploring Gill's contribution. Choosing progressivity over halting progressivity to attend to factual content may be beneficial for persons with dementia and allow them to actively participate in social interaction. It is, however, not always an easy task to just go along with a conversation regardless of whether an already initiated sequence is finished or not. In this case, the carer pursues the question, and this time gets an explicit explanation that Gill does not remember the location of the cottages. From her response to the initial question, it might just have been a confusion about what the carer was asking for and not a memory problem, and posing the question one more time in this situation very much follows common conversational practices where a question should get an answer (Schegloff, 2007). When Gill claims that she does not remember where the cottages were located, the carer immediately provides a general suggestion of where the cottages might have been in the form of a question, thereby providing Gill with an easy way of closing this topic without any additional face threat. In this way, Gill and the carer can move on and close the topic in a smooth way.

In contrast to asking factual questions, our material shows some examples of carers and relatives posing questions about feelings and attitudes in relation to the conversational material in the applications. Unlike factually oriented questions, there are no right or wrong answers to these kinds of questions, and they do not to the same extent highlight problems associated with a dementia disease. Extract 3 shows another sequence from the conversation between Lee and his daughter.

Excerpt 3
R=relative, L=Lee (person with dementia)

```
01   R:   du har du vart fantast utav Abba har du gillat dom
          were you been a fan of Abba did you like them
02   L:   ja dom va bra
          yea they were good
03   R:   dom va bra du har gillat dom va
          they were good you have liked them right
04   L:   ja o ja dom va bra
          oh yea they were good
05   R:   har du- va du- har du sett nått uppträdande med dom
          have you- were you- have you ever seen any performance with
          them
06        (1.7)
07   L:   ja har nog sett uppträdande med dom ja
          I have probably seen a show with them yea
08   R:   det har man vart på nått
          one has been to some
```

Asking about feelings, attitudes and opinions is less common in our material compared to asking more factually oriented questions. As we can see in the example here, however, talking about feelings, attitudes and opinions might actually be a lot easier than talking about personal experiences of actual events, and will provide grounds for exploring personal topics that move beyond more general and unspecific conversations in the same way as descriptions of experiences of events do, thus promoting involvement by the person with dementia. In this example, the conversation moves smoothly when the topic concerns Lee's opinions about Abba and their music, but when asked about whether he has been to any of their performances, it becomes evident that this is a much more difficult domain for him to talk about. The problems in answering this question are demonstrated by the 1.7 second pause in line 6, and also by the use of the pragmatic particle 'nog/probably' (line 7). The relative's generalizing response in line 8, may be aligning with Lee's uncertainty, by refocusing the discussion on any person going to any concert.

Having difficulties remembering and recognizing what a picture or a video clip shows is common in our data, and whether or not this becomes a problem for the participants in many ways depends on responses to and uptakes of such difficulties. Extract 4 shows a situation where a person with dementia has obvious problems with recognizing what a photo depicts and thinks that a puppy included in the CIRCA materials is her own puppy.

Extract 4
C=Carer, E=Eva (person with dementia)

```
01   C:   nu valde jag lite där ska vi se va de är
          now I chose some here let's see what it is
02   C:   ((changes picture)) ↑oj du
                              look at that
```

```
03    E:    e de min hundvalp
            is that my puppy
04          (0.2)
05    C:    har du haft en ↑sån?
            have you had one like that?
06    E:    *ja*
            *yea*
07          (0.7)
08    E:    [hon var sådär preci] s [samma]
            [she was just like tha] t [the same]
09:   C:    [jaha:              ]   [va     ]
            [yea:               ]   [what:  ]
10          (.)
11    C:    va hette den?
            what was it called
```

Since the participants in Extract 4 are using CIRCA (the application with generic material), it is obvious for the carer that the puppy in the picture is not Eva's puppy. When Eva suggests that they are looking at her puppy (line 3), this is, however, not something the carer explicitly addresses in her response. Instead, she picks up an aspect of Eva's response and directs the conversation toward Eva's experiences with puppies (line 5). In doing this instead of responding to Eva's question regarding whose puppy it is, the carer smoothly continues the conversation without explicitly addressing the uncertainty about the puppy. While not explicitly addressing Eva's inquiry about the ownership of the puppy, the carer's response could be seen to implicitly address Eva's question in her response 'have you had one like that'. Her 'one like that' implies that the puppy in the picture is not Eva's puppy, but the turn is not focused on this topic and instead asks about Eva's previous life with dogs. By avoiding explicitly addressing Eva's uncertainty with the puppy, that is choosing not to disrupt the progressivity of the talk to address its factual content, the conversation can continue without Eva losing face, but also without the conversation being built on a misconception that the puppy in the picture is Eva's puppy. As is shown in Eva's contributions when she continues her story, she acknowledges that the puppy in the picture is not her puppy by comparing the puppy in the picture with the puppy she used to own, 'she was just like that' (line 8).

We now move on from the use of questions to the second focal point for this chapter: the way materials in the applications are used and managed in interaction, also with a focus on promoting participation and involvement of persons with dementia. What material is displayed on the tablets in many ways directs the conversation. In Extract 5, Isa is talking to a carer using CIRCUS. They are talking about a house where Isa lived as a child, and she is describing differences between the house now and what it used to look like when she lived there.

Extract 5
I=Isa (person with dementia), C=carer

```
01  I:   [m] du förstår att (0.3)
         [m] you see (0.3) ((points toward the picture))
02  I:   de fanns ju inge (0.3) rödfärg på huset eller (0.3) nånting
         ((hawks)) there was no (0.3) paint on the house or anything
03  I:   eller elektriskt
         or electricity
04  C:   nä nä
         no no
05  I:   nä
         no ((hawks))
06  I:   senare år så de ha ju tillkommit (0.8) på på
         recent years so that's an addition (0.8) in in
07  C:   yea okay yea
         ja okej ja
08       (0.5)
09  I:   de f- e ju en
         it is a ((points to the picture))
10  I:   lam- (0.5) elektrisk lampa där (0.6) över verandan
         lam- (0.5) electric lamp there (0.6) over the porch
11  C:   ja: de kanske det är ja (.) ↑ja   [ ja]
         yea: maybe there is yea (.) ↑yea [yea]
12  I:                                    [m:]
13       (0.6)
14  C:   .hja
         .yea
15       ((C changes picture))
16  I:   men ↑ja ha ju växt ↑upp (1.0) i: (0.7) de här huset
         but ↑I grew ↑up (1.0) in (0.7) this house
17       ((C changes back to the previous picture))
18  C:   M: (.) hur många rum var de
         m: how many rooms were there
19       (0.4)
20  I:   ja de va inte mer än två
         well there were no more than two
```

At the beginning of the extract Isa is leading the conversation, describing changes made to the house after she moved out, and the carer is mainly providing short acknowledging responses during Isa's telling (lines 1–7). Having pointed out an electric lamp on the house in the photo as one of the new additions to the house (line 10), there is a short silence, after which the carer adds a quiet 'yea' while breathing in, something that in Swedish can be seen to be finishing off a topic, and a transition to something new (Hoey, 2020). There is then a new, longer silence during which the carer also changes the material displayed on the tablet. However, as becomes apparent in line 16, Isa has not finished the topic of her childhood home and continues to talk about the house from the previous picture. Even though the carer has already changed the material and signalled that she is ready to move on to the next topic, she then quickly changes back to the picture of Isa's previous home and continues the topic by asking a question about the house (line 18). By being sensitive to Isa's topic preferences and by quickly going back to a previous photo, the conversation about Isa's house continues for several turns. This demonstrates how the management of the device may contribute to promoting the engagement of the person with dementia. One way to understand this interaction is in terms of the conversation itself being prioritized over looking at the pictures. As soon as Isa adds a new turn related to a previous picture, the carer abandons her project to change the material (and the topic) and goes back to display the photo of Isa's house that is related to the conversational topic Isa is continuing. This behaviour shows that the carer is sensitive to the conversational trajectory of the person with dementia.

In Extract 6 Jon and a carer are using CIRCA in their conversation, and as the transcript shows, management of the material is quite different from Extract 5. In this extract the carer quickly moves from picture to picture, creating a much more task-oriented conversation than in Extract 5.

Extract 6
C=carer, J=Jon (person with dementia)

```
01 C:  nu kom de mer bilde=
       now there are more pictures
02 J:  =Cassius Clay
03     (1.0)
04 C:  a::
05 J:  (Mohammad Ali en) boxaren värsmästarn
       (Mohammad Ali a) the boxer world champion
06 C:  aa precis
       yea:: exactly
07     (5.8) ((C changes pictures))
08 J:  e de Tage Elander
       is it Tage Erlander
09 C:  aa (1.7) han va- va han statsminister?
       yea (1.7) he wa- was he prime minister?
10 J:  ja=
       yes
11 C:  =aa
       yea
12     (2.8) ((C changes pictures))
13 C:  ja lär mig också på de här vet du
       I learn too when doing this you know
14 J:  (xx) fotbolls vm femtiåtta)=
       (xx) football World Cup fifty-eight
15 C:  =a:
       yea:
16 J:  de va ju: gick dom ju långt i
       that was, they got on well there
17 C:  m:
18     (1.2)
19 J:  de va femtiåtta (eh:) ja tro de va de
       it was fifty-eight (eh.) I think it was
```

As the excerpt begins, Jon and the carer are presented with a picture of Muhammad Ali, or Cassius Clay as he was originally called, a person Jon immediately recognizes and names. After a silence of about 1 second (line 3), the carer provides an acknowledgement token but does not expand on the topic. Jon then uses the name 'Mohammad Ali' to refer to the picture and adds that he was a world champion boxer – a turn that immediately gets an affirmative response from the carer 'yea exactly' (line 6). As the caption for the picture is indeed 'Muhammad Ali' and not 'Cassius Clay', one way to understand this short exchange is that the carer becomes uncertain when Jon first calls the person in the picture 'Cassius Clay' when in fact the caption used in CIRCA says 'Mohammad Ali'. It may also be the case that the carer does not know that Mohammad Ali's original name was Cassius Clay. While Jon shows clear recognition of the person in the picture, the carer does not pick up on this and instead changes to a new photo, this time of former Swedish prime minister Tage Erlander. This person is also recognized by Jon, who provides the name in the format of a question, indicating that he is requesting confirmation of the name (line 8). The carer confirms that it is Tage Erlander (this name is also provided in the caption to the picture, which is visible to both participants) and after some silence she asks Jon if Tage Erlander used to be prime minister, which Jon can confirm (lines 9–11). Again, Jon shows recognition of the person in the photo being viewed, and again the carer decides to move on to a new picture while stating that she, too, learns from the activity. Jon, however, has already moved on to the new photo showing the Swedish football team from 1958. As for the previous pictures, Jon recognizes the people depicted and adds some additional information about the events.

The pattern in Extract 6 is both clear and stable: the carer shows a picture, Jon recognizes who is in the picture and adds some additional information, and the carer then moves on to the next picture. In contrast to Extract 5, here the specific content of the pictures seems to be prioritized over conversation around related topics, as demonstrated by the fact that the participants look at each picture for a shorter amount of time. The fact that the carer does not pick up on or expand on any of the potential topic-starters provided by Jon also indicates that she is not attuned to Jon's conversational trajectory. There are arguably several opportunities to explore Jon's knowledge and experiences of what is shown in the pictures that are not employed by the carer. While Jon and his carer get to see a lot of pictures, they do not go into any detail on any of the pictures or explore potential associations, experiences and memories related to the pictures. This may of course also be due to the fact that the pictures are of a more generic character and not as personal as in Extract 5.

While changing pictures before a topic is ended may be viewed as constraining the possibilities to engage in conversation, there are also examples where changing materials in the middle of a topic could be argued to be a way of moving a conversation forward. In our last example, a carer is talking to Gudrun using CIRCA. Gudrun used to have a cat when she was younger, and this is something she recurrently talks about.

Extract 7
C= carer, G= Gudrun (person with dementia)

```
01  C:  här då?
        this then? ((looks at the tablet where a dog is shown))
02  G:  oh jössenamn
        oh my gosh
03  C:  vilka färger
        look at the colours
04  G:  jaa (0.4) vi- vi har ju alltid haft hund
        yea (.4) we- we always had a dog
05  C:  ja juste
        yea that's right
06  G:  men (0.9) en helig birma hade vi
        but (0.9= we had a Holy Birman
07  C:  just de en liten        [katt]
        that's right a little [cat]
08  G:                          [ a::]
09  G:  å sen (1.8) ja:
        and then (1.8) yea:: ((C changes pictures))
10  C:  mm har ni haft sånhärna då?
        mm have you had any of these? ((shows a picture on the tablet))
11  G:  [ nej]
        [no]
12  C:  [ nåt] akvarium?
        [any] aquarium
13  G:  nähe det har vi inte haft
        no that we didn't have
```

When looking at a picture of a dog, Gudrun mentions that she used to have a cat, a Holy Birman. In our recordings we have examples where Gudrun tells the carer about her cat and where he helps to fill in details, and it is reasonable to believe that the carer has heard this story several times. In this example, however, the carer does not elaborate on Gudrun's initial mentioning of her cat, but instead marks the topic as something he already knows about in line 7 ('just det/that's right). Gudrun continues with something that seems to be an initiation of a story related to this (line 8, 'å sen/and then'), but before she manages to start her telling, the carer has changed to a new picture and initiates a new topic about aquariums. By showing Gudrun a new picture and posing a question related to this, the carer directs the conversation away from a potentially upcoming story of Gudrun's cat. Throughout the data Gudrun often tells the story of her cat. As we have also seen in Extract 6, introducing a new picture into the conversation is a powerful tool for changing the topic. Given the fact that the story about Gudrun's cat has appeared several times in the data, we would suggest that in this example the carer uses this strategy to avoid a story he has heard many times before. Interrupting an upcoming story by changing the topic is often considered to be both impolite and a violation of conversational norms. Therefore, it is reasonable to assume that the carer does this in order to move the conversation forward. In interaction with people with dementia, repetitive behaviours, such as telling the same story over and over again, is often considered a behavioural problem by conversational partners (Hydén, 2018; Searson et al., 2008). In conversations where a digital communication support is used, changing the picture being displayed is not just a powerful way of guiding the conversation in a new direction; it could potentially also be a less face-threatening way of interrupting an ongoing topic than verbally disrupting an ongoing story.

13.7 Discussion

As the results have demonstrated, asking questions in interaction with people with dementia can be challenging but also interactionally rewarding. As demonstrated in Extracts 1 and 2, asking the person with dementia factual questions about a picture generates personal stories from them, albeit in different ways. If the person with dementia remembers what is in the picture, they may tell a story about this. It is also the case that if the person does not provide recollections associated with the content of the picture, a somewhat more far-fetched story may be generated. In Extract 3 the person with dementia is asked about his feelings and opinions on what is depicted in the application, which seems to be beneficial for avoiding the potential face threat that might have occurred if he had been asked, for example, to name who was in the picture. This also happens in Extract 4, where the carer turns the sequence into a more general conversation rather than focussing on the specific content of the picture. How the interaction will proceed following a specific question is dependent on several factors that are difficult to foresee and control. Whether or not to ask questions, or whether certain types of questions are better than others, is, from our experience, not possible to determine. Rather, what we think may be learnt from the analysed examples is that an awareness of potential problems associated with certain types of questions and a readiness to handle difficulties that might occur are important competences in interaction involving people with dementia in order to promote their participation and involvement in the best possible way.

As regards the management of the material in the applications, we have demonstrated that compliance with the associations of the person with dementia, by, for example, changing the pictures back and forth, following the conversation, and being sensitive to the conversational trajectory initiated by the contributions of the person with dementia, may be beneficial for the development and the expansion of a topic. In support of this argument, we have also shown that in Extract 6 changing pictures too rapidly, or turning the activity into a naming task, may hamper expansion of topics and a more varied conversation, since it is clear from that extract that a rapid change of pictures does not elicit any expansions from the person with dementia. However, there is no simple way of advising how to manage the material, since Extract 7 demonstrates that changing the picture in the middle of someone's talk may actually be beneficial for the progression of the conversation.

The main implications of our findings regarding care and assessment of people with dementia are that in order to promote participation and involvement, it may be beneficial to choose to prioritize moving on in conversation rather than focussing on facts, and to be sensitive to the conversational trajectory initiated by the contributions of the person with dementia. In many countries, in policy documents for care and support for people with dementia, person-centred care is emphasized. The use of strategies that promote participation and involvement in conversation could contribute to the implementation of this. Our findings also point to the fact that the use of communication support may contribute to enhancing active participation and engagement in conversation involving people with dementia if the users are aware of how management of it may affect the outcome of its use.

References

Alm, N., Astell, A., Ellis, M., Dye, R., Gowans, G. and Campbell, J. (2004) 'A cognitive prosthesis and communication support for people with dementia.' *Neuropsychological Rehabilitation*, 14(1/2): 117–134. doi: 10.1080/09602010343000147.

Alzheimer's Society. (2007) *Home from Home: A Report Highlighting the Opportunities for Improving Standards of Dementia Care in Care Homes*. London: Alzheimer's Society.

Astell, A. J. and Parsons, M. S. (2010) 'CIRCA: Technology to prompt reminiscing and conversation between residents in care homes and care staff.' *Gerontechnology* 9(2): 68–69. doi: 10.4017/gt.2010.09.02.049.00.

Astell, A. J., Ellis, M. P., Alm, N., Dye, R., Campbell, J. and Gowans, G. (2004) 'Facilitating communication in dementia with multimedia technology.' *Brain and Language,* 91(1): 80–81.

Astell, A. J., Ellis, M. P., Bernardi, L., Alm, N., Dye, R., Gowans, G. and Campbell, J. (2010) 'Using a touch screen computer to support relationships between people with dementia and caregivers.' *Interacting With Computers*, 22(4)(Supportive Interaction: Computer Interventions for Mental Health): 267–275. doi:10.1016/j.intcom.2010.03.003.

Astell, A., Gradisek, J., Bizjak, J., Gjoreski, H., Gams, M., Goljuf, K., Cabrera-Umipierrez, M. F., Montalva, J. J., Karavidopoulou, Y., Panou, M., Toulioue, K., Kaklanise, N., Stavrotheodorose, S., Tzovarase, D., Kaimakamisf, E., Laakso, K., Buchholz, M., Derbring, S., Samuelsson, C., Ekström, A., Garcia, A., Chamorro Matak, J., Smith, S. K., Stephen Potter, S., Tabak, M., Dekker-Van Weering, M., Cossu-Ergecern, F. and Black, B. (2018) 'IN-LIFE – Independent Living Support Functions for the Elderly: Technology and Pilot Overview.' In I. Chatzigiannakis, Y. Tobe, P. Novais and O. Amft (eds.) *Intelligent Environments 2018: Workshop Proceedings of the 14th International Conference on Intelligent Environments*. Amsterdam: IOS, pp. 526–535. doi:10.3233/978-1-61499-874-7-526.

Azuma, T. and Bayles, K. A. (1997) 'Memory impairments underlying language difficulties in dementia.' *Topics in Language Disorders*, 18(1): 58–71.

Baker, R., Angus, D., Smith-Conway, E., Baker, K., Gallois, C., Smith, A. and Chenery, H. J. (2015) 'Visualising conversations between care home staff and residents with dementia.' *Ageing and Society*, 35(2): 270–297.

Bayles, K. A. (2001) 'Understanding the neuropsychological syndrome of dementia.' *Seminars in Speech and Language*, 42(4): 251–260.

Bayles, K. A. and Tomoeda, C. K. (2014) *Cognitive-Communication Disorders of Dementia : Definition, Diagnosis, and Treatment*. San Diego, CA : Plural Publishing, Inc.

Beukelman, D. R., Fager, S., Ball, L. and Dietz, A. (2007) 'AAC for adults with acquired neurological conditions: A review.' *Augmentative and Alternative Communication*, 23(3): 230–242.

Bourgeois, M. S. and Hickey, E. M. (2009) *Dementia: From Diagnosis to Management—A Functional Approach*. New York: Psychology Press.

Brooker, D. and Duce, L. (2000) 'Wellbeing and activity in dementia: A comparison of group reminiscence therapy, structured goal-directed group activity and unstructured time.' *Aging & Mental Health*, 4(4): 354–358.

Burgio, L. D., Allen-Burge, R., Roth, D. L., Bourgeois, M. S., Dijkstra, K., Gerstle, J., Jackson, E. and Bankester, L. (2001) 'Come talk with me: Improving communication between nursing assistants and nursing home residents during care routines.' *The Gerontologist*, 41(4): 449–460.

Cook, C., Fay, S. and Rockwood, K. (2009) 'Verbal repetition in people with mild-to-moderate Alzheimer disease: A descriptive analysis from the VISTA Clinical Trial.' *Alzheimer Disease and Associated Disorders*, 23(2): 146–151.

Ekström, A., Ferm, U. and Samuelsson, C. (2017) 'Digital communication support and Alzheimer's disease.' *Dementia*, 16(6): 711–731.

Evans, S., Fear, T., Means, R. and Vallelly, S. (2007) 'Supporting independence for people with dementia in extra care housing.' *Dementia*, 6: 144–150.

Finnema, E., Dröes, R. M., Ribbe, M. and Van Tilburg, W. (2000) 'The effects of emotion-oriented approaches in the care for persons suffering from dementia: A review of the literature.' *International Journal of Geriatric Psychiatry*, 15(2): 141–161.

Fried-Oken, M., Rowland, C., Daniels, D., Dixon, M., Fuller, B., Mills, C. and Oken, B. (2012) 'AAC to support conversation in persons with moderate Alzheimer's disease.' *Augmentative and Alternative Communication*, 28(4): 219–231.

Gowans, G., Campbell, J., Alm, N., Dye, R., Astell, A. and Ellis, M. (2004) 'Designing a multimedia conversation aid for reminiscence therapy in dementia care environments.' In *CHI'04 Extended Abstracts on Human Factors in Computing Systems.* New York: ACM, pp. 825–836.

Guendouzi, J. and Davis, B. H. (2014) 'Dementia discourse and pragmatics.' In Davis, B. H., Guendouzi, J. and Morón, R. G. (eds.) *Pragmatics in Dementia Discourse.* Newcastle upon Tyne: Cambridge Scholars Publishing, pp. 1–28.

Heritage, J. (1984) *Garfinkel and Ethnomethodology.* Cambridge, MA: Polity Press.

Higginbotham, D. J., Shane, H., Russell, S. and Caves, K. (2007) 'Access to AAC: Present, past, and future.' *Augmentative and Alternative Communication*, 23(3): 243–257.

Hitch, D., Swan, J., Pattison, R. and Stefaniak, R. (2017) 'Use of touchscreen tablet technology by people with dementia in homes: A scoping review.' *Journal of Rehabilitation and Assistive Technologies Engineering*, 4. doi: 10.1177/2055668317733382.

Hoey, E. M. (2020) 'Waiting to inhale: On sniffing in conversation.' *Research on Language and Social Interaction*, 53(1): 118–139.

Hydén, L-C. (2018) *Entangled Narratives. Collaborative Storytelling and the Reimagining of Dementia.* Oxford: Oxford University Press.

Jansson, G. (2016) '"You're doing everything just fine": Praise in residential care settings.' *Discourse Studies*, 18(1): 64–86. doi: 10.1177/1461445615613186.

Johansson, M. (2015) *Cognitive Impairment and Its Consequences in Everyday Life.* Doctoral dissertation, Linköping University Electronic Press.

Murphy, J. and Boa, S. (2012) 'Using the WHO-ICF with talking mats to enable adults with long-term communication difficulties to participate in goal setting.' *Augmentative and Alternative Communication*, 28: 52–60.

Murphy, J., Oliver, T. M. and Cox, S. (2010) 'Talking mats and involvement in decision making for people with dementia and family carers'. Full report, Joseph Rowntree Foundation. www.talkingmats.com/wp-content/uploads/2013/09/Dementia-and-Decision-Making-full-report2.pdf.

Örulv, L. and Nikku, N. (2007) 'Dignity work in dementia care: Sketching a microethical analysis.' *Dementia*, 6: 507–525.

Perkins, L., Whitworth, A. and Lesser, R. (1998) 'Conversing in dementia: A conversation analytic approach.' *Journal of Neurolinguistics*, 11(1–2): 33–53.

Prince, M. and Jackson, J. (2009) World Alzheimer's report. www.alz.co.uk/research/world-report/.

Sacks, H. (1992) *Lectures on Conversation*, Vol. I and II. Oxford: Blackwell.

Sacks, H., Schegloff, E. A. and Jefferson, G. (1974) 'A simplest systematics for the organization of turn-taking for conversation.' *Language*, 50(4): 696–735.

Schegloff, E. A. (2007) *Sequence Organization in Interaction: Volume 1: A Primer in Conversation Analysis* (Vol. 1). Cambridge: Cambridge University Press.

Searson, R., Hendry, A. M., Ramachandran, R., Burns, A. and Purandare, N. (2008) 'Activities enjoyed by patients with dementia together with their spouses and psychological morbidity in carers.' *Aging and Mental Health*, 12(2): 276–282.

Small, J. A. and Perry, J. (2005) 'Do you remember? How caregivers question their spouses who have Alzheimer's disease and the impact on communication.' *Journal of Speech, Language, and Hearing Research*, 48(1): 125–136.

Small, J. A., Gutman, G., Makela, S. and Hillhouse, B. (2003) 'Effectiveness of communication strategies used by caregivers of persons with Alzheimer's disease during activities of daily living.' *Journal of Speech, Language, and Hearing Research*, 46(2): 353–367.

Smith, S. and Astell, A. J. (2018) 'Technology-supported group activity to promote communication in dementia: A protocol for a within-participants study.' *Technologies*, 6(1): 33. doi: 10.3390/technologies6010033.

Swan, K., Hopper, M., Wenke, R., Jackson, C., Till, T. and Conway, E. (2018) 'Speech-language pathologist interventions for communication in moderate–severe dementia: A systematic review.' *American Journal of Speech-Language Pathology*, 27(2): 836–852.

Upton, P., Jones, T., Jutla, K. and Brooker, D. (2011) Evaluation of the impact of touch screen technology on people with dementia and their carers within care home settings. Department of Health West Midlands, University of Worcester. http://79.170.44.96/lifestorynetwork.org.uk/wp-content/uploads/downloads/2012/11/evaluation-of-the-impact-of-the-use-of-touchscreen-technology-with-people-with-dementia-.pdf

Wray, A. (2010) '"We've had a wonderful, wonderful thing": Formulaic interaction when an expert has dementia.' *Dementia*, 9(4): 517–534.

Yasuda, K., Kuwabara, K., Kuwahara, N., Abe, S. and Tetsutani, N. (2009) 'Effectiveness of personalised reminiscence photo videos for individuals with dementia.' *Neuropsychological Rehabilitation*, 19(4): 603–619.

14 "It's More than Eating, It's a Social Situation"
Video Analysis and Professional Vision in Dementia Care

*Camilla Lindholm and Tuula Tykkyläinen**

14.1 Introduction

Dementia is a prominent challenge for public health today and is one of the most frequent reasons for admitting older adults to institutional care. Even if the health care policies in many countries aim to enable people with dementia to remain in their own homes as long as possible (Verbeek et al., 2012), at some point during the disease the care needs of the person with dementia exceed the resources available at home. In such cases, professional long-term care is required. Traditionally, the care of the aged was influenced by a medical model that focused on the disease, its symptoms, and the lost abilities of the person with dementia. In line with this model, a body of research has identified a disparity between the task-focused agenda of professional care staff and the socially oriented interests of residents (for an overview, see Ward et al., 2008). A contrast to the disease- and task-oriented perspective is the approach of person-centered care developed by Kitwood (1997). Person-centered care is defined as having a holistic caregiving culture in supporting the personhood of people with dementia. Person-centered care is inherently relational and interactional. In personhood support, positive interactions are key, and the supportive functions of these interactions work by facilitating deep and mutually empathetic relationships between people (Kitwood, 1997; Brooker, 2007).

Therefore, the concept of person-centered care and its role in improving the quality of life of people with dementia have been established in dementia care since the late 1990s. Recently, there has been growing research interest in mealtimes and dining as an important aspect of person-centered care. Indeed, most studies have stressed the importance of food and mealtimes in dementia care (Berg, 2006), describing eating as the most social of all daily activities (Amella, 1999). Food remains an enduring pleasure, and the taste and smell of food are associated with memory. Eating is also an aspect of life over which a

---

* We thank participants on the panel *Technologies to Participate – the Role of Material Objects in Communication Impairment* at IIEMCA in Kolding, August 2015, and the editors of this volume for their valuable contributions. This work was supported by The Academy of Finland (project no. 256792) and by Jan-Magnus Janssons stiftelse.

person with dementia can maintain some control. In many studies, autonomy, choice, control, and particularly dignity are linked to notions of personhood and quality of life (Kane et al., 2003; Mittal et al., 2007; Degenholtz et al., 2008; Robinson & Gallagher, 2008; Venturato, 2010). In work focusing specifically on mealtimes in long-term care homes, Reimer and Keller (2009) outline four aspects of person-centered mealtime care – providing choices and preferences, supporting independence, promoting the social side of eating, and showing respect.

This chapter demonstrates how a community of professional caregivers change their view of a mealtime situation during a session of video guidance (see Section 14.2 on Data for a description). Using data from this session, the study shows how the professional caregivers' view of mealtimes and the activity of "having a meal" was transformed during the intervention session. The chapter focuses on how the professional guide uses practices such as hypothetical questions and reformulations of previous contributions to redirect the group's focus toward the interaction between the professional caregiver and the person with dementia in the video. It is demonstrated how the session of video guidance creates awareness of the ability of the person with dementia to communicate through embodied practices, and the caregivers' capacity to respond to this embodied behavior. The notion of *professional vision* (Lave & Wenger, 1991; Goodwin, 1994; Pilnick & James, 2013) is of particular importance. In this case, the intervention is demonstrated to facilitate professional caregivers' particular "socially organized ways of seeing and understanding events that are answerable to the distinctive interests of a particular social group" (Goodwin, 1994: 606).

14.2 Data and Methods

The data analyzed in this chapter were collected in an extensive project on dementia and interaction.[1] The project was approved by the social services and health care division in the municipality in which data were collected. Written consent was sought from participants (health care providers, people with dementia, and/or their family members or legal guardians). Participation in the project was voluntary. In all research reports, personal and identifiable items have been changed to protect the anonymity of the research subjects.

The context of the data is a guidance session introducing a Finnish communication intervention model called OIVA (Koski et al., 2010; Burakoff & Martikainen, 2015), which is targeted at professional communities and aims to enhance interaction between people with complex communication needs

---

[1] The title of the project is *Dementia and Interaction – Intersections between Research and Communication Training*, and it is funded by the Academy of Finland (project no. 256792).

(due to, for example, dementia) and their communication partners. The duration of the OIVA training process is ten months, and it includes five meetings focusing on video interaction guidance led by a trained OIVA guide. In this study, we focus on a 90-minute video guidance meeting between the OIVA guide and five staff members from a group home for older adults with dementia. The session analyzed in this study is the third meeting out of five in the OIVA process of a particular organization.

In OIVA, videos are used as tools to stimulate discussion and reflection. The staff members film everyday interactions and meet with a trained OIVA guide to discuss scenarios from their videos. Because the OIVA approach is solution-focused, the guide chooses a video clip of successful interaction for further reflection. Concentrating on the successful aspects of interactions serves to advance communication. The aim is to empower the professional community and render its resources and successful experiences visible.

The 90-minute video guidance meetings have a three-part structure. The meeting starts with an opening phase in which the group reflects on the aims and goals of their previous meeting before the topic of the day and the group's questions to the guide are introduced. The main part of the meeting is the video analysis phase, during which the group watches the chosen video several times. After watching the whole video once, the group discusses their general thoughts. After the focus has been (re-)defined, the group watches the video in short clips and discusses these clips with the guide. During the video analysis, someone in the group acts as a secretary and makes notes of the most important discussion points. In the closing phase, the group's findings and the secretary's notes are summarized, and the group decide upon a so-called concrete act that is related to the question posed in relation to the video. The group decides to try out a new way of performing an action, and the outcome of this change in professional behavior is evaluated in the next session.

In the 90-minute guidance session studied in this chapter, the group members analyze the interaction in a 3-minute video in which a caregiver helps a resident with no preserved spoken language to begin eating. Six people participate in the guidance session, five staff members and the guide. The staff members come from a professional community in residential dementia care, and the guide is in charge of the OIVA intervention program in which the professional community participates.

The methodological approach utilized in this chapter is ethnomethodological conversation analysis (Sacks et al., 1974; Schegloff, 2007); the video data is analyzed using this micro-analytic approach. In addition, we also have access to some written documents in which the OIVA guide describes her experience of the guidance session. These ethnographic data provide complementary results to the conversation analytic findings.

14.3 Analysis

Even if previous research (Fukkink, 2008) has demonstrated that interventions involving video guidance can be an effective means of rehabilitation, we still lack knowledge about how change may arise as a result of micro-level interactional practices observed in video guidance. We illustrate how change in professional vision is facilitated through the practices of the guide and how the process unfolds from the beginning to the end of the conversation. The following account presents how the group proceeds from a task-oriented view of mealtimes to an interactional focus on dining via the analysis of embodied practices. Simultaneously, the group becomes more aware of their good caregiving practices.

14.3.1 Defining the Question: Eating as an Individual Task vs. Interaction-Seeking Behavior

As mentioned above, the professional caregivers film their daily work and decide upon an issue to be analyzed in the video guidance session. They hand in a video addressing this issue, and the guide selects a short clip of successfully attuned interaction to be discussed. We show how the guide and the staff members work on a 3-minute clip of a professional caregiver (Annika) assisting an elderly lady (Sarah) when starting to eat her daily lunch.

Our first example was preceded by the guide asking the caregivers about their reasons for choosing this mealtime situation for further discussion. Extract 1 illustrates how the caregivers describe the mealtime in the opening phase of their guidance session. Even if the institutional frame of the intervention program they are participating in is related to interaction, and the caregivers are aware of this, they initially focus on how the resident performs the task of having her daily lunch. Nurse Annika, who provides an account for the choice of a mealtime situation, defines Sarah's eating as "challenging" (line 3) and indirectly describes the eating as non-fluent by referring to "spreading food" (line 3). Further, Annika describes the videotaped situation as an opportunity to evaluate to what extent Sarah is capable of independent eating in contrast to feeding. Thus, Annika seemingly describes the discussion of the videotape as an opportunity to assess and address the challenges related to Sarah's independent eating.

Extract 1 Seeking interaction (A, L, E = Annika, Laura, Eva, nurses; G = OIVA guide); X = unclear

```
01   A:    piti sitte (0.8) (.nf) (0.4) keksii joku ja (.) no
           had to (0.8) (.nf) (0.4) come up with something and (.) well
02         (.) ruokailutilanne on Saaran kans suht koht
           (.) mealtimes with Sarah are rather
```

```
03            haasteellinen (-) levittelee sitä ruokaa (0.5)
              challenging (-) spreads the food (0.5)
04            ympäristöön ja sitte (0.3) päälle se
              all over the place and then (0.3) on herself
05            (hyvin paljon syödessä)
              (very much when eating)
06            (0.3)
07      G:    joo
              yes
08            (0.4)
09      A:    että on aika (0.3) pitkälle syötetty
              so we used to (0.3) feed her quite often
10            (1.3) siinä nyt sitte(hh) (0.5) halutt[iin]
              (1.3) there we now then(hh) (0.5) wan   [ted   ]
11      X:                                            [mm    ]
12      A:    se että (1.0) että miten (1.2) miten hän ite
              this that (1.0) how (1.2) how she herself
13            (0.5) pystyy ja miten paljon
              (0.5) is able and how much
14            #pystyy ite syömään ja (.) tämmöstä#
              # is able to eat herself (.) and such#
15      G:    joo?
              yes?
16            (0.7)
17      X:    [(-)       ]
18      L:    [kyl       ] niinku ihan niinku san- sanallises- tai ei niinku
              [Well] like like ver- verball- or not like
19            (0.7) ainakaan lauseilla keskustele et hän ei         [(-)]
              (0.7) at least doesn't speak with sentences so she not[(-)]
20      G:                                                          [mm ]
21      L:    [se ]mmosia vuorovaikutuksei (.) mut kyllä ihan selväst-
              [tho]se interactions (.) but really clearl-
22      G:    [mm]
23      L:    kyllä hän niit vuorovai- kyllä hänellä (0.4) kyllähän
              she does interaction- she has (0.4) well she
24            siinä videollakin näki et siinä on (.) [ (ihan) hakee
              on the video you saw that here (.)     [really seeks
25      A:                                           [((coughs))
26      L:    semmost vuorovaikutusta siinä (.) <niinkun>
              this interaction there (.) <like>
27            (0.4)
28      G:    joo (0.5) (.hh) ja toi on    [ihan   ] <totta> että tehän
              yes (0.5) (.hh) and that's   [really] true that you
29      X:                                 [(-)    ]
30      G:    näätte tuolla nyt sitte (0.8) ja tota: m- muunki ku
              see on the video there (0.8) and erm: o- other things than
31            vuorovaikutuksen näkökulmal:tsta nii esimerkiks just sitä
              from an interaction perspective for example the
32            syömistä siis ihan[niinku] (.hh) mut et se (.) et nyt te
              eating like       [this  ] (.hh) but that it (.) that now you
33      E:                      [mm    ]
34      G:    (0.6) varmaan eli sitä tottakai (.) pystytte
```

```
              (0.6) for sure so of course (.) you can
35            havainnoimaan (.hh) niin sä olit kirjottanut tähän (.)
              observe (.hh) and you wrote here (.)
36            tähän että tota (0.5) et Saara ei kommunikoi
              here that erm (0.5) that Sarah doesn't communicate
37            <keskustelemalla> niin tota (0.3) ja sit et e-e-
              <by discussing> so well (0.3) and then that e- e-
38            jotenki siihen et (.) miten se sitte (1.1) [ sekö   ] (.)
              in some way that (.) how does she then (1.1)[did she ] (.)
39    L:                                                 [mm      ]
40    G:      olikse niinku mä (.) mä nyt ymmärsin täs[tä] et
              was it like I (.) I now understood th    [is ] like
41    X:                                               [mm ]
42    G:      eikö mekin mietitty jo se et no millä tavoilla
              didn't we already think that in which ways
43            se sit se (.) tavallaan se keskustelu (.nff) (0.5)
              the then the (.) in a way the discussion (.nff) (0.5)
44    L:      mm
45            (.)
46    G:      sujuu
              works out
47            (.)
48    A:      mm
49            (.)
50    G:      kun se ei oo tällaist perinteistä (.)
              when it isn't a traditional (.)
51            puheella >keskustelua olinko mä onks mä< (.)
              discussion >with speech did I did I< (.)
52    G:      [yh ] tään oikeeseen suuntaan ettiny sielt videolta sitä,
              [at ] all search the video for the right things
53    L:      [joo]
              [yes]
```

When discussing Sarah's performance, there is, however, a contrast between the account provided by caregiver Annika and the description given by Laura, who was the person in charge of filming the situation and who therefore can perhaps be seen as having a special responsibility for the videos. In line 18, Laura enters the conversation and changes the topic; instead of focusing on how Sarah performs the eating task, she begins to describe Sarah's communication impairment. She evaluates Sarah as being non-verbal and unable to produce sentence-level language (lines 18–19). In contrast to this, she then makes an attempt to describe Sarah's preserved communication skills. Laura's attempts are, however, cut off and syntactically disfluent (lines 21, 23, 24), and she ends up by stating that Sarah clearly seeks interaction (lines 24, 26). Thus, the focus changes from Sarah's interaction skills to her motivation to interact.

Caregivers Annika and Laura present different perspectives on the importance of videoing the mealtime situation. When the guide takes her turn, she relates to both perspectives. Initially (lines 30–32, 34), she refers to Annika's perspective by acknowledging that there are of course other dimensions than the interaction visible on the video, such as matters related to the activity of eating. In line 35, the guide then leads the topic toward the interaction-related issue that the group has talked about in a cover letter accompanying the video. She makes explicit reference to the cover letter written by Laura ("and you wrote here", line 35) and asks (lines 40, 42–43 and 46) the staff members to confirm her interpretation of the central question the group wants to discuss with her. To create and formulate a mutual understanding between the staff members and herself is apparently of great importance to the guide. In her contribution, she acknowledges the practical, task-oriented perspective of mealtimes presented by Annika, but then she continues by focusing on the interaction perspective. Note that both Annika and Laura, the people who presented the different perspectives on the video, respond with the rather weak acknowledgment *mm* (lines 44, 48). This is perhaps the reason why the guide (lines 50–52) asks whether she has understood the group's point of interest correctly.

14.3.2 From Task Orientation to Embodied Practices: Video Analysis

Earlier we noted how one of the caregivers initially focused on independent eating, whereas another staff member emphasized the preserved interaction skills and the interactional behavior of the resident. The task-oriented focus demonstrated by nurse Annika in Extract 1 is, as the video analysis and conversation proceed, transformed into an analysis of the embodied behavior of the participants, and later into a more interaction-focused perspective on the mealtime, as explicated by the caregivers. We now proceed to demonstrate three various practices used by the guide to induce the analysis of the participants' embodied behavior. These three practices are so-called "speech bubble" metaphors, hypothetical questions, and formulations. Later, we show how the staff members change their way of speaking about the mealtime situation from a task-oriented view to a person-centered view during the guidance session.

14.3.2.1 Speech Bubble Metaphors

The video analysis phase consists mostly of a detailed microanalysis in which the guide asks the staff members to identify and define the interactional initiatives and responses produced by the caregiver and the resident on the videotape. In this phase, the guide utilizes various practices to promote reflection. The first of these practices are speech bubble metaphors. In Extract 2 we enter the guidance session at a point where the guide, through questions and interpretations, has done extensive work to change the staff members' perceptions of the resident with dementia as a conversational partner. She has pointed out the resident's embodied initiatives and even explicitly stated that Sarah is a person not only with the capacity to recognize the initiatives produced by others but is also capable of taking initiatives herself. In Extract 2 the staff members are asked to redefine Sarah's actions. The guide points toward the still picture of Sarah on the screen behind her and poses a question to the caregivers (line 1). The picture features Sarah looking straight into the camera, with her mouth slightly open.

Extract 2 What would Sarah say (O, L, E = Olivia, Laura, Eva, nurses; G = OIVA guide)

```
01    G:    no jos tos ois nyt (0.9) puhekupla (0.9)
            well if there was now a (0.9) speech bubble (0.9)
02          (nii) mitähän Saara (.) sanois?
            (then) what would Sarah (.) say?
03          (2.0)
04    O:    (£kohta aloitetaan)   syömi  [s:tä      ]
            (£soon we'll start)eat:       [ing       ]
05    G:                                 [*mm*      ]
06          (0.3)
07    L:    £(että) ↑jaahas, mitäs ruokaa
            £(that) ↑well, what food do we have
08          tääl(hehe       [he)£
            here(hehe[he)£
09    E:                    ([*↑nii, ruokaa*)
                            ([*↑yeah, food*)
10          (0.4)
11    G:    *että* @alampa syödä.@= ((imitoi)) ((ojentaa kätensä))
            *like* @I'll start eating.@= ((imitates)) ((reaches her
            hand))
12    L:    =nii (hehehhe)
            =yeah (hehehhe)
```

The guide's question is hypothetical (Peräkylä, 1995) and contains a speech bubble metaphor; the caregivers are asked to add a speech bubble to the still picture of Sarah visible on the screen. Because Sarah is looking straight into the camera with her mouth slightly open, it is easy to think that she is either saying something or is about to say something. With this metaphor, the guide invites the staff to engage in comparing Sarah's embodied interaction practices with the verbal initiatives of speakers with preserved spoken language. Thus, the speech bubble metaphor is closely related to how the guide defines the overall question related to the video as identified by the guide in Extract 1 – that is, to investigate how the interaction unfolds when one participant is a resident with very little preserved language production. Learning to identify the resident's subtle, embodied initiatives has a central role in this process.

The guide's question is followed by responses from several staff members. Both Laura (line 7) and Eva (line 9) respond and laugh, which might be a sign of mutual agreement on finding words for the resident's embodied activity. In her response in line 11, the guide rephrases the staff members' previous contributions. The falling prosody in line 11, in combination with the gesture with which the guide imitates Sarah's manner of handling the spoon, indicates that her response is a confirmation of the caregivers' previous utterances.

The use of the speech bubble metaphor is a recurring pattern in our data set and apparently has the function of normalizing the interaction of the person with little spoken language and facilitating the staff members' capacity to interpret the resident's initiatives as meaningful actions. In addition, the metaphor apparently has the function of assigning motives or actions to participants. This metaphor is used to encourage the group to engage in a guessing activity regarding what is going on in a participant's head. The speech bubble metaphor also expands the everyday understanding of communication as primarily based on spoken language. The metaphor underlines the meaning of nonverbal communication seen in the video as an important part of "talking."

14.3.2.2 Hypothetical Questions
Another guidance practice used to initiate reflection is hypothetical questions, with which the guide introduces the topic of successful professional practices already in use. Before Extract 3, the guide asked the staff members how they made the interpretation that Sarah was having problems with the food because it was too warm. The caregivers explained how they analyzed Sarah's embodied practices to make this interpretation. In response, the guide states that the caregivers are proficient in interpreting Sarah's embodied behavior because of their familiarity with Sarah. In her hypothetical question in lines 1–2, the guide asks the staff members how they would make this tacit knowledge explicit to a new member of the professional community.

Extract 3 If I came to work for you (A, E, O = Annika, Eva, Olivia, nurses; G = OIVA guide)
```
01    G:    (hh) miten te tota (0.5) nyt jos mä tulisin teille töihin
            (hh) how would you like (0.5) now if I came to work for you
02          nii miten te tän mulle selittäsitte ((katselee ympärilleen))
            then how would you explain this to me ((looks around))
03          (4.0)
04    E:    (*mitenkö*)
            (*how*)
05          (0.2)
06    A:    *j(h)aa:*
            *let's s(h)ee:*
07          (0.3)
08    G:    (£hhheh [heh£)
09    E:            [((hh heh))=
10    O:    =(kyllä    [Saara       ] [sitten)      [((heh heh))
            =(I'm sure [Sarah       ] [will then)   [((heh heh))
11    E:                                [(£-aa-)£   ]
```

```
12   G:                  [((    heh[heh     )
13   E:                          [((hehee))
14   A:              [£odotetaan
                [£we'd probably wait
15           että ite huomaat tän as(h)ian£ ((heh))
                for you to notice th(h)is by yourself£ ((heh))
```

Extract 3 contains various signs of the difficulties the staff members perceive in answering the guide's hypothetical question. For example, the long pause in line 3 indicates that nobody immediately finds an answer. After the long pause, there are various pauses and tentative reactions (lines 4–9) produced with a laugh. When Olivia finally produces a more elaborated response (line 10), it is done in a joking manner and is accompanied by laughter. The other staff members produce additional laughter particles, and Annika's utterance in lines 14–15 is a more explicit elaboration of Olivia's response (line 10); she confirms that probably nobody would think of informing a new staff member about Sarah's embodied practices.

Three caregivers out of five respond to the guide's hypothetical question in a joking manner. The use of jokes and laughter seemingly indicates that the question initiated a perspective the group was previously unfamiliar with. Further, the responses carry a tone of slight embarrassment. It is worth noting that this session was the third meeting out of five in the process, as mentioned above, and the group and the guide had already established a safe relationship. The guide would not necessarily have challenged the group in this manner in the beginning of the process. The guide's hypothetical question apparently has the function of promoting verbalization of the staff members' silent knowledge about Sarah, but the staff members are unable to provide an explanation of Sarah's behavior. Thus, Extract 3 demonstrates a common pattern in the data: the guide uses various practices to promote staff members' reflections about their silent knowledge, and the staff members have difficulty coming up with answers. During the analyzed conversation, however, there is a change, which is illustrated in this chapter.

14.3.2.3 Formulations
In addition to speech bubble metaphors and hypothetical questions, the guide uses formulations as a guidance tool during the video analysis, which is illustrated in Extract 4. Formulations are a well-investigated phenomenon in the literature on institutional interaction (Heritage & Watson, 1979; Davis, 1986; Buttny, 1996; Hak & te Boer, 1996; Vehviläinen, 2003; Weiste & Peräkylä, 2013). They are defined as paraphrases of some prior statement that preserve relevant features of the prior utterance while also recasting it and are usually connected to the institutional agenda represented by the professional. This is also the case in our data, where the professional uses formulations to highlight certain aspects of the foregoing conversation, usually related to either

the preserved skills of the individual with dementia (as in Extract 4) or the role of the professional community in supporting the person with dementia in interactions.

Extract 4 Sarah has many skills left (A, L, O = Annika, Laura, Olivia, nurses; G = OIVA guide)

```
01   O:   ja minusta vielä (s-) (se sai selville mitä Annika tahtoo)
          and I think (-) (she made out what Annika wants)
02        sit sehän kiinnostuu mitä siellä tapahtuu
          then she gets interested in what's happening there
03        (tästä sai selvää mutta) mitä
          (this she made sense of but) what
04        siell           [on ((naurahtaa))
          what's          the[re ((laughs))
05   L:                   [nii.
                          [yeah.
06             (0.3)
07   G:   nii et Saaralla on itse asias aika paljon taitoja (.)
          so Sarah has in fact many skills (.)
08        jä[ljellä]
          le[ft    ]
09   O:     [mm    ]
10   L:     [mm    ]
11   A:   nii
          yeah
```

The staff members have been discussing Sarah's interactional behavior. The guide's formulation (lines 7–8) initiates a change; the staff members' perceptions of the interactional features change into a statement of the preserved skills of the resident with dementia. That a change from more specific observations of Sarah's embodied interactional practices to a more general statement is taking place is signaled by the linguistic features of the contributions. In lines 1–5, the nurses are referring to how Sarah responded to Annika's initiatives in the video clip they watched, but the guide's formulation (lines 7–8) indicates a general truth about Sarah's skills. This is the first time the notion of Sarah's skills is initiated in the conversation, so the formulation does not exactly highlight an aspect of the previous conversation but instead for the first time reveals new aspects of the resident with dementia as a person with various preserved skills. Thus, the formulation directs the group toward a new perspective of the person with dementia. The formulation is followed by various responses (lines 9–11), in which nurses Olivia, Laura, and Annika demonstrate agreement with the statement proposed in the guide's formulation. However, it is worth noting that both Olivia and Laura (lines 9 and 10) respond with the semantically neutral particle *mm*, which can be considered a rather weak indication of agreement. However, at the end of the conversation (not shown in the extract) nurse Olivia notes that Sarah is in constant interaction with her environment, even though she does not take the initiative in interacting. In this statement, Olivia uses the word *skill* to describe Sarah's ability to participate in interaction. Thus, the formulation used in Extract 4 apparently had an impact on the professional caregivers' view of Sarah in the later phases of the conversation.

14.4 The Mealtime as a Social Occasion

Section 14.3 illustrated how the guide uses certain practices during the video analysis to invite and draw the staff toward a focus on embodied interaction instead of task orientation. The following account demonstrates how the analysis of embodied behavior is transferred to a multifaceted, interaction-focused view on the mealtime situation.

Extract 5 is preceded by a hypothetical question posed by the guide in which she asked the caregivers how they think Sarah would have felt if nobody had responded to her initiatives. The staff members responded to the guide's question in two different ways. Whereas several caregivers answered that the lack of response probably would have no impact on Sarah, others considered the caregivers' uptake as significant for Sarah's well-being. In response, the guide showed the video clip again and asked the staff members to discuss how they think Sarah felt in the interaction using the hypothetical expression *if you were Sarah* (line 1). Thus, this utterance seems to have the function of facilitating empathy with Sarah and her needs. Olivia (line 3) provides a rather general response, indicating that Sarah enjoys having company when she is eating. Olivia's response is followed by two long pauses (lines 5, 7) and the guide's minimal response tokens (lines 6, 8). This indicates that Olivia's response is treated as insufficient, and the guide is expecting more responses from the staff members. At this point, nurse Laura explicitly states (lines 9–10) that having lunch not only provides nutrition but also social stimulation for Sarah.

Extract 5 More than eating (L, O, E = Laura, Olivia, Eva, nurses; G = OIVA guide)

```
01   G:   jos te oisitte ite Saarana ((katselee ympärilleen))
          If you were Sarah ((looks around))
02        (3.0)
03   O:   [(see on mukava olo hänellä ja semmonen et joku on mukana)
          [(she is feeling comfortable and that someone is with her)
04   G:   [(- -)
05        (2.4)
06   G:   mm
07        (4.4)
08   G:   [[m ((katsoo Lauraa ja nyökkää))
          [[m ((looks at Laura and nods))
09   L:   [[se tuo on niiku Saaralle enemmän kuin syömistä vaan et
          [[it's like more than eating for Sarah
```

```
10            et   [se on nii        ] ku semmonen sosiaalinen tilanne
                   it's[it's li      ]ke a social situation
11      O:         [(-joo)     ]
                   [(-yes)     ]
12      L:         [et se      ] haluaa et me ollaan (niiku tässä näin)
                   [that she   ] wants us to be (here like this)
13      E:         [nii        ]
                   [yes        ]
14                 (2.6)
15      G:         (.h) niin itseasias varmaan on
                   (.h) in fact I guess that's the case
16      O:         mm
```

Laura formulates a new view of the mealtime as a social occasion for Sarah (line 10) and that Sarah enjoys the company of others at the lunch table (line 12). Laura's responses are topically related to Olivia's previous response (line 3), but she gives more detail. Olivia (line 11) and Eva (line 13) respond to Laura by agreeing using minimal acknowledgment tokens (lines 13, 15). The guide confirms Laura's statement (line 15) by saying *in fact I guess that's the case*. Her confirmation seems to claim epistemic authority (Heritage & Raymond, 2005) and thus upgrades Laura's prior statement. It is important to note that several of the other participants confirm Laura's formulation. This shows the first stage in a process where the idea about mealtimes as social occasions turns into "common property", that is something the group agrees on. Extract 6 illustrates how this process continues; Laura's utterance about mealtimes as social events is soon followed by a similar statement by Eva (line 1).

Extract 6 More than feeding (A, E = Laura, Annika, Eva, nurses; G = OIVA guide)

```
01      E:     se on enemmän kuin syöttäminen se tilanne
               that situation is more than feeding
02      G:     joo
               yes
03      E:     se o:n niiku tämmönen     s[osiaalinen kanssakäyminen
               it i:s like a kind of s[ocial interaction
04      A:                               [((clears throat))
05             (0.3)
06      G:     joo
               yes
```

In contrast to Laura, who defined the situation as being *more than eating* (Extract 5, line 1 -> 9), Eva focuses on the action of the caregiver; she defines the situation as being more than *feeding* (line 1). Rather than speaking about how the resident perceives the situation, she highlights the relationship between the resident and the caregiver; the caregiver is described as not only feeding the resident but also as engaging in a social interaction with her (line 3). Eva also

14 "It's More than Eating, It's a Social Situation"

implicitly states that the situation on the video is not only feeding but a social situation that can be enjoyed by both the resident and the caregiver.

In Extracts 5 and 6, two different caregivers provide elaborate formulations of mealtimes as opportunities for social interaction with Sarah. Thus, we can see the group of professional caregivers moving toward a collective understanding of meals as occasions of great social importance. The discussion continues for a while, with a focus on how Sarah engages in interaction with her co-residents at mealtimes. Finally, the discussion is summarized by the guide (Extract 7, lines 1–3).

Extract 7 More than a meal (L, E = Laura, Eva, nurses; G = OIVA guide)

```
01 G:  nii jos aattelee sitä just että tää on
       yes if one thinks about that that this is
02     niinkun tilanteena (.) niinku te sanoitte et tää on
       as a situation (.) like you said that this is
03     enemmän   kuin   ruokailu[tilanne
       more than   a     meal [time
04 E:                           [niin on niin[on ehdottomasti
                                [yes that's  [definitely right
05 L:                                        [mm
```

The guide connects her summary to the previous discussion by using the formulation *like you said* and by rephrasing the gist of the previous discussion of the situation on the video being *more than a mealtime* (line 3), which is strongly confirmed by nurse Eva. Epistemics seem to play an important role here; because the guide referred to the staff members as the source of the idea of eating as social interaction ("like you said", line 2), this may have encouraged Eva to take a strong epistemic position. At this point, the importance of this thought has been established and highlighted. This is additionally confirmed in the closing phase of the conversation, where Laura, who has been acting as a secretary, sums up the central points (lines 1–3) discussed during the video analysis.

Extract 8 Social situation (L = Laura, nurse; G = OIVA guide)

```
01 L:  sit mä laitoin viel >tos et< (.) ku ruokailutilanne on
       then I wrote >there< (.) that mealtime is
02     Saaralle tämmönen s-sosiaalinen tilanne (.)
       a s- social situation for Sarah (.)
03     *ainakin nyt tässä ihan selkeesti*
       *at least here very clearly*
04     (2.0)
05 G:  joo
       yeah
```

The notion of the mealtime as a social event for Sarah thus gets the status of being in the secretary's written summary of the discussion of the video clip.

The summary of Laura's notes is followed by a phase in which the staff members and the guide negotiate the so-called concrete act, that is what they will change in their interaction with Sarah based on their previous discussion. As their concrete act, the staff members decided to add a social aspect to mealtime situations involving Sarah. The concrete act, as formulated by the guide, is the following:

(9) The concrete act as decided upon in the guidance meeting January 23, 2012
    Every day the meals start with quality time: The caregiver
    - sits down next to Sarah
    - observes her gaze, facial expressions, gestures, use of voice, presence, and actions
    - responds to her messages by talking and using facial expressions, gestures, and actions
    - has a small conversation with Sarah
    - helps her to begin eating her meal

Thus we can see how the caregiving task of helping Sarah to start her meal is combined with verbal and embodied interaction. The social aspects of the mealtime discussed by the group are in the concrete act transferred into detailed aspects of interaction. The general notion of mealtimes as social events is transferred into concrete interactional details, initiating verbal language, and paying attention to the resident's sometimes subtle messages.

14.5 Excursus: Successful Interaction as the Caregivers' Achievement

In Section 14.4 we saw during the video analysis phase how the group moved toward the analysis of embodied behavior and then toward a more interaction-oriented understanding of a mealtime situation. As an excursus, we want to compare how the group assessed the interaction video in the opening phase of the consultation (as outlined in Extract 1) and how the video is described in the closing phase of the guidance session. Several staff members (Annika, Laura, and Eva) participate in summarizing the interaction on the video.

Extract 9 It was a success (A, L, E = Annika, Laura, Eva, nurses; G = OIVA guide)

```
01 A:  se: onnistu hyvin
       i:t was a success
02     (0.4)
03 G:  [joo
       [yeah
```

```
04  L:  [mm mä sanoin [heti sen jälkeen et tää oli
        [mm I said    [straight after that this was
05  G:                [mm
                      [mm
06  L:  [iha:na täs oli niku ihan selkee(*tämmönevuorovaikutus*)=
        [won:derful had like a really clear (*sort of interaction*)=
07  G:  [.nii
        [yeah
08  E:  =(nii oliha meillä  [se toinenki video)  ]
        =(yeah we had       [that other video too)]
09  L:                      [(et <aivan>         iha]na)
                            [(so like <just> wonde]rful)
10      (.)
11  L:  ↑ni[i (-)
        ↑ye[ah (-)
12  E:     [(joka onnistu tosi hyvin)
           [(that turned out good very good)
13      (.)
14  G:  *te o-*   [↑te [ootte nii hyvii↑
        *you a-*  [↑you['re so talented↑
```

Annika's general evaluation, *it was a success* (line 1), is followed by an assessment by Laura (lines 4, 6) of the interaction in the video discussed during the guidance meeting. It is worth comparing Laura's evaluation with her assessment produced in the opening phase of the guidance meeting (Extract 1, lines 18−26). In both cases, Laura makes positive evaluations, but her focus has moved from the participant with complex needs, who initially was described as seeking interaction and having some preserved skills, to the interaction situation as a whole, which is assessed as *wonderful* and having *clear interaction* (line 6). In addition, Eva makes a reference to another video (line 8), which is also described as successful (line 12). At this point, the guide draws a more general conclusion, as she states "you're so talented" (line 14). In this conclusion, she relates the occurrence of successful interaction situations to the overall competence of, and especially the good practices of caregiving used by, the staff members seen in the video. This apparently aims at empowering the staff members and making them aware of their own role as participants in interaction involving participants with complex communication needs.

The change in focus from the skills of the individual to the interaction as a mutual achievement can be compared with the conversation analytic way of regarding interaction as a collective production in which meaning is co-constructed in co-operation between conversationalists through dynamic processes. This change in view provides the guide with the opportunity to relate the successful interaction situations to the professional community; she utilizes the references to various successful situations to empower the professional caregivers and make them aware of their interaction skills.

14.6 Discussion

The goal of this study was to demonstrate how the staff members' view of a mealtime situation and their professional vision changes during one session of video guidance. In the opening phase of the session there was a discrepancy between how various staff members explained the choice of the eating situation to be discussed in the guidance session. Whereas one staff member described the interest in the eating situation as originating from the challenges related to the eating as a caregiving task, others took the communication with a resident with very little preserved spoken language as their point of departure, treating the mealtime merely as an illustration of an opportunity to interact with a resident who does not use speech. In the phase of video analysis, the initial multifaceted perspective involving aspects of both task orientation and interaction orientation is transformed into a focus on embodied practices. Through various guidance practices, such as hypothetical questions and reformulations of the caregivers' prior contributions, the guide directs the focus toward the embodied behavior of the participants in the interaction video. The guide's practices work to create a parallel between the embodied behavior of Sarah and the spoken language used by people for whom this channel is still intact and to make the caregivers aware of their capacity to respond to Sarah's often subtle communication attempts. Thus, the video analysis creates awareness of both Sarah's ability to communicate through embodied practices and the professional community's tacit knowledge of their clients.

As a result of the guide's work, the professional community changes its way of viewing the mealtime. The changes indicate that more diverse perspectives become accessible in addition to the original views of the professional community. As the guidance session proceeds, the caregivers advance from perceiving the mealtime as a caregiving task and a showcase for the individual resident's communication abilities to defining it as a social occasion. The group's reflection upon the mealtime as a social situation takes the resident's perspective as its point of departure; we can see the group adapting the position of the resident in the manner outlined by the guide's so-called speech bubble metaphors during the video analysis. In addition, the speech bubble metaphor reveals and expands the view of nonverbal/embodied communication as a way of talking despite the lack of speech. The significance of mealtimes as social opportunities is addressed with regard to both the professional caregivers and the co-residents, and the discussion results in concrete measures with the aim of strengthening the social dimension of Sarah's meals. Speaking within the framework of person-centered care, the altered view on mealtimes might decrease the risk of objectifying the client during mealtimes (see Reimer, 2012).

As described above, the professional caregivers in our study altered their vision toward viewing interaction as an integrated part of routine caregiving tasks. Previous findings have reported that interventions around everyday tasks of caregiving had positive effects on communication outcomes: "Care staff can improve their communication with residents with dementia when strategies are embedded in daily care activities" (Vasse et al., 2010: 199). For a successful outcome of interaction, it is critical that communication and daily care are treated as intertwined processes. There is a need to rethink the foundations of dementia care, outlined by Ward et al. (2008), as an area of current importance. Even if the biomedical model of dementia has been challenged by the person-centered framework for the last 20 years, there is still a need to re-evaluate the significance of communication for high-quality dementia care. Therefore, we need to think of *communication as care* (Wilkinson et al., 2014) and to consider communication both as work and as an important element of care.

What, then, can be achieved by a more interaction-oriented manner of accomplishing routine caregiving tasks? The well-being and dignity of residents with dementia is, of course, a central objective. Communication is key for the development and improvement of dementia care (Ward et al., 2008), and an interaction-oriented view on daily caregiving improves residents' opportunities to participate and to be heard in interaction, despite their impaired language skills. There is, however, another aspect to this question. In their influential study on job crafting, Wrzesniewski & Dutton (2001) discussed how changing the quality and amount of interaction with others in a job had a positive effect on their job satisfaction. In line with this finding, learning to see work as something more than a daily sequence of tasks (Ward et al., 2008) may provide a remedy for the frequent lack of job satisfaction in dementia care (Vernoij-Dassen et al., 2009). This topic is of relevance for further research in the field of dementia care.

References

Amella, E. J. (1999) 'Factors influencing the proportion of food consumed by nursing home residents.' *Journal of the American Geriatric Society*, 47(7): 879–885.

Berg, G. (2006) *The Importance of Food and Mealtimes in Dementia Care: The Table Is Set.* London and Philadelphia: Jessica Kingsley Publishers.

Brooker, D. (2007) *Person-Centred Dementia Care. Making Services Better.* London: Jessica Kingsley Publishers.

Burakoff, K. and Martkianen, K. (2015) 'OIVA – supporting staff for better interaction with people with complex communication needs.' In H. Kennedy, M. Landor and L. Todd (eds.) *Video Enhanced Reflective Practice. Professional Development through Attuned Interaction.* London: Jessica Kingsley Publishers, pp. 136–146.

Buttny, R. (1996) 'Clients' and therapist's joint construction of the clients' problems.' *Research on Language and Social Interaction*, 29(2): 125–153.

Davis, K. (1986) 'The process of problem (re)formulation in psychotherapy.' *Sociology of Health & Illness*, 8(1): 44–74.

Degenholtz, H., Rosen, J. Castle N., Mittal V. and Liu, D. (2008) 'The association between changes in health status and nursing home resident quality of life.' *The Gerontologist*, 48(5): 584–592.

Fukkink, R. G. (2008) 'Video feedback in widescreen: A meta-analysis of family programs.' *Clinical Psychology Review*, 28(6): 904–916.

Goodwin, C. (1994) 'Professional vision.' *American Anthropologist*, 96(3): 606–633.

Hak, T. and te Boer, F. (1996) 'Formulations in first encounters.' *Journal of Pragmatics*, 25(1): 83–99.

Heritage, J. and Raymond, G. (2005) 'The terms of agreement: Indexing epistemic authority and subordination in talk-in interaction.' *Social Psychology Quarterly*, 68(1): 15–38.

Heritage, J. and Watson, R. (1979) 'Formulations as conversational objects.' In G. Psathas (ed.) *Everyday Language: Studies in Ethnomethodology*. New York: Irvington Press, pp. 123–162.

Kane, R. A., Kling K. C., Bershadsky B., et al. (2003) 'Quality of life measures for nursing home residents.' *Journal of Gerontology*, 58A: 240–248.

Kitwood, T. (1997) *Dementia Reconsidered: The Person Comes First*. Buckingham: Open University Press.

Koski, K., Martikainen, K., Burakoff, K. and Launonen, K. (2010) 'Staff members' understandings about communication with individuals who have multiple learning disabilities: A case of Finnish OIVA communication training.' *Journal of Intellectual and Developmental Disability*, 35(4): 279–289.

Lave, J. and Wenger, E. (1991) *Situated Learning. Legitimate Peripheral Participation*. Cambridge: University of Cambridge Press.

Mittal, V., Rosen, J., Govind R., Degenholtz, et al. (2007) 'Perception gap in quality of life ratings: An empirical investigation of nursing home residents and caregivers.' *The Gerontologist*, 47(2): 159–168.

Peräkylä, A. (1995) *AIDS Counselling: Institutional Interaction and Clinical Practice*. Cambridge: Cambridge University Press.

Pilnick, A. and James, D. (2013) '"I'm thrilled that you see that": Guiding parents to see success in interactions with children with deafness and autism spectrum disorder.' *Social Science & Medicine*, 99: 89–101.

Reimer, H. D. (2012) *Providing Person-Centred Mealtime Care for Long Term Care Residents with Dementia*. Unpublished thesis in Family Relations and Applied Nutrition. Ontario, Canada: University of Guelph. https://atrium.lib.uoguelph.ca/items/4d0d4564-9972-4577-9d30-de2fe1748fae.

Reimer, H. D. and Keller, H. H. (2009) 'Mealtimes in nursing homes: Striving for person-centered care.' *Journal of Nutrition for the Elderly*, 28(4): 327–347.

Robinson, G. and Gallagher, A. (2008) 'Culture change impacts quality of life for nursing home residents.' *Topics in Clinical Nutrition*, 23(2): 120–130.

Sacks, H. Schegloff, E. A. and Jefferson, G. (1974) 'A simplest systematics for the organization of turn-taking for conversation.' *Language*, 4(1): 696–735.

Schegloff, E. A. (2007) *Sequence Organization in Interaction: A Primer in Conversation Analysis*. Volume 1. Cambridge: Cambridge University Press.

Vasse, E., Vernooij-Dassen, M., Spijker, A., Rikkert, M.O. and Koopmans, R. (2010) 'A systematic review of communication strategies for people with dementia in residential and nursing homes.' *International Psychogeriatrics*, 22(2): 189–200.

Vehviläinen, S. (2003) 'Preparing and delivering interpretations in psychoanalytic interaction.' *Text*, 23(4): 573–606.

Venturato, L. (2010) 'Dignity, dining and dialogue: Reviewing the literature on quality of life for people with dementia.' *International Journal of Older People Nursing*, 5: 228–234.

Verbeek, H., Meyer, G., Leino-Kilpi, H., et al. (2012) 'A European study investigating patterns of transition from home care towards institutional dementia care: The protocol of a RightTimePlaceCare study.' *BMC Public Health*, 12: 68.

Vernoij-Dassen, M., Faber, M. J., Olde Rikkert, M. G., et al. (2009) 'Dementia care and labour market: The role of job satisfaction.' *Aging & Mental Health*, 13(3): 383–390.

Ward, R., Vass, A. A., Aggarwal, N., Garfield, C. and Cybyk, B. (2008) 'A different story: Exploring patterns of communication in residential dementia care.' *Ageing and Society*, 28(5): 629–651.

Weiste, E. and Peräkylä, A. (2013) 'A comparative conversation analytic study of formulations in psychoanalysis and cognitive psychotherapy.' *Research on Language and Social Interaction*, 46(4): 299–321.

Wilkinson, E., Randhawa, G., Brown, E. A., et al. (2014) 'Communication as care at end of life: an emerging issue from an exploratory action research study of renal end-of-life care for ethnic minorities in the UK.' *Journal of Renal Care*, 40(Suppl. 1): 23–29.

Wrzesniewski, A. and Dutton, D. E. (2001) 'Crafting a job: Revisioning employees as active crafters of their work.' *The Academy of Management Review*, 26(2): 179–201.

15 Social Quizzes for People Living with Dementia
How Enactment Impacts Interaction

*Joe Webb**

15.1 Introduction

Support offered to people living with dementia is often done in group settings. In these groups, activities such as quizzes are often played and/or promoted as good practice (for example, see Swan, 2004; Light & Delves, 2011; Graty, 2013). Given that dementia is likely to affect memory and communication, it is easy to see why such an activity could have positive effects in encouraging/supporting use of recall but may also carry with it inherent difficulties for the players. For example, previous conversation analysis research has outlined difficulties people with dementia may have in responding to certain types of question formulation (Jones et al., 2016; Williams et al., 2019). Despite the prevalence of 'social quizzes' for people with dementia, there has been little research focusing on the interactional enactment of such activities (see Lindholm & Wray, 2011; Webb et al., 2020 for exceptions). The term 'enactment' is used throughout this chapter to refer to the different ways quizzes are organized in practice. For example, how players are seated, how players are selected (or are able to self-select) to talk, and how the design of the initiating question can impact the subsequent interaction (i.e., questions with one possible answer or questions with multiple possible answers).

Quizzes are based on the activity of answering questions, often relying on memory and recall. Jones et al. (2020) have shown how the delivery and variation of question design within medical assessments affects how people living with dementia may respond. In that research, the focus was on a test (Addenbrooke's Cognitive Examination) to help inform dementia diagnoses. Despite the aim and function of social quizzes and dementia diagnosis tests being vastly different, both can entail a person without dementia asking a person living with dementia questions which rely on memory, recall and functional cognition to answer. The work of Jones et al. (2020; Chapter 2 this

---

* This research was part of a large grant, 'Tackling Disabling Practices: Co-production and Change', funded by the Economic and Social Research Council (ESRC) ES/M008339/1, led by Val Williams. Thank you to Val for her thoughts and feedback on this chapter and for being such a wonderful person to work with. Thanks to all staff and people living with dementia who allowed me to learn more about them and their lives. It was a privilege.

volume) brings into sharp focus the need to examine turn design and understand the interactional context in which these activities are built. 'Quizzes' are often treated in the literature as a uniform activity. This chapter explores the interactional enactment of quizzes and seeks to outline the variability in quiz enactment, demonstrating the interactional (and social) consequences for those involved, specifically regarding the degree of institutionality and possible threats to the 'face' of the players.

15.1.1 Epistemics, Deontics and Face Work in Quizzes

Questions typically occur in initiating position, and often mark the institutional rights of the speaker; as Hayano (2012, p. 395) comments, 'questions are a powerful tool to control interaction: they pressure recipients for a response, impose presuppositions, agendas and preferences', and their occurrence make an answer conditionally relevant (Schegloff & Sacks, 1973). Many institutional practices are constructed by question–response sequences (see Jones et al., Chapter 2 this volume). Questions also shed light on how epistemic issues are managed in interaction. In many situations, a question may mark the speaker's lack of knowledge on a subject (or K- stance: see Heritage, 2012) whereby they treat the questionee as being more knowledgeable (or K+) about the matter at hand. However, there are certain institutional situations, such as quizzes, in which the questioner asks 'known answer questions' (Schegloff, 2007), typically forming a three-part sequence: test question and response, with the third turn evaluating whether the question has been answered correctly. Quizzes are thus an epistemic activity and may reveal the epistemic status of participants in relation to the question. For example, an answer may be deemed to be correct by the questioner or may reveal a K- stance from the questionee (e.g., 'I don't know the answer to that one').

Questions can also play a deontic function in interaction, as they are a public way of initiating a new sequence and action (see Svennevig & Stevanovic, 2015). Quizzes are both an epistemic activity, testing players' memories and ability to recall, and a deontic activity, in which a quiz master directs the course of action. It is unsurprising that managing and saving 'face' may be entangled in these deontic and epistemic dimensions.

'Face work' is central to the organization of social interaction, motivated by the individual's desire for face preservation/restoration (Goffman, 1967), and all interactions carry the risk of face threatening acts (Brown & Levinson, 1987). I take the view that 'face' is 'the relationship two or more persons create with one another in interaction' (Arundale, 2010, p. 2078) and is an emergent phenomenon, negotiated between participants in interaction. I build on face work while focusing on the different ways quizzes are enacted, and the consequences these different iterations have for staff and players alike.

Epistemic and deontic dimensions (see Heritage, 2012; Stevanovic & Peräkylä, 2012) may occasion threats to face during quizzes. Asking a quiz question puts the player under a degree of pressure and carries a threat to face. Potentially being unable to answer or giving an incorrect answer brings face work to the interactional fore (the epistemic domain). Being able to answer the question correctly can be seen as fulfilling the 'positive face wants' of affirmation and acceptance (Brown & Levinson, 1987). Additionally, asking a question imposes an implied future course of action on players and implies a primary right to direct action (the deontic domain: see Stevanovic & Peräkylä, 2012). Should players resist playing the game or answering the question, this could be seen as impacting their negative face wants and desire to remain unimpeded (Brown & Levinson, 1987). I examine these issues below.

15.2 Data and Method

This chapter draws on video data from a corpus of 10 hours of naturally occurring interactions between 28 people living with dementia and staff. It includes 10 quizzes led by staff members, held in 4 settings (2 memory cafes, an activity group and a day centre). The data were collected as part of a larger study about disabling and enabling social practices (Williams et al., 2023) for people with different types of disabilities in different settings. It was not the intention of the project to collect quiz data involving people living with dementia. Rather, the aim was to find out whether Conversation Analysis (CA) of video recordings of natural interactions could be useful in creating change in the practices of support staff and carers. To gather the data, collective spaces for people living with dementia were visited. It happened that in every group that was visited, quizzes were put on by the staff members for the service users.

The study followed a strict protocol approved by the Social Care Research Ethics Committee in the UK to ensure that people assessed as lacking capacity to consent had personal consultees who could advise on their behalf. Each quiz was transcribed according to the detailed conventions common in CA (Jefferson, 1984). All names are anonymized.

CA was used to identify and explore how different ways of enacting quizzes impacted the types of possible interactions within them. I aim specifically to describe how these differing interactional frameworks impact players and their threats to face, and how players and staff alike marshal deontic and epistemic strategies to do the activity of quizzing.

15.3 Findings

As previously mentioned, quiz questions in these institutional contexts can be a way to control interaction (Hayano, 2012): they require a response, and limit the parameters of that response, impose presuppositions and preferences, and can be potentially face-threatening. Unlike ordinary question and answer sequences where the questioner may be uninformed and the questionee is often assumed to be knowledgeable about the matter at hand (Heritage, 1984), in a quiz often the person asking the question already knows the answer (an occurrence which is echoed in the data from Chapter 9 of this volume by Muntigl & Hödl). This can be seen from the evaluative third turn in the sequence organization of quizzes.

Take the following example from a quiz in a day centre. The extract features Richard, a quiz player living with dementia, and S1 and S2 who are both staff members.

Extract 1: RIC=Richard; S1=Staff Member; S2=Staff Member

```
1   S1:    Okay Richard. ((Clears throat)). Okay. What      Question
2          colour (0.2) is a New York taxi.
3          ((Another player says something quietly)))
4          (4.0)
5   RIC:   A mustardy colour                                Answer
6   S2:    Mmnahh yeah that's ↑right                        Evaluation
7   S1:    Well done ↑Ri:chard.
```

We will return to this extract in more detail later. For now, it is enough to note that a news receipt (e.g., 'oh') is appropriately absent in third position and thus instantiates an epistemic hierarchy. The initial third turn component ('yeah') treats the response as 'correct information' (Mehan, 1979), while the following turns ('that's right' and 'well done') praise Richard's achievement in answering correctly. This basic structure tells us that the activity of 'doing a quiz' is an institution that can impose particular roles and restrictions on speakership, and that there is a preference and social value to answering the question correctly. This can be seen most obviously in examples where quiz players answer the question incorrectly, which I will address later in the chapter.

Whilst all quizzes shared the sequence outlined here, no quiz was enacted in quite the same way. Next, I outline the distinct features of these different approaches, and what effect this has on the interactions within the framework imposed by the different quizzes. The chapter ends with some thoughts on how these approaches impact the 'face' of the participants, and relatedly the degree of agency afforded to participants in each quiz variation.

15.3.1 Full Group Quizzes where Players Self-Select to Answer

One approach to implementing a quiz was to treat everyone present as having the potential to answer. These questions were typically posed by a member of staff. In this scenario, seated players with dementia are asked a series of questions *en masse*. The people living with dementia were collected from their homes by minibus and dropped off at an activity group which runs for the day, once a week.

Extract 2 is taken from an activity group for people living with dementia. The group was run in a large social room with chairs and tables in a residential home. The people living with dementia were sitting on three large tables. Most of the attendees had early to mid-stage dementia. There were four staff present and twenty service users. However, as it was close to lunch two staff members left to prepare food, leaving two staff members with a small window of time to fill before lunch. They had some pre-prepared questions that had been printed off from an internet quiz resource. There had been a few questions before Extract 2, and the previous question had led to people talking amongst themselves.

Rianne (staff member) began by announcing they would do a quiz. The people with dementia were asked questions by Rianne, who stood in the middle of the room, and any person could self-select to answer. Although there were twenty service users, only three appear in the extract as the rest were silent: Rianne (staff member), Jim (service user) and Bob (service user).

Extract 2

```
1   RIA:   Now come on then guys what president did Marilyn
2          Monroe sing for?
3          (1.6)
4   BOB:   The Kenne[dys]
5   JIM:            [JF ] K.
6          (0.8)
7   RIA:   John FK yep
```

Lines 1–2 see the staff member make explicit the 'newness' of the upcoming activity by using the discourse marker 'now' to start. The turn initial 'now' functions as a transition marker to introduce a new topic and change the direction of the discourse (Stenström, 1994), in this case that there is a new question sequence being launched. That it is intended for all present to participate (and therefore for any extraneous talk to stop) is underlined by Rianne's use of the plea, 'come on then guys', which reinstates collective action before she asks a question, to which Bob gives a fitted answer in line 4 ('The Kennedys'). Jim then gives a more specific answer in line 5, which is confirmed as correct by the staff member in an evaluative third turn (line 7). It would be typical of a positive evaluation to come immediately after a correct answer, without delay. There is however a 0.8 second gap following the answers (line 6). This is likely to deal with the fact that two answers were given in overlap, the second more accurate than the first. The quiz master therefore has to decide which answer to give a positive evaluation to: the one which came first, which was *somewhat* correct but lacking specificity, or the one that came second but was more accurate. In the end, Rianne's confirmation does not pick out Jim or Bob for praise as is sometimes the case (e.g., 'well done, Janet!'), and therefore manages the potential threat to face of giving a high-grade evaluation to only the second of two answers given by players.

Next we will see another quiz enacted in the same way – where all players are addressed and must self-select if they want to answer the question set by the staff member. However, a correct answer may not be immediately forthcoming. In Extract 3 players are sitting in a semi-circle facing a staff member. In this instance, the quiz takes place in between songs in a music session. After each song, the staff member asks the service users questions related to the song.

Extract 3

```
1    STA:    Who sang that on sta:ge >can you remember<?
2    BOB:    What?
3    STA:    Who sang that so:ng on[the sta ] ge
4    LYN:                          [(person)]
5    RIT:    ↑Oh I
6    LEN:    Oh what a beautiful morning
7    STA:    Howard,
8            (0.5)
9    BAR:    [Ke[el.]
10   TON:    [Ke[el.]
11   SHE:       [Kee]l.=
12   STA:    =↑Keel °yeah
```

In line 1 the staff member (STA on the transcript) poses a quiz question to the group related to the song they have just sung: 'Oh What a Beautiful Morning'. However, he does not name the song in the question, referring to it as 'that'. The staff member explicitly topicalizes memory in the first instance ('>can you remember<?'). Bob initiates an open class repair initiator (Drew, 1997) to which the staff member reformulates the question, including a missing piece of information that it is the song that is the subject of the question, but he again does not name the song (line 3). Lyn and Rita then both make utterances that are not attended to. Lyn's turn overlapping the staff member's seems to acknowledge that the missing piece of information he is asking about is a person (line 4). Len then names the song, but not the person who sang it (line 6). As with the turns by Lyn and Rita, this is not attended to or acknowledged by the staff member. This is in line with the broader trend of large group quizzes in which players' turns which do not progress the overarching activity, or are not in alignment with the question posed, are frequently treated as if they were not spoken (Webb et al., 2020). Instead, the staff member treats the absence of an answer as in need of a prompt ('Howard' on line 7 is the first name of Howard Keel, the correct answer to the question). This turn reveals that the staff member is asking a question that the quiz

participants know the answer to, whilst 'can you remember' in line 1 shows how the staff member frames their knowledge of it as contingent upon their memory. After a gap of 0.5 seconds, three players give the correct answer in overlap (lines 9, 10 and 11), which in turn elicits the staff members' confirmatory third turn (line 12).

As in Extracts 1 and 2, this turn design represents the quiz as a form of institutional interaction, displayed through the way players are given hints (see also Chapter 9 this volume by Muntigl & Hödl), and through the evaluative third turn, which reveal the staff member to be asking a known answer question (Schegloff, 2007). Likewise, turns that do not further the overarching activity of answering correctly (see Webb et al., 2020 for further work on progressivity and quizzes) are not responded to or acknowledged (lines 4, 5 and 6), as in Extract 2. Here we see an interactional structure which shows participants with specific goal orientations tied to institutional identities made present through the talk: quiz master and quiz players (Drew & Heritage, 1992). These involve constraints on what is treated as allowable contributions.

This style of quiz is an efficient way of organizing the interactional space, requiring only one staff member for many players (there were 17 in this case). However, in practice this often meant most of the group members did not say anything. Whilst this allows players agency in joining in, it also means that many players are not guaranteed a turn. A different iteration of the whole group quiz was to ask each player in turn a question, so that each person was assured equal attention. We will explore this in Section 15.3.2.

15.3.2 *Mediated Turn Allocation Quizzes*

Another variation on quiz enactment were quizzes in which players were chosen in order, by name, to answer a quiz question. Other-selection of the next speaker is a feature of multi-party institutional interaction (see e.g. Heritage & Greatbatch, 1989). The turn-taking system can be navigated in such interactions by means of 'mediated turn-allocation procedures' (Heritage & Clayman, 2011), wherein a central authority figure (teacher, chairperson or quiz master in this case) decides who speaks next and allocates them an interactional slot.

Extracts 4a and 4b are taken from a day centre for people living with dementia, in which the service users are playing a different kind of quiz than in Extract 1. Note that here, instead of being asked a general knowledge question, players are asked to provide an answer that meets *two* conditions: a food beginning with the letter R. Here, each player is asked in turn to name something from a category that begins with a letter chosen by the quiz master. The extract features a staff member asking the questions and two players, Julie and Richard.

15 Social Quizzes for People Living with Dementia

Extract 4a
```
1   STA:    Moving on, Rich:ard. Can you think of a
2           food, beginning with R:.
3           (1.8)
4   JUL:    Radish (.) huh huh ↑ha hugh huh
5           (1.7)
6   RIC:    .hh hh #Po↑tatoes
7           (2.0)
8   STA:    Not quite have another go,
```

In line 1 Richard is selected by the staff member to answer a quiz question ('can you think of a food beginning with R'). Julie provides an answer 'out of turn' (line 4) which is not responded to by the staff member. Richard gives an incorrect answer to the question, and this is followed by a silence, a typical feature of a response to a dispreferred turn (Pomerantz, 1984). Following this silence, the staff member confirms the inadequacy of the answer, and instructs the player to 'have another go' (line 8). This is still an evaluative third turn, as 'not quite' effectively evaluates Richard's turn as incorrect. However, it also softens the blow and potentially face-threatening act of indicating a wrong answer (Goffman, 1967). Goffman notes, 'when a person volunteers a statement or message [he] ... places everyone present in jeopardy' (p. 37), thus in this instance it is down to the quiz master to save the player's face (e.g., line 8). For Goffman (1967, pp. 10–11) people are expected 'to go to certain lengths to save the feelings and the face of others present', which could account for the staff member giving Richard a second turn to answer the question (line 8). However, there are clear signs that Richard is unable to produce a relevant response (the delay in lines 2 and 5, and the incorrect answer in line 6). Despite the attempt to save face by responding with 'not quite' instead of an outright 'no', giving Richard a second chance to answer also puts him in a vulnerable and face-threatening position when the prior sequence suggests he is struggling to answer.

It is worth reflecting on the response to an incorrect answer in this extract compared with the response to a correct answer, as seen in Extract 1 (see Jones, Chapter 12 in this volume for responses to incorrect answers). This can be seen most notably in the silence that follows an incorrect answer (line 7, Extract 4a), as well as the staff member giving the quiz player with dementia another turn, demonstrating a social preference for a correct answer to be given. This is in contrast to the positive evaluative third turn, delivered without hesitation after a correct answer (line 7, Extract 1). In these ways, we can see the central features of preferred and dispreferred responses to quiz questions (Pomerantz, 1984).

Having noted these differences in response to correct and incorrect answers, and therefore a marked preference for correct answers, we return to Extract 4b, which gives the full transcript of this interaction. Extract 4b also features other quiz players living with dementia: Julie, Jennifer and Tim.

Extract 4b (continued)
```
1    STA:   Moving on, Rich:ard. Can you think of a
2           food, beginning with R:.
3           (1.8)
4    JUL:   Radish (.) huh huh ↑ha hugh huh
5           (1.7)
6    RIC:   .hh hh #Po↑tatoes
7           (2)
8    STA:   Not quite have a[nother go,]
9    JEN:                   [  (    )  ]
10   TIM:   h↑mm #rump steak
11   STA:   Food beginning with R::
12          ((S draws an R in the air with his finger))
13   RIC:   Oh ↑sorry[huh huh huh huh huh]
14   STA:            [That's alright car]ry on?,
15   JUL:   O:hh[me back]
16   ?          [(     )]
17          (8)
18   ?      O:h ↑woo ↑woo ↑↑woo
19          (2.1)
20   ?      ((clears throat))
21          (2.2)
22   TIM:   Come ##o:n
23   RIC:   [ehuh huh huh] [huh huh] huh
24   TIM:   [Huh huh     ] [rice   ]
25   JUL:   Huh huh huh
26          (0.6)
27   RIC:   No=
28   STA:   =No? Okay th:en let's move on to ↑Sa::l
```

Immediately after the staff member pursues a response from Richard, another participant produces a 'correct' answer (line 10) that is again ignored (as in line 4). Here, as in many other examples in our data, non-sanctioned turns taken outside allocated turns are ignored as if they were not spoken. This is perhaps not surprising, as to acknowledge the correctness of the answer would potentially mean invalidating the turn of the selected speaker, as well as encouraging (or implicitly sanctioning) self-selection in a mediated turn allocated speech system. This sequential deletion of 'out of turn' answers corresponds to Drew and Heritage's (1992) argument that institutional interactions are distinctive because they often involve participants with specific goal orientations which are tied to their institutional identities (i.e., quiz master and quiz player/staff member and service user), and they normally involve constraints on what will be treated as allowable contributions. These 'out of turn' correct answers in this extract could of course be understood as working to help Richard, who is not able to answer. However, Richard does not treat them as such and does not repeat or use one of the multiple correct answers as his own. Perhaps because as others have self-selected to answer, the answers are no longer 'available' for Richard.

The staff member once more reformulates the question and gives Richard another turn; the conditions of the question are reiterated (line 11), removing all linguistic packaging ('food beginning with R::') to aid comprehension of the task by 'deleting' an already articulated element (Schegloff, 2013). Richard's 'oh' prefaced turn on line 13 seems to acknowledge the new information (Heritage, 1984). The placement of laughter matters, in this case, as it comes after an apology and apparent recognition of a misunderstanding or mishearing that the answer should begin with R (line 13). This could also indicate a recognition of having transgressed by answering incorrectly. It is noteworthy here that Richard laughs alone; his laughter is not reciprocated or treated as an invitation to laugh. As Sacks (1992, p. 571) notes, when one interlocutor laughs and the other does not, perhaps they are committing a violation. Here, the violation is of an intersubjective nature; Richard either did not hear or did not understand the quiz master's instructions. The staff member's lack of laughter in response aligns to the delicacy of the situation. To laugh in response to Richard could be construed as laughing at Richard, and risks producing a face-threatening action, even if occasioned by Richard himself (Haakana, 2001).

Richard's long silence (lines 14–23) shows that answering the question remains difficult. Richard sits motionless for 15 seconds, in which time the silence is punctuated by an off-topic interjection from Julie (line 15). Silences in response to questions are normatively treated as accountable (Sacks et al., 1974). This may explain Tim's utterance ('come on'), which is hearable as a rebuke for Richard holding up the game. This elicits Richard's laughter particles in response (line 23), which can be seen as managing his inability to supply an appropriate response, and how that might seem to his interlocutors. Again, Richard laughs alone to deal with a delicate interactional slot (Haakana, 2001), this time after an admonishment highlighting a perceived transgression; Richard has taken too long with his go and has held up the game for others. Due to Richard being selected, and his slot being held open, his turn is protected. However, the responsibility and pressure to provide what is a preferred answer is also increased. He is 'put on the spot', a situation he deals with by laughter at the points at which a fitted response is notably absent (Lindholm, 2008). Thereafter, he cedes his turn (line 27).

While Richard's turn was 'safeguarded' as other responses were elided by the staff member, this mediated turn allocation system also carries with it the possibility of the player failing to respond correctly. Mediated turn allocation also forestalls some social interaction; other players stepping into Richard's turn space are not acknowledged, which shows that the preference for a response from the selected speaker trumps progressivity of the sequence. We found that the strictness of the mediated turn allocation system, and the social desirability to fulfil the allotted interactional slot, could not only place players on the spot, but could also be used as the basis for overriding players' decisions to opt out of the quiz altogether in one case (not shown here – see Webb et al., 2020).

We have seen how quizzes can be enacted when staff members ask questions they know the answers to. Next we will examine what difference it makes if a staff member plays *with* the person living with dementia as a co-player.

15.3.3 Small Group Quizzes with Staff Members as Players

All previous examples have shown staff members in positions of authority, asking questions of players with dementia and assessing the competency and correctness of their answers through evaluative third turns. In this sense, we may say staff are, or reveal themselves to be, in a position of knowledge (K+ in Heritage's (2012) terms) relative to the players living with dementia. Additionally, we have shown that staff members also control access to the interactional floor as turns outside the procedural order may be ignored or sequentially deleted. In this last section we briefly examine how playing in small groups/teams rather than as individuals affects the interactional space and opportunities for participation.

In Extract 5 there were three teams with five to six players with dementia and one staff member. Janet, Gina, Fred, Barbara, Mary and a staff member are sitting around a table playing a team quiz. The staff member has the categories and blank answer spaces on a piece of paper in front of her.

In Extract 5 Fred uses his turns to accomplish a different kind of activity to quizzing: storytelling. The staff member is in the position of potentially having to satisfy both the role of story recipient and her role as quiz member and 'team captain'. Here we examine how that interactional dilemma plays out.

Extract 5

```
1      STA:    Okay let's move on then number ten. A weapon.
2              A weapon beginning with tee.
3              ((Staff member signs the letter T using her hand
4              and a pen))
5      BAR:    Ooh umm=
6      STA:    =Mmm
7              ((Staff member taps pen on table))
8              (4)
9      STA:    °A weap[on°
10                    [((Staff member taps pen on table))
11             (3.4)
12     BAR:    °I can't think of one°
13     STA:    No:::.
14     JAN:    A torped(h)o(h): heh.
15     STA:    Ye[ah
```

```
16   JOE:   [Yeah
17   ?      A[tee]
18   STA:   [Exc]ellent Ja↑[net   ]
19   GIN:                  [Which]
20          (0.3)
21   STA:   A tor↑pe↓do
22   GIN:   ↑Oh ↑↑[yeah]
23   STA:         [Tor ]↑pe↓do
24          ((STA writes on the pad of paper))
25          (0.6)
26   FRE:   My- my brother[was in the na]vy.
27   STA:                 [Oh well done ].
28          ((STA is looking at JAN))
29   STA:   (Good[answer)]
30   FRE:        [He w    ]as torpedoed,
31   STA:   Wa[s he? ]
32   FRE:     [In the] m↑ed
33   STA:   Oh[wo:w.]
34   GIN:     [Mmm  ]
35          (0.6)
36   STA:   That must have been ↑frightening Fred?
37          (1)
38   FRE:   Yeah he was interned in Tun↑isia.
39   STA:   Yeah?
40          (1.5)
41   STA:   And was[that in the war?]
42   FRE:          [A-a- a (W       ]ater convoy)
43   STA:   Yeah. Yeah.
44          (0.7)
45   STA:   Wo:w.
46          (0.8)
47   STA:   That's a↑mazing yeah,
48          It's a↑mazing ↑isn't it what people,
49          you know, (0.8) ha-have done.
50          (0.5)
51   STA:   .HH >Alright okay number eleven<. .tch ↑Things
52   STA:   that are ro:und
```

Lines 1–24 make up the recognizable base sequence of a quiz: question – possible answer/response – evaluation of answer that we have seen in previous extracts. Note that in this iteration the staff member still poses the question (lines 1–2) and provides the confirmation (line 15) and positive evaluation (line 18). In lines 1–25 the staff member asks the players to name a weapon beginning with T (lines 1 and 2), which Janet does (line 14), and the answer is confirmed by the staff member (line 18). Gina then initiates a sequence to repair understanding/intersubjectivity, as she apparently did not hear the answer (lines 19–24).

However, it is not the base sequence that I focus on in this extract, but rather what happens afterwards. Following the answer of 'torpedo', Fred launches a storytelling sequence ('My- my brother was in the navy', line 26). Upon receiving no response to his turn, Fred produces an increment ('he was torpedoed'), with continuing intonation forecasting further talk. Once the link between the quiz answer and Fred's turn has been established, the staff member treats Fred's turns for the action they were seemingly intended to accomplish: a story announcement. This casts the staff member in the role of story recipient, and she duly attends to her recipient role ('was he?', line 31). Fred adds a turn increment, ('In the m↑ed', line 32), further specifying the location of the torpedo attack in the Mediterranean sea, which the staff member responds to with a news receipt + high-grade assessment ('Oh wo:w', line 33) (Goodwin, 1986). The staff member's turns in second position (high-grade assessments, continuers, yes preferring follow-up questions) attend to her role as story recipient, and in doing this interactional work, she steps momentarily out of the part she has played in progressing the quiz itself. The more relaxed approach to turn-taking and rights to speakership in this quiz iteration appear to give Fred agency to self-select to do something other than quizzing. More than this, unlike in other quiz iterations, Fred's turn is attended to by the staff member. The staff member then prompts further information with an 'and-prefaced' turn (line 41), to which Fred talks in overlap giving further information (line 42). Likely because Fred does not continue his story, the staff member produces a high-grade assessment. After another silence (line 46), the staff member again reiterates her high-grade assessment of the story, followed by a kind of non-specific summary/gist formulation (Heritage & Watson, 1979) of Fred's story (lines 47–49). After a further silence of 0.5 seconds, the staff member produces a first pair part action which reinstates the activity of the quiz by prefacing her turn with 'alright' and 'okay', both single lexical items which show a readiness to shift to subsequent matters, followed by the declaratively formed next quiz question ('things that are round'). Fred's turns are validated and attended to; it is only when no further increments or talk are forthcoming that the staff member reinstates the interactional framework of the quiz. The staff member aligns with Fred to maintain his role as a storyteller, before drawing on her deontic status to reinstate the overarching activity through a gist summary of Fred's story and a single lexical item prefaced turn to shift topics/activities.

I found this a common occurrence in team quiz activities; players who may find it difficult to give an answer were able to produce topically relevant, but not task relevant, actions related to the quiz answer. This may not correspond to fulfilling the overarching activity of completing the quiz (Webb et al., 2020), but is topically relevant to the subject at hand. Fred's anecdote at that point in the sequence (1) transforms the current activity from quiz into (topically related) talk about biographical events (what happened to his brother in the war); (2) shows that he can remember events related to their current conversational topic; and (3) shows that for these participants, the activity is

15 Social Quizzes for People Living with Dementia

not rigid but permeable and fluid, allowing people to enter and exit into other language games. There was space and opportunity in the more informal set up for this to happen. We will see a further example of how players can use their interactional skills to expand on a topic introduced as a quiz answer below.

Extract 6 involves the same quiz team as the previous extract. We join the quiz players after an answer 'telegram' had been given to the question 'name a form of communication beginning with T'. The extract features Fred, Barbara, Mary and the staff member.

Extract 6

```
1    STA:   What one do you like, team? What one shall we
2           go with?
3    FRE:   Thread.
4    STA:   Yeah. Thread. (.) I think telegram, because
5           they might not-[the other team-
6    FRE:                  [Telegram, yeah.
7    STA:   Yeah, telegrams. Let's go with that,
8           because that's an unusual one.
9    BAR:   Yeah.
10   FRE:   Yeah, my father had a- (used telegrams)
11   STA:   So you remember getting telegrams. You
12          don't see that any more nowadays, do you,
13          people[don't send telegrams.
14   FRE:         [No, they- but-
15   BAR:   Yeah, they would knock on the door with
16          a telegram, your[heart started beating=
17   STA:                   [Really?
18   BAR:   =and you .hh heh heh
19   STA:   Yes, yeah, you[wondered=
20   BAR:                 [what's wrong
21   BAR:   [heh heh heh heh heh heh
22   STA:   [=what it was, yeah. If it
23          was going to be bad news.
24   BAR:   Yeah.
```

In lines 1–2 the staff member attempts to elicit a collective decision regarding which one of the previously given possible answers they should choose. Fred offers a new possible answer in line 3 ('thread'), which does not straightforwardly satisfy both criteria for the question (a form of communication that begins with T). The staff member acknowledges Fred's turn but proffers an alternative opinion, foregrounding her own epistemic rights (Heritage, 2012), and begins to give a reason for her choice, which is possibly abandoned when Fred agrees with her in overlap (line 6). The staff member once more affirms the reasoning behind her choice (lines 7–8), displaying an awareness of the delicacy around her drawing on her status (Stevanovic & Peräkylä, 2012) to decide on answers for the group. Following Barbara's agreement (line 9), this could have been the end of the matter, having completed the question–answer–evaluative sequence. In line 10 Fred initiates a new action not related to the overarching activity of quiz-completion, informing the group that his father had used telegrams. This piece of information is treated as the beginning of a story, with the staff member probing Fred for additional information (line 11) whilst making an observation about telegrams within her own epistemic territory ('You don't see that any more nowadays, do you, people don't send telegrams'). Fred's initiation of topicalizing telegrams leads to Barbara sharing her own recollections about what it meant to receive a telegram when its content could be life-altering (lines 15–16, 18), which the staff member collaboratively completes (lines 19, 22, 23).

Here then we have two players self-selecting to reminisce, building on the topic of the quiz to share aspects of their lives. So, whilst quizzes impose an overarching interactional agenda characterized by a base question–answer sequence, in group quizzes played as a team there are more opportunities to command the interactional floor. Players could, and often did, use their turns to do actions which did not expedite the completion of the quiz but were of social value to them. This suggests that quizzes in these contexts may create opportunities for this kind of 'divergent' talk, but rather than being an obstacle to progressivity, it can be an opportunity to make the social occasion a bit richer.

Small group quizzes tended to allow players more agency in initiating actions in first position, rather than only responding in second position. Additionally, players could profess to not know an answer but continue to be involved in the interaction, as opposed to mediated turn allocation quizzes, in which not knowing the answer meant losing one's right to the interactional floor.

Whilst most group quizzes enabled players with dementia to be more included, even if their turns were not strictly related to the quiz activity, there was a deviant case. I observed that when the players without dementia outnumbered the players with dementia, the project of quiz completion could again be prioritized.

Extract 7 took place in a memory cafe. Pat, who is in her early 80s and has dementia, is doing a quiz with her visiting daughter Mel and her 'dementia navigator' Anne, both of whom are sitting on Pat's right. We join the group as they engage in a quiz about famous crimes and criminals throughout history. The extract begins with the group discussing a possible answer to a question about the location of a famous historic prison. Lynne, a service centre organizer, walks over behind them and leans over the table between Mel and Anne. All three pore over the quiz sheet.

Extract 7

```
1    MEL     So. (1) let's have a think about this other prison then.
2            (1.5)
3    MEL:    Is there one in Fra:nce
```

```
4          (15.4 )
5          ((LYN walks over and stands between PAT and ANN))
6   LYN:   It's °a ↑rea↓lly hard quiz I
7          (2.8)
8          ((MEL turns over the quiz paper. LYN bends
9          down to look at the paper))
10  MEL:   ( )
11  LYN:   I think you're probably right with number eight
```

At the start of the extract, Pat is in a leaning-in posture that she adopts throughout the next few minutes, and from which she occasionally looks up in apparent readiness to be addressed by another member of the group. This does not happen. There is no need to show the entire transcript, since at no point does anyone around the table – Pat's daughter, Mel, the dementia navigator, Lynne the service manager – address Pat or look towards her. Eventually she simply slumps back in her chair and turns her head away.

Pat's slumping does not appear as a response to a specific prior turn, but rather a cumulative disengagement borne out of a response to her fellow quizzers' numerous prior turns that exclude Pat. Pat can in fact speak and engage in conversation. Indeed, on the same day she was involved in a different type of quiz – equally hard, but the other participants made sure she was included. Here, the other participants keep the quiz sheet too far away, and effectively the other quizzers prioritize getting the answers right over including Pat in the game. The drive for progressivity as the overall activity to which the participants' turns at talk orient can work against the ostensible therapeutic purpose of this type of quiz: facilitating social interaction (Antaki & Webb, 2019). Thus, moving the activity on licensed the exclusion of the sole player with dementia, as completing the activity took precedence over inclusion. Quizzes rely on the cooperation of everyone involved to *remain* involved. In some cases, speakers may also have to take initiative to remain involved. However, this can be difficult to do if physical resources (being on the edge of the group, other group members turning away from the person, lack of eye gaze, the quiz sheet being out of sight) and mutual epistemic resources (knowing the answer to the question and being treated as someone who *may* know the answer to the question) work to make participation more difficult. This was particularly the case when players without dementia outnumbered players with dementia.

15.4   Discussion

This chapter began by observing that social quizzes impose an interactional framework driven by a triad sequence (question–answer–evaluation) which marks this type of structure out as institutional. Like the boundaries demarcating institutional talk from everyday talk that Drew and Heritage (1992) observed, the quizzes that were observed were distinctive because they involved the participants in specific goal orientations which are tied to their institutional identities (quiz master – quiz player/staff member – service user), and the interactional frameworks of quizzes often involved special constraints on what will be treated as allowable contributions to the business at hand. Exceptions to this were demonstrated in Section 15.3.3 (small group quizzes), although it should also be noted that actions and turns that were not relevant to progressing the activity of the quiz, whilst treated as allowable in that quiz configuration, were nevertheless temporary diversions to the quiz, after which activity-progressivity was always reinstated (Webb et al., 2020). Analysis also demonstrated that correct answers were treated as preferred, whilst incorrect answers were treated as dispreferred.

While quizzes are often mentioned in research looking at collective spaces for older people and/or people living with dementia, the specific way the quiz is enacted is often absent. Although quizzes are often promoted as a fun activity to do with groups of people living with dementia (for example, see Swan, 2004; Light & Delves, 2011; Graty, 2013), there are many variations in the way they are performed, all of which have an impact on the players and access to the interactional floor. This chapter has sought to begin exploring three examples of potential iterations and their impact on players. For example, in mediated turn allocation quizzes, talk delivered outside a designated turn was mostly ignored, or at least not attended to. The three quiz examples analysed can be seen as imposing different degrees of responsibility for participants to answer. In 'whole group quizzes', an entire group is addressed and therefore players choose whether to 'self-select' to answer. Here the interactional spotlight does not fall so brightly on any one individual, but correspondingly this also means many of the players do not get a turn. In mediated turn allocated quizzes, individual players are under an increased amount of expectation and pressure to provide an answer to the question, but all players are guaranteed a turn (sometimes even if they do not want one). In small group quizzes players again self-select to answer, but also initiate 'non-activity-completing' actions such as telling stories and discussing topical aspects of the answers. However, it was shown that where completing the activity took priority, players with dementia could be left out.

Quizzes are a particular interactional activity where face-threatening acts, such as issues around cognitive processes, memory and appropriate participation, can become interactionally relevant. This was particularly present in mediated turn allocation quizzes. Elements of 'face work' include solo laughter from players where an answer should occur in the sequence and the work done by staff to reduce threats to face in these extracts, such as offering another turn to get a right answer. However, this need not be the case; two extracts where the staff member did not know the answer at the outset (Extracts 5 and 6) also occasioned the most group interaction with people self-selecting to talk. Indeed, a low epistemic stance and status encoded in questions from the staff members proved to be an effective way of eliciting talk in general (Williams et al., 2019). Team quizzes contained fewer moments of people being put 'on the spot', and so it might be expected that fewer face-threatening situations arise in that context. This is especially important given that these types of quizzes are (a) put on for fun, (b) intended to facilitate social interaction, and (c) attended by people at different stages of dementia and with different communicational and cognitive abilities and challenges. Because speakership is more fluid and less constrained than mediated turn allocated quiz formats, there is more space for people living with dementia to initiate actions (such as storytelling) that do not correspond to the overarching goal of quiz completion, but which do serve an important interpersonal function.

In Extracts 5, 6 and 7 the player(s) without dementia asked questions to be answered by the team, to which the answer was not already known. It could therefore be presumed that this would ameliorate epistemic asymmetries, and therefore threats to face. However, in the case of Extract 7 it also licensed the exclusion of the sole player with dementia, as completing the activity took precedence over inclusion. This should remind us that whilst the interactional framework imposed by the quiz has important implications for the possible agency and inclusion of players, the quality of the relationship is the paramount task for staff. Staff/players without dementia are often the gatekeepers of activities such as quizzes and likely to be the driving force behind them, both in choosing to enact them in a social care setting and, mostly, taking turns in first position and driving the interaction forward according to their own agenda.

It is important to note that the players with dementia themselves showed us that the question–answer sequence is not the only way to promote memory and recall. As shown in Section 3, players with dementia built on a topic introduced by the quiz question answer to not only self-select to elaborate on it, but also to show interactional and cognitive competency by recalling personal facts related to the topic. Whilst this did not further the quiz, it could be argued that it served an important personal and social function. This was in stark contrast to the other kinds of quiz, in which out-of-turn or non-quiz progressing activities were commonly ignored and sequentially deleted. The flexibility afforded by a more communal approach to the quiz enabled players greater opportunity to initiate story-telling sequences about their life, and to thus reshape the activity from an institutional one to a conversational, and personal, one. This chapter has shed light on how this may be possible, taking into account how different quiz enactment impacts the interactional space, and how threats to face are occasioned by the activity, and navigated in situ.

A communication training interactive video about quizzes made in collaboration with co-researchers with dementia can be accessed on the following link:

www.youtube.com/watch?v=eInXlF_bzes

References

Antaki, C. and Webb, J. (2019) 'When the larger objective matters more: Support workers' epistemic and deontic authority over adult service-users.' *Sociology of Health & Illness*, 41(8): 1549–1567.

Arundale, R. B. (2010) 'Constituting face in conversation: Face, facework, and interactional achievement.' *Journal of Pragmatics*, 42(8): 2078–2105.

Brown, P. and Levinson, S. C. (1987) *Politeness: Some Universals in Language Usage* (Vol. 4). Cambridge: Cambridge University Press.

Drew, P. (1997). '"Open" class repair initiators in response to sequential sources of troubles in conversation.' *Journal of Pragmatics*, 28(1): 69–101.

Drew, P. and Heritage, J. (eds.) (1992) *Talk at Work: Language Use in Institutional and Work-Place Settings*. Cambridge: Cambridge University Press.

Goffman, E. (1967) *Interaction Ritual: Essays on Face-to-Face Interaction*. Oxford: Aldine.

Goodwin, C. (1986) 'Between and within: Alternative sequential treatments of continuers and assessments.' *Human Studies*, 9(2–3): 205–217.

Graty, C. (2013) *Taking Part: Activities for People with Dementia* (Vol. 14). London: Alzheimer's Society.

Haakana, M. (2001) 'Laughter as a patient's resource: Dealing with delicate aspects of medical interaction.' *Text – Interdisciplinary Journal for the Study of Discourse*, 21(1–2): 187–219.

Hayano, K. (2012) 'Question design in conversation.' In J. Sidnell and T. Stivers (eds.) *The Handbook of Conversation Analysis*. Malden, MA: Blackwell Publishing Ltd, pp. 395–414.

Heritage, J. (1984) 'A change-of-state token and aspects of its sequential placement.' In J. M. Atkinson and J. Heritage (eds.) *Structures of Social Action: Studies in Conversation Analysis*. Cambridge: Cambridge University Press, pp. 299–345.

(2012) 'Epistemics in action: Action formation and territories of knowledge.' *Research on Language and Social Interaction*, 45(1): 1.

Heritage, J. and Clayman, S. (2011) *Talk in Action: Interactions, Identities, and Institutions* (Vol. 44). Hoboken: John Wiley & Sons.

Heritage, J. and Greatbatch, D. (1989). 'On the institutional character of institutional talk: The case of news interviews.' In P. A. Forstorp (ed.) *Discourse in Professional and Everyday Culture*. Linkoping: Department of Communication Studies, University of Linkoping, Sweden, pp. 47–98 [Reprinted in D. Boden and D. H. Zimmerman (eds.) *Talk and Social Structure*. Berkeley: University of California Press, pp. 93–137.

Heritage, J. and Watson, D. R. (1979) 'Formulations as conversational objects.' In G. Psathas (ed.) *Everyday Language: Studies in Ethnomethodology*, pp. 123–162.

Jefferson, G. (1984) 'Transcription notation.' In J. M. Atkinson and J. Heritage (eds.) *Structures of Social Action: Studies in Conversation Analysis*. Cambridge: Cambridge University Press, pp. 9–16.

Jones, D., Drew, P., Elsey, C., Blackburn, D., Wakefield, S., Harkness, K. and Reuber, M. (2016) 'Conversational assessment in memory clinic encounters: Interactional profiling for differentiating dementia from functional memory disorders.' *Aging & Mental Health*, 20(5): 500–509.

Jones, D., Wilkinson, R., Jackson, C. and Drew, P. (2020) 'Variation and interactional non-standardization in neuropsychological tests: The case of the Addenbrooke's cognitive examination.' *Qualitative Health Research*, 30(3): 458–470.

Light, D. and Delves, J. (2011) 'A guide to setting up a memory café.' *REPoD (Rotarians Easing Problems of Dementia)*. www.repod.org.uk/downloads/REPoD-mc-guide.pdf.

Lindholm, C. (2008) 'Laughter, communication problems and dementia.' *Communication & Medicine*, 5(3): 3.

Lindholm, C. and Wray, A. (2011) 'Proverbs and formulaic sequences in the language of elderly people with dementia.' *Dementia*, 10(4): 603–623.

Mehan, H. (1979) *Learning Lessons: Social Organization in the Classroom.* Cambridge, MA: Harvard University Press.

Pomerantz, A. (1984) 'Agreeing and disagreeing with assessments: Some features of preferred/dispreferred turn shapes'. In J. M. Atkinson and J. Heritage (eds.) *Structures of Social Action: Studies in Conversation Analysis.* Cambridge: Cambridge University Press, pp. 57–101.

Sacks, H. (1992) *Lectures on Conversation* (Vol. 2), ed. G Jefferson. Oxford: Blackwell.

Sacks, H., Schegloff, E. E. and Jefferson, G. (1974) 'A simplest systematics for the organization of turn-taking for conversation.' *Language*, 50: 696–735.

Schegloff, E. A. (2007). *Sequence Organization in Interaction: A Primer in Conversation Analysis* (Vol. 1). Cambridge: Cambridge University Press.

(2013) 'Ten operations in self-initiated, same-turn repair.' *Conversational Repair and Human Understanding*, 30: 41–70.

Schegloff, E. A. and Sacks, H. (1973) 'Opening up closings.' *Semiotica*, 8(4): 289–327.

Stenström, A-B. (1994) *An Introduction to Spoken Interaction.* London: Longman

Stevanovic, M. and Peräkylä, A. (2012) 'Deontic authority in interaction: The right to announce, propose, and decide.' *Research on Language and Social Interaction*, 45(3): 297–321.

Stevanovic, M. and Svennevig, J. (2015) 'Introduction: Epistemics and deontics in conversational directives.' *Journal of Pragmatics*, (78): 1–6.

Swan, J. (2004) 'The value of recreational activities within a care setting.' *Nursing and Residential Care*, 6: 440–442.

Webb, J., Lindholm, C. and Williams, V. (2020). 'Interactional strategies for progressing through quizzes in dementia settings.' *Discourse Studies*, 22(4): 503–522.

Williams, V., Gall, M., Mason-Angelow, V., Read, S. and Webb, J. (2023) 'Misfitting and social practice theory: Incorporating disability into the performance and (re)enactment of social practices.' *Disability & Society*, 38:776–797.

Williams, V., Webb, J., Dowling, S. and Gall, M. (2019) 'Direct and indirect ways of managing epistemic asymmetries when eliciting memories.' *Discourse, Studies* 21(2): 199–215.

Index

Account, 43–45, 67, 79, 226
  ethnographic, 79, 93
  inability, 44, 277
Accountability, 48, 229, 232
Accountable, 27, 137, 147, 229, 239, 345
Acknowledgment, 37
  minimal, 58–59
  neutral, 37
  third-turn, 40
Action
  embodied, 180, 232, 235
  social, 6, 50, 152
Activity, 11, 16
  deontic, 337, *See* Deontics
  epistemic, 337, *See* Epistemics
  institutional, 16
  joint, 30, 137
  routine, 110, 113
  seek and find, 201
  task-based, 117
  testing, 27
Advice, 15, 37, 177
  giver, 252
  giving, 153, 177, 250, 252
  recipient, 252
  sequence. *See* Sequence
Affective stance, 134, 147
Affiliation, 68, 133, 138, 255
Agency, 170, 177–178, 353
  distributed, 191
Agenda, 50
  action, 178, 189
  institutional, 325
  topical, 10, 175, 178, 189
Agreement, 57, 67, 152–153, 159, 171
  pro-forma, 133
Aid
  communication, 12
  digital, 292
  memory, 295
Albury, C., 51

Alignment, 133
Alzheimer Europe, 93
Alzheimer's disease, 3, 106, 232, 269
  amnestic, 179
Answer
  out of turn, 344
Answering without knowing, 259, 289
Antaki, C., 11, 27, 73, 177, 189, 249
Applications, 15
  CIRCA, 296
  CIRCUS, 296
  digital, 293
Assertion, 157
Assessment, 157
  clinical, 13
  cognitive, 26
  high grade, 348
  interpreter-mediated, 13
  medical, 27
  multilingual, 77
  psychiatric, 68
  self, 50
  third position, 214
Astell, A.J., 292, 295
Awareness, 3, 68, 231, 311, 317
  cultural, 94

Backhaus, P., 175
Barnes, R.K., 69
Blame, 272
  rhetoric of, 68
Blame-worthy, 167
Brain scan, 51, 67
Brown, P., 171, 337

Call opening, 274
Care
  equity in, 94
  inequity in, 73
  intercultural, 73

Index

long-term, 316
residential, 12, 76, 272
Care home
  residential, 299
  specialist, 271
Caregivers
  formal, 148, 175
  informal, 131, 143, 175
Choi, K.T., 147
Coercion, 166
Cognition, 6, 123, 131, 137, 146–147, 269–270, 289
Cognitive process, 270, 352
Cognitive state, 250, 269, 271
Cognitive test, 28, 67
  feedback, 68
Communication as care, 333
Communication support, 292, 312
  digital, 292
  traditional, 292
Communicative projects, 175, 177–178, 191
Compensatory practices, 122–123
Competence
  cognitive, 137, 158
  interactional, 45, 154, 171, 249, 275
  social, 45, 147, 275
Complaint, 134, 164
  cognitive, 33
  implicit, 282
Compliment, 144
Confirmation, 9, 159, 208
  check, 40
  extended, 53
contingencies, 199
Contingencies, 199
Conversation Analysis
  applied, 11, 73, 249
  interventionist, 11, 75
  multimodal, 232
  social problem-oriented, 75
Conversation Analysis (CA), 4
Couper-Kuhlen, E., 199
Coupland, J., 249
Coupland, N., 249

Declarative syntax, 9
Deficit, 7, 105, 122–123
  cognitive, 6, 191, 289
Deontics, 8–10
  deontic authority, 30
  deontic congruence, 143
  deontic force, 169
  deontic order, 170
  deontic rights, 153
  deontic stance, 9

deontic status, 9
Directives, 10, 122, 199, 205
  attention-focus, 212, 217
  emphatic, 116
  explicit, 117
  find X, 201
  first postition, 215
  infantile, 106
  precise, 120
Disaffiliation, 134, 205
Disagreement, 59, 133, 138, 179–185, 231
Dispreference, 133, 137–138
Diversity
  ethnic and cultural, 75
Dooley, J., 4, 29, 52
Drew, P., 26, 37, 104, 169, 186, 199, 250

Education
  level of, 91
  limited, 76
Edwards, D., 269
Ekström, A., 104, 292
Elaboration, 36, 184
Elderspeak, 154, 168, 170
Elsey, C., 4, 29, 171
Embodied
  behavior, 317
  practices, 16, 104, 317
  resources, 190
Emotion, 32
  negative, 32
  social, 105
Emotional
  behavior, 105
  burden, 45
  engagement, 68
  functioning, 197
  labour, 27
  order, 157, 170
  territory, 171
Empathic displays, 275
Enactment, 16, 155, 336
  quiz, 342
Encouragers, 207, 214
Enfield, N.J., 146, 177
Enquiry, 273–274, 285
Epistemics, 198–199
  epistemic authority, 30
  epistemic domain, 8, 15, 170, 197–198, 229, 245
  epistemic order, 170
  epistemic primacy, 230, 262, 279
  epistemic stance, 8, 152, 189, 198, 229
  epistemic status, 15, 176, 229, 250
  epistemic territory, 350

Epistemics (cont.)
  epistemic trespassing, 162, 170
  [K−], 9, 337
  [K+], 9, 199, 205, 337
Ethnic
  group, 73
  majority, 76
  minority, 73, 94
Ethnicity
  minority ethnic group, 73, 76
Ethnographic
  fieldnotes, 108
  interviews, 79
  observations, 78, 106–107, 249
  study, 26, 107
Ethnography, 76
Expectations, 50, 67, 176

Face, 27
  face work, 337, 352
  face-protective responses, 27
  face-saving act, 244
  face-saving practices, 227
  face-saving strategies, 13, 69
  face-threating activity, 296
  facework, 10, 66
  negative face, 171
  positive face wants, 338
  preservation/restoration, 337
  save, 45, 50
  threat, 10, 231
  threatening, 205
Family communication, 15, 270
Fanshel, D., 8, 198, 229
Fishing devices, 199
Footing, 204
Formulaic
  expressions, 294
  sequence, 131, 135
Formulation
  gist, 348
  locational, 38, 40, 45
Formulations, 325
Foster, R.M.G.L.W., 135
Frontotemporal dementia, 3, 154, 220, 231
  behavioral variant, 13
  byFTD, 105, 197

Glenn, P., 254–255
Goffman, E., 10, 167, 204, 228
Goodwin, C., 88, 147, 227–228, 232, 244, 317
Goodwin, M.H., 88, 228, 244
Granularity, 207, 209
Guendouzi, J., 5

Haakana, M., 58, 345
Hamilton, H.E., 5–6, 176, 249
Harré, R., 5
Hepburn, A., 151
Heritage, J., 4, 8, 12, 28, 62, 151, 270
History-taking, 28, 40, 51, 92
Home, 271–273, 316
Houtkoop-Steenstra, N.C., 26, 37
Hydén, L-C., 5, 104, 130, 297

Identity, 147, 254
  construction, 130, 134, 147
  cultural, 73
  self-identity, 50, 57, 66
Informing, 143
  turn, 146
Institutional
  interaction, 325, 344
  setting, 3, 11
  talk, 352
Interpreter
  proficient, 79
  trained, 76
Interpreting
  prima vista, 80, 91
Interrogative
  clause, 151
  tag, 151
  wh-, 200–201
  yes/no, 152
Intersubjectivity, 106, 347
Intervention, 11, 13, 15, 91
  early, 3
  ecologically valid, 12
  healthcare, 12
  music-based, 129

Jansson, G., 76, 178
Jefferson, G., 4, 137, 141, 261
Jones, D., 4, 6–7, 27, 77

Keady, J., 11
Kendrick, K.H., 120, 187, 190
Kindell, J., 4, 103, 155, 256
Kitwood, T., 5, 177, 249, 316
Kitzinger, C., 283
Knowables, 8
  Type 1, 229–230, 245
  Type 2, 229
Knowledge
  access, 198, 227, 229
  access to, 245
  A-event, 8, 10, 198–199, 229
  asymmetry, 154, 230
  B-event, 8, 198, 229

Index

domain, 245
lifeworld, 198
rights to, 245

Labov, W., 8, 198, 229
Landmark, A.M.D., 10, 154, 176, 226
Laughable, 254
Laughter, 6, 242, 255
  laughing at, 255
  laughing with, 255
  speaker-invited, 138, 140
  volunteered, 138
Levinson, S.C., 4, 152, 171, 220
Lewy Bodies, 3
Life story
  books, 221
  sequences, 252
Lifeworld, 9, 159, 170
Lindeberg, S., 30
Lindholm, C., 4, 88, 175–176, 184, 242
Lindley, L., 249, 251
Linell, P., 178, 230
Literacy
  limited, 76
Longitudinal
  analysis, 6
  case study, 123
  insight, 289
  study, 6, 13
  work, 107
Luckmann, T., 230

Majlesi, A.R., 4, 104
Markova, I.S., 50
Marlaire, C.L., 26, 37
Maynard, D.W., 26, 28, 40, 68
McCabe, R., 51
Memory clinic, 7, 26, 50–51, 67
Memory loss, 15, 50, 232, 270, 288
Memory retention, 272
Mikesell, L., 4, 104
Milne, A., 50
Mirroring, 209, 215
Misalignment, 50–51, 69, 178
Mok, Z., 249
Mondada, L., 200, 227
Multimedia systems, 296
Multimodal
  analysis, 227
  notations, 78
  resources, 15, 178
Müller, N., 5, 249
Muntigl, P., 147, 199

National Dementia Declaration, 7
Neuropsychiatry, 77
Next-turn proof procedure, 299
Nielsen, T.R., 77, 92, 96
Nilsson, E., 4, 199, 230
Nonalignment, 137

Örulv, L., 5
Other-attentive, 31, 273
Over-suppose and under-tell, 222

Participation framework, 228, 244
Peel, E., 68
Personhood, 5, 249, 316
Peräkylä, A., 9, 28, 153, 338
Plejert, C., 4, 92
Poetics, 137
Policy proposal, 91, 94
Pomerantz, A., 8, 129, 198, 229, 343
Positioning, 228
  interactional, 228, 238, 246
  sequential, 108
Post-expansion
  minimal, 37–38
  sequences, 43
Potter, J., 151, 269
Preference, 133
Presupposition, 337, 339
  embedded, 273, 281
Professional vision, 317, 319, 332
Proposal, 10, 153, 199

Question, 6, 337
  and-prefaced, 39
  confirmation-seeking, 8, 234
  design, 336
  exam, 204–205
  hypothetical, 317, 322, 324, 332
  information-seeking, 8
  multiple tag, 54
  quasi-scripted, 33
  tag question, 14, 32, 151
Quizzes, 336

Rasmussen, G., 130, 154
Raymond, G., 32, 151, 226, 259
Raymond, W.C., 77
Recipient design, 27, 31
Recommendation, 94
  treatment, 28, 65, 68
Recruiting assistance, 120, 177, 180, 190
Reminiscence, 250, 254, 259, 295
Reminiscing, 292, 296
Repair, 6, 77, 112, 230, 279
  initiator, 217

Repair (cont.)
  open class repair initiator, 186, 341
Repetitive
  behavior, 130, 311
  first actions, 191
  verbalizations, 295
Requests, 10, 153, 199
  explicit, 177
Resistance, 68, 178
Response
  polar, 32
Response cry, 66, 167
Response pursuit, 212, 221
Reuber, M., 28, 35
Robinson, J.D., 151

Sabat, S., 5–6, 250
Sacks, H., 8, 27, 110, 151, 299
Samuelsson, C., 4, 130
Schegloff, E.A., 36, 38, 178, 209, 217, 345
Schrauf, R.W., 10
Self-talk, 110, 118
Semantic dementia, 154
Sequence
  confirmation-seeking, 213
  question–answer, 33, 353
  question–answer–comment, 205
  three-part, 16
Sequence closing thirds, 215
Sidnell, J., 4, 200
Skill, 8, 105, 122–123, 289, 331
Smith, M.S., 10
Social relationships, 4, 272, 293
Solicitous, 273
Sorjonen, M.L., 39, 153
Stance accretion, 147
Standardization, 25, 27
  in surveys, 26
  -in-interaction, 26
  non-, 27
Standardized test, 13, 39
Stevanovic, M., 8, 30, 157, 184, 338
Stigma, 3, 60, 68
Stivers, T., 4, 28, 69, 191
Stokoe, E., 12

Surprise, 283
Svennevig, J., 8, 176, 182

Tablets, 306
  touchscreen, 295
Task orientation, 327, 332
te Molder, H., 269
Technology
  in dementia care, 295
  digital, 292
  touchscreen, 295
Third-turn
  position, 37
  receipts, 238
  response, 36
  responses, 40
  utterances, 37
Token
  acknowledgement, 54, 83, 184
  change-of-state, 186
  minimal, 256
  non-lexical, 32
  response, 285
Topic proffer, 162, 180
Treatment
  acceptance of, 68
  resistance to, 68
Try-marking, 207
Tsekleves, E., 11
Turn design, 153, 169, 231, 337
Turowetz, J., 26
Tykkyläinen, T., 11

Under-suppose and over-tell, 222

Vascular dementia, 3, 131
Video guidance, 317–319, 332

Watson, D.R., 348
Webb, J., 4, 189
Wilkinson, R., 7, 28, 88, 168, 283
Williams, K., 154
Williams, V., 353
Wittgenstein, L., 269
Working diagnosis, 30, 35–37, 45
Wray, A., 294, 336

www.ingramcontent.com/pod-product-compliance
Lightning Source LLC
Chambersburg PA
CBHW071223180125
20471CB00041B/171